# THE FERTILITY FORMULA

TAKE CONTROL OF YOUR REPRODUCTIVE FUTURE

Dr Natalie Crawford

**flightbooks**

FLIGHT BOOKS

UK | USA | Canada | Ireland | Australia
India | New Zealand | South Africa

Flight Books is part of the Penguin Random House group of companies
whose addresses can be found at global.penguinrandomhouse.com

Penguin Random House UK
One Embassy Gardens, 8 Viaduct Gardens, London SW11 7BW

penguin.co.uk

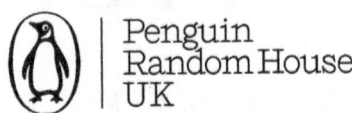

First published in the USA by Penguin Life in 2026
First Published in the UK by Vermilion in 2026

1

Copyright © Dr Natalie Crawford 2026

The moral right of the author has been asserted.

Penguin Random House values and supports copyright.
Copyright fuels creativity, encourages diverse voices, promotes freedom
of expression and supports a vibrant culture. Thank you for purchasing an
authorised edition of this book and for respecting intellectual property laws
by not reproducing, scanning or distributing any part of it by any means without
permission. You are supporting authors and enabling Penguin Random House to
continue to publish books for everyone. No part of this book may be used or reproduced
in any manner for the purpose of training artificial intelligence technologies or systems. In
accordance with Article 4(3) of the DSM Directive 2019/790, Penguin Random House
expressly reserves this work from the text and data mining exception.

Typeset by Six Red Marbles UK, Thetford, Norfolk

Printed and bound in Great Britain by Clays Ltd, Elcograf S.p.A.

The authorised representative in the EEA is Penguin Random House Ireland,
Morrison Chambers, 32 Nassau Street, Dublin D02 YH68

A CIP catalogue record for this book is available from the British Library

ISBN 9781785045592

Penguin Random House is committed to a sustainable future
for our business, our readers and our planet. This book is made
from Forest Stewardship Council® certified paper.

# Praise for *The Fertility Formula*

"Dr Natalie Crawford has written the book I wish every woman had from the very beginning of her reproductive life. *The Fertility Formula* is not just about getting pregnant—it's about understanding your body, your hormones, your health, and your options. She hands us the agency we have always deserved, guiding us toward a future where we can make informed choices for ourselves. This book is power. This book is permission. This book is a lifeline for women who are ready to take control of their own story."

—Jen Hatmaker, five-time *New York Times* bestselling author and host of the *For the Love Podcast*

"In *The Fertility Formula*, Dr Natalie Crawford dismantles outdated myths about reproductive health and presents a compelling case for an anti-inflammatory approach to fertility. This book will change your life."

—Rebecca Fett, author of the bestselling fertility book *It Starts with the Egg*

"Fertility isn't luck. It's knowledge, awareness, and empowerment. In *The Fertility Formula*, double board–certified OB-GYN and reproductive endocrinologist Dr Natalie Crawford breaks down what every woman should know about her hormones, cycle, and reproductive health but was never taught. Grounded in science and empathy, this book gives you the tools to understand your body, protect your fertility, and take control of your future."

—Dr Mary Claire Haver, board-certified OB-GYN and bestselling author of *The New Menopause*

"*The Fertility Formula* makes a powerful case for a proactive, anti-inflammatory approach to fertility—and to health itself. Dr Natalie Crawford shows how healing the gut, calming inflammation, and syncing your rhythm can help you take control of your reproductive future. A bold and necessary road map for thriving reproductive health and overall well-being."

—Dr Will Bulsiewicz, gastroenterologist and New York Times bestselling author of *Plant Powered Plus*

"As a surgeon and longevity doctor, I've long believed that our menstrual cycle is not a mystery to be endured but a vital sign—one of the clearest indicators of our metabolic health, hormonal balance, and overall well-being. In *The Fertility Formula*, Dr Natalie Crawford demystifies this truth with science-backed clarity, compassion, and deeply practical steps that every woman deserves to know. Her evidence-based approach to optimizing reproductive health fills a gap that has existed for far too long, and I can honestly say I would have loved to have a book like this when I was hoping to have children. Dr Crawford has created a truly empowering guide that helps women understand their bodies and take confident action in one of the most important aspects of their health."

—Dr Vonda Wright, board-certified orthopedic surgeon and *New York Times* bestselling author of *Unbreakable*

"In *The Fertility Formula*, Dr Natalie Crawford makes it clear how to assess and optimize your reproductive and hormone health. The road map she provides is based on her extensive clinical experience with thousands of patients, each of whom came to her with different histories, hopes, and needs. *The Fertility Formula* is not only crucial for those who are planning to have children; it should be read by every woman—regardless of age or reproductive goals—because of the close relationship that exists between hormone and general health, especially in women. *The Fertility Formula* is going to vastly improve and indeed save countless lives, and surely create many new ones as well!"

—Dr Andrew Huberman, associate professor of neurobiology and ophthalmology at Stanford School of Medicine and host of the *Huberman Lab* podcast

"A comprehensive guide to the science behind hormones and conception, including the role of lifestyle factors such as nutrition, exercise, and sleep. *The Fertility Formula* is an absolute must read for anyone looking to understand and optimize their fertility!"

—Dr Karen Tang, author of *It's Not Hysteria*

"Dr Natalie Crawford's *The Fertility Formula* is an empowering, science-backed guide that every woman deserves. She brilliantly bridges medical expertise with compassion, helping women truly understand and optimize their fertility at every stage. This book is a must read for anyone seeking clarity and control over their reproductive health."

—Kayla Barnes-Lentz, longevity expert and host of *The Longevity Optimization* podcast

"For any woman wanting to conceive, *The Fertility Formula* offers insights to help dismantle the complexities and fears of the journey, and gives actionable advice and hope. Dr Natalie Crawford shines as an expert clinician, but with the human softness to unpack the confusion and create clarity for all. I highly recommend this book to the many women (and their partners) who are seeking answers and guidance from a true, compassionate expert."

—Dr Stacy T. Sims, coauthor of *Roar* and *Next Level*

"I am so excited to be able to refer my readers to *The Fertility Formula* by Dr Crawford. It's such an accessible guide, not just for those dealing with fertility issues but for those wanting to be proactive with their family building. By using a holistic approach to diagnosing the root cause of a problem, she covers the overall health of both women and their partners, including evidence-based recommendations about nutrition and other complementary therapies that really should be part of any excellent clinician's therapeutic options. I also love her use of analogies to explain complicated principles. And the fact that she was so honest about her own fertility challenges makes her that much more credible and sensitive to the concerns of her readers and patients. Kudos for a fabulous book!"

—Toni Weschler, author of *Taking Charge of Your Fertility* and cocreator of the cycle tracking app Cyclisity

"Dr Natalie Crawford has written the book I wish every patient—and every clinician—had years ago. *The Fertility Formula* is honest, practical, and deeply empowering, giving readers the knowledge and confidence they need to understand their bodies and advocate for their fertility with clarity and compassion. *The Fertility Formula* provides a fertility road map that is both an actionable checklist and a deeply evidence-based guide. She helps readers understand the 'why' behind every recommendation, helping women truly understand—and take control of—their fertility."

—Dr Lora Shahine, board-certified OB-GYN and reproductive endocrinologist, author, and host of the *Brave & Curious* podcast

"Women are taught to treat fertility like a coin toss—something you get lucky with or not. In *The Fertility Formula*, Dr Natalie Crawford makes clear just how culturally harmful this thinking is. Crawford gives women the language and agency to approach their fertility with care and control—amen to that!"

—Dr Pooja Lakshmin, psychiatrist and author of *Real Self-Care*

"*The Fertility Formula* goes far beyond getting pregnant—it teaches you to understand your body so deeply no one can dismiss your experience again. With expert clarity and genuine allyship, Dr Crawford breaks down hormones, cycles, and reproductive health in a way every woman deserves. If you've ever felt dismissed or told to 'just relax,' this practical and empowering guide is your antidote to confusion, shame, and silence."

—Dr Kelly Casperson, board-certified urologist and author of *The Menopause Moment*

*To Campbell and Rhett,*
*The road to you shaped who I am. Chase your dreams fearlessly,*
*and always find your way home.*

*To the worst club with the best members—every woman who*
*has doubted her future, questioned her health, and longed for answers.*
*This is for you. I see you.*

# Contents

*Author's Note* .................................................................. *xi*
*Introduction: Are You Leaving Your Fertility to Chance?* ............ *xiii*

## PART I

## THE TRUTH ABOUT FERTILITY

1. How Inflammation Hijacks Your Fertility ........................... 3
2. Decode Your Hormones and Menstrual Cycle ..................... 19
3. Your Biological Clock ................................................. 39

## PART II

## PREPARING FOR CONCEPTION

4. Getting to the Root Cause of Abnormal Cycles .................. 65
5. Mastering Cycle Tracking ........................................... 105
6. Trying to Conceive .................................................... 127
7. Navigating Infertility ................................................. 151

## PART III

## NATURALLY BALANCE YOUR HORMONES AND IMPROVE YOUR FERTILITY

8. Create a Strong Foundation: Stress, Sleep, and Exercise ..... *191*
9. Eat to Boost Fertility ..... *213*
10. Reduce Exposure to Endocrine-Disrupting Chemicals and Toxins ..... *247*

## PART IV

## THE FERTILITY FORMULA ROAD MAP

A Guide to Optimizing Your Fertility ..... *273*

## PART V

## THE FERTILITY FORMULA RECIPES

Eating Your Way to Better Fertility ..... *319*

*Acknowledgments* ..... *345*
*Appendix: Navigating Your Fertility Appointments* ..... *349*
*Notes* ..... *361*
*Index* ..... *385*

# Author's Note

Fertility is nuanced and personal. The information presented in this book is intended to educate you and help you advocate for your own care. However, medicine is complex, and all treatment decisions should be individualized. Always discuss your symptoms with your healthcare provider. If you do not have a doctor you trust, get a second opinion and find someone who can help guide you on your journey.

Throughout this book, patient cases will be used to help explain difficult scenarios. Although case studies may be similar or based on my clinical experience, no case is about a single patient and all names and identifying information have been modified.

For the sake of simplicity, female/woman/she/her refers to someone born with female reproductive organs (ovaries, uterus), and male/man/he/him refers to someone who is born with male reproductive structures (testes). Some people are born without "normal" reproductive organs or lose them as a result of medical problems. I take care of patients who may identify with a gender incongruent with their reproductive organs or patients who do not have typical reproductive ability for their gender. No part of this book is meant to discriminate or make you feel unworthy. Please take this disclaimer as my note that reproductive biology is complex, and there is something in this book for you no matter how you identify.

Not everyone who needs reproductive assistance has a partner. I have patients who are single, in a same-sex relationship, or in a partnership with someone who doesn't have full reproductive abilities. These are circumstances where donor egg, donor sperm, donor embryo, and/or a gestational carrier may be needed. When discussing the diagnosis and evaluation of infertility, I will often refer to a partner to represent the full evaluation needed for most patients. If you do not have a partner or are pursuing a different path to parenthood, please know this book is still for you. I tell patients every single day that a family is much more than genetics.

I know there are many different scenarios that may lead you to pick up this book or walk into a fertility clinic. No matter who you are, how you identify, or what your goals are, you deserve to learn about your fertility. This book will help you understand your own body and become a better advocate for your reproductive health.

INTRODUCTION

# Are You Leaving Your Fertility to Chance?

Most of us don't think about our fertility until we are ready to get pregnant. We spend half our reproductive life actively trying to prevent pregnancy until one day we decide to start trying. "Trying" usually means stopping contraception, having unprotected sex, and trusting nature to do its thing. Fertility is a matter of chance, we think. We either get pregnant or we don't.

When I was ready to have children, that's what I believed. I stopped my birth control and started trying without thinking about what to do. My husband and I called this "not trying but not preventing." I was sure that after preventing pregnancy for so long, getting pregnant would be easy.

The reality was a lot harder and more complicated than I'd ever expected. I struggled to get pregnant, and I experienced three miscarriages and an ectopic pregnancy, resulting in a fourth loss. This journey was emotionally difficult. I felt a lot of shame and guilt. I know what it is like to question your future.

I'm a double board–certified OB-GYN and Reproductive Endocrinologist. I'm one of the true hormone and fertility experts. My entire career is dedicated to helping women understand how their hormones and bodies work so they can set themselves up for pregnancy when the time is right for them. I've built an online community that helps women understand their fertility and advocate for their health. I've worked with thousands of patients, many of whom have been dismissed by prior physicians and told they would never conceive or have a family.

But fertility was glossed over throughout my OB-GYN training. I never asked my patients, "Do you want to have kids one day? When do you plan to start trying? How many kids do you see yourself having?" Instead, contraception was the priority. I asked every patient, "What are you doing to prevent pregnancy? Are you interested in birth control?" We reviewed contraceptive choices at every annual exam, every postpartum visit, and even as patients were leaving the hospital just after giving birth. But we never asked about their future plans for a family, or even tried to help them understand how their hormones—the entire blueprint for fertility—worked.

Unfortunately, the medical field has been taught to take a reactive approach to fertility. Care is centered around medications, procedures, and treatment instead of education. Most doctors aren't taught the essential facts about fertility, from how female anatomy and hormones actually work, to what happens to fertility as we age, and what a normal menstrual cycle looks like and how to track it. Even if your medical provider does know these facts, they don't always have time to answer your questions—and by the time you get an answer, it may be too late.

Even though I was an OB-GYN resident when my husband and I decided to start trying to conceive, I didn't know what to do after I stopped my birth control. I didn't know how to check to see if I was ovulating or time intercourse with my fertile window. Then when I had miscarriage after miscarriage, I was desperate, frustrated, and convinced that something was wrong. When I went to see my own doctor, I was told it was just "bad luck."

But fertility is not a matter of luck. It's not about luck at all. It is the net sum of choices you make throughout your life, choices that either set you up for a successful pregnancy or impede your ability to conceive.

As you will learn in this book, fertility is much more than the ability to reproduce. It is a marker of your health and proper hormonal function. We need to start seeing our fertility not as separate, but as an integral part of our overall health.

My mission is to educate women about their fertility, their bodies, and how their hormones work so they are empowered to make the choices that are right for them, whatever those choices may be—when to start trying to conceive, what to do if things aren't working, and how to optimize their hormones throughout their life, regardless of whether children are part of the plan. I strongly believe that it should not be a lack of information that makes those choices for you.

If you picked up this book because you want to have a child, are ready to start trying, but don't know where to start; are struggling to get pregnant; or are deeply frustrated by a diagnosis of infertility and unsure of what to do, you are not alone. So many of us have the shared experience of uncertainty and loss of control on the fertility journey.

In my online community, I hear from thousands of women asking the same questions every single week:

*Why am I losing pregnancies?*
*When is the best time to have intercourse?*
*What is a normal period?*
*Are my hormones balanced?*
*When am I ovulating?*
*How do I track my cycle?*
*What should I do next?*
*How can I help improve my fertility?*

Understanding your fertility is the single most important thing you can do for your reproductive future. In a world where misinformation is rampant, it is more imperative than ever that you take ownership of your own body. It is time to start prioritizing your hormonal health and talking about how to plan for the future. The current wait-and-see approach to your fertility no longer works.

At the end of the day, your fertility story is your own. I understand that sometimes we are faced with situations that are out of our hands. But oftentimes, there is more we can do than we think. More than a decade after I struggled with my own infertility, I was diagnosed with celiac disease. It turns out my unexplained pregnancy losses had an explanation after all. It wasn't bad luck. There were things I could have done.

I don't ever want you to sit in a doctor's office saying what I hear patients say every day: "I wish I had known this sooner. I could have made different choices." No one action will cause or cure infertility. Our reproductive health is complex. But choosing to focus on what you can do—by modifying your lifestyle and understanding your body—will benefit your fertility now and down the road.

## BEFORE WE BEGIN

*The Fertility Formula* is divided into five parts. In part I, I explain what you should have learned about your fertility but never did. You'll learn how inflammation hijacks your fertility, the role of hormones, how your menstrual cycle should really work, and the truth about your biological clock: the foundation of fertility. In part II, we put all this knowledge into action, reviewing cycle tracking, natural family planning, best practices for "trying" to conceive, fertility testing, and infertility. In part III (my favorite), we dive into everything you can do—starting now—to prepare your body for conception and take charge of your fertility, from nutrition, supplements, and toxins, to sleep, stress, and exercise. Part IV will put all this information together in an actionable plan to optimize hormonal health and fertility. And finally, part V offers recipes for easy, real-life, and hormone-friendly meals, based on what my family makes every day.

I knew there was no book like this because I looked for it when I needed it, and it didn't exist. I wrote the first version of this book years ago and was passionate that it would go beyond stating facts in order to provide a plan to improve your health. I truly believed this book needed to exist, but the world didn't believe me at first. For years, I was told there was no market for a fertility book, that readers didn't want to read about "depressing" topics like infertility.

*The Fertility Formula* is for all of you. You proved them wrong. By engaging on social media, sharing my videos, downloading podcast episodes, and watching hours of YouTube videos, you changed their minds. You proved that women are invested in understanding their bodies, their health, and their fertility.

Lack of proper information hinders you from making the best decisions about your fertility. In a time when the future of reproductive access is uncertain, it is more important than ever that you prioritize your reproductive health. My hope is that women pick up this book earlier in their life, and we collectively continue to spread the message that fertility matters well beyond pregnancy. It is an important part of our overall well-being.

When it comes to your health, hormones, and fertility, you deserve to be the one in control of your future. I'm not asking you to do this alone. I'm giving you the road map and walking you through what you need to know in order to make the best choices for yourself.

It is time for you to take control of your fertility.

PART I

# THE TRUTH ABOUT FERTILITY

# 1

# How Inflammation Hijacks Your Fertility

During my last year of OB-GYN residency, I was the senior resident in charge of a busy labor and delivery (L&D) unit. We had women laboring in the hallways (yes, the hallways), and it wasn't uncommon on a night like that to not eat, not sit, and to be on the move through my entire shift. As the senior resident, my job was to manage all the patients in labor, but I was six weeks pregnant myself.

My OB-GYN residency program was the largest and busiest in the country, with eighty residents. Despite managing pregnancies every single day, we never talked about our own family plans. There was no discussion about miscarriage or infertility, even though female physicians have double the rate of infertility.[1] The shame and stigma of infertility exists even for the doctors who help you get pregnant. Infertility impacts us all.

Nobody knew I was pregnant—or that this was actually my second pregnancy. My first pregnancy ended in a miscarriage very early. I remember telling my husband, "It's OK," after that first pregnancy loss, reciting stats and medical facts just as I did to patients. "It's no big deal. It wasn't meant to be. We should be happy that things didn't get further along."

I felt more "pregnant" this pregnancy; my symptoms were stronger, and I was convinced everything would be great. But in the middle of that busy night on L&D, I started cramping. I ran to the bathroom trying to hold back the tears, but I was bleeding. There was nothing I could do. This was another pregnancy that wasn't going to be the child I wanted to hold in my arms.

I was devastated and alone, and I couldn't tell anyone. Nobody knew I was pregnant, so how could I go and tell them I was having a miscarriage? I ignored my bleeding and went back to work. I scrubbed into four C-sections that night, showed each family their brand-new baby, all while losing mine.

These are the things people don't prepare you for or explain to you unless they've been there. Infertility is isolating and full of self-blame and doubt. I had no control over what was happening to me, and I am a person who likes to be in control. I went on to miscarry my next pregnancy and then had an ectopic pregnancy. Four losses. I started to give up. Would I be a fertility doctor who could not have her own children? I felt like a failure. My body was betraying me. I didn't understand what I could do or how I could help myself.

I know the questions that go through your head when you start doubting your body. I searched the internet and tried to find answers—even though I was an expert on pregnancy! I eventually received the diagnosis that nobody wants: unexplained infertility. When I asked my own doctor what I could do to help improve my chances of keeping a pregnancy, I was told to "just keep trying and don't stress about it."

This advice is ridiculous anytime, but especially if you're in medical training. I was working thirty-six-hour shifts, eating whatever junk food I could find (crackers and peanut butter from the nurses' station), and drinking after my shifts to unwind. Weren't there things I should be doing that could help me? I couldn't believe that the answer was no.

After completing my residency, my husband and I moved to North Carolina so I could start a fellowship in Reproductive Endocrinology and Infertility (REI). I was pregnant when we bought our house, and I knew exactly which room would be the nursery. By the time we moved in, I had lost my third pregnancy. I didn't even want to walk into the room, as it was an obvious reminder of what we were missing.

Convinced that it couldn't be just bad luck, I became passionate about researching natural fertility. I completed my thesis on the luteal phase. I published research about natural fertility, cycle tracking, and lifestyle exposures. Throughout my research, I kept seeing the same word over and over: *inflammation*.

## YOUR INFLAMMATORY BURDEN

Inflammation is a normal part of our body's immune system. In response to injury or illness, inflammation is short-lived (known as acute) and helpful for healing and recovery. However, constant activation of the immune system can lead to what is known as chronic inflammation, ultimately impairing our body's ability to heal or handle normal cellular functions. Many disease states harm our body via an inflammatory pathway. But the most shocking data I kept finding throughout my research showed that our environment and lifestyle choices—everything from stress and diet to our sleep quality, exercise, and exposure to toxins—can also create inflammation within our bodies. This is called the inflammatory burden.

Our body reacts to the world around us. So I began to wonder, "Do our daily life choices impact our fertility?"

The answer is a resounding yes.

I like to explain it to my patients like this: Imagine your brain is your air traffic control center. It is constantly receiving and sending signals to keep everything functioning smoothly, but there are many moving parts that contribute to flying and landing the plane:

1. Brain: the control center
2. Ovaries: the plane
3. Uterus: the runway
4. Inflammation: the weather

If the control center can't send or receive signals, the plane can't take off (you won't ovulate). If the plane has mechanical issues, you won't depart on time (irregular ovulation). If the runway is damaged, the plane won't be able to land (a pregnancy can't implant). And we all hate when our flight gets canceled (pregnancy loss and infertility).

Consider inflammation inside your body a terrible hailstorm. The longer the storm lasts, the more damage there will be to the planes and the runways. Even after the weather clears, the damage remains. Just imagine if you could change the weather—it may not fix everything, but you certainly have a higher chance of landing the plane with clear skies.

We can't control the weather, but we can control how much inflammation we take on. The data is clear that inflammation is silently harming your body in more ways than you know, especially when it comes to your hormones and reproductive health.[2] Inflammation hijacks your fertility in multiple ways—decreasing egg quality, preventing ovulation, interfering with hormone production, and decreasing implantation rates.[3] Women who have infertility are at risk for other significant health conditions later in life.[4] Sometimes, infertility can be a sign of an underlying autoimmune condition. You have one body; everything is connected.

There are many causes of infertility, many of which you can't control—and we'll talk about them in the pages to come. But we can all agree it is harder to fly a plane in bad weather. After helping thousands of people with infertility navigate the difficult road of IVF, I know that everyone wishes they could rewind the clock and make different choices to lower inflammation. The choices you make all the years you aren't trying to conceive do matter.

Unfortunately, many of the signs and symptoms of inflammation—from fatigue and bloating to brain fog and weight gain—are vague and frequently dismissed by medical professionals. Women often say that this is just "how their body is." Despite knowing something is wrong, nobody will take them seriously. As a fertility physician, I see the ramifications of this daily. More people than ever are struggling to get pregnant.

## THE TRUTH ABOUT RISING INFERTILITY RATES

Infertility is defined as the inability to conceive after twelve months of regular, unprotected intercourse. Ten years ago, one out of eight couples had infertility; that rate has now increased to one out of six.[5] In fact, 20 percent of couples in the US who are trying to conceive their first child will now have infertility.[6] Over 186 million people are currently living with infertility.[7]

There are several factors contributing to rising infertility rates. Your odds of pregnancy decrease the longer you have been trying, regardless of your age. Seventy-two percent of people get pregnant in the first six months of trying, while only 13 percent get pregnant between months six and twelve.[8] (If you are worried about your fertility and wonder if you should keep waiting before getting an evaluation, the answer is no.) Another factor is that people are waiting longer to have children.[9] As fertility and age are tightly connected, the odds of having infertility increase directly with maternal age.[10] We'll talk about all this in depth in chapter 3.

However, it is no coincidence that infertility rates are rising just as our lifestyle choices and the world around us are becoming more inflammatory. Think about the Western diet, lacking whole foods and high in artificial ingredients, which is directly associated with an increase in inflammation.[11] We also consume more plastic and are exposed to chemicals in our food that increase our inflammatory burden.[12] Even chronic daily stress directly increases inflammation inside our body.[13]

Inflammation alters everything from egg quality, hormone production, and ovulation to your uterine environment. We are born with all the eggs we will ever have, but long before we enter menopause, there is a distinct decrease in the ability to get pregnant as we age. This is because our eggs are exposed to the wear and tear of daily life, resulting in more abnormal eggs over time—meaning that age-related infertility is more than just running out of eggs. As our society becomes more inflammatory, more women are being diagnosed with low egg counts.[14] Miscarriage rates are increasing even in young populations.[15]

Sperm are particularly sensitive to inflammation. One of the most startling pieces of data to reveal the debilitating effects of inflammation is the global change to male fertility. There has been a consistent decrease in testosterone levels in men over the past forty years.[16] This drop was observed even when individual variables such as obesity and smoking were accounted for. Over this same time period, sperm counts decreased 52.4 percent worldwide, with the most dramatic drop seen in North America, Europe,

Australia, and New Zealand.[17] Even more concerning, when looking at data after 1995, sperm counts decreased at almost twice the rate as the earlier time period of the study. Put simply, even when controlling for personal health, the world around us is causing an exponential decline in male fertility.

Our lifestyle is contributing to our inflammatory burden. This means that decreasing inflammation is the key to improving fertility and taking control of our hormonal health.

## THE INFLAMMATION CONTINUUM

In order to understand how to decrease inflammation, you first must understand what inflammation does to your body—specifically to your fertility.

Our immune response is a continuum:

1. Acute inflammation—a good process
2. Chronic inflammation—a bad process
3. Autoimmune disease—a toxic process

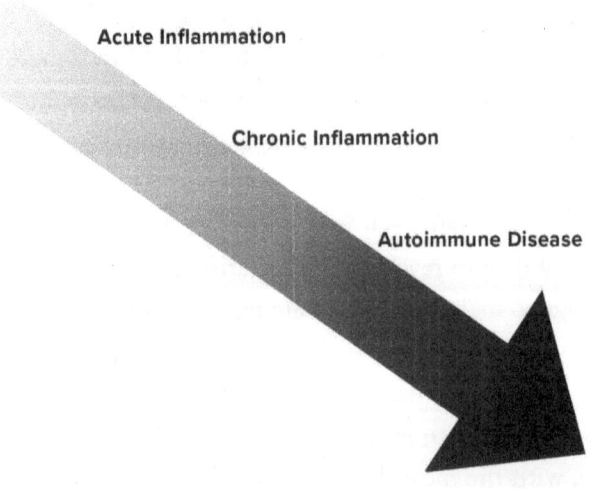

Inflammation Continuum

Acute inflammation is a normal part of your immune system, important in healing and overall health. When you cut your hand, your body sends out immune cells to help heal the cut. Acute inflammation results in increased blood flow to bring immune cells to the damaged area of the body to initiate the process of cellular repair. Local, acute inflammation is also essential for reproduction, including egg growth and maturity, ovulation, and implantation.[18]

However, your body is not meant to be in a constant inflammatory response state. The shift from a temporary immune response to a continuous one results in an overworked immune system and what is known as chronic inflammation. When your immune system can never rest, your cells are never able to fully repair. Chronic inflammation leads to oxidative stress, DNA damage, and impaired healing.[19] You can't see inflammation happening at a cellular level, but chronic inflammation is extremely harmful to your cells, your body, and your fertility.

The first symptom of chronic inflammation is often fatigue, a general sense of being unwell or intrinsically tired. Fatigue is a sign that your body is worn down and trying to get time to heal. Fatigue is your body asking you to pay attention. But there are many other symptoms, including brain fog, insomnia, mood swings, increased irritability, weight gain, and digestive issues, which can all point to chronic inflammation.

When I run through these symptoms with my patients, I always try to elicit what has changed from the norm or when certain symptoms may be present. Keeping a daily journal can be extremely helpful to track your symptoms, food, exposures, and more. Ultimately, your healthcare team can only make medical connections based on the information you present to them. When you say everything is fine, but everything is not fine, you are doing yourself a disservice.

Review the list of chronic inflammation symptoms and think about how many you mark "yes" for. If you mark fewer than five symptoms, your inflammation levels are likely in a healthy range. If you mark yes for six to fifteen symptoms, you may be experiencing mild inflammation, and if the symptoms persist or are clustered around one organ system you should check in with your doctor. Sixteen or more symptoms is a sure sign that inflammation is impacting your health and quality of life, and now is a good time to look closer at your lifestyle and seek a medical evaluation.

## CHRONIC INFLAMMATION SYMPTOMS

- Fatigue
- Apathy
- Restlessness
- Hyperactivity
- Headaches
- Fainting
- Lightheadedness
- Insomnia
- Poor memory
- Confusion
- Brain fog
- Decreased coordination
- Slow decision-making
- Poor attention
- Stuttering or slurring speech
- Difficulty learning
- Mood swings
- Increased irritability
- Depression
- Anxiety
- Binge eating or drinking
- Food cravings
- Compulsive eating
- Water retention
- Weight gain
- Weight loss
- Weakness
- Stiffness
- Arthritis
- Joint or muscle pain
- Watery, itchy eyes
- Swollen or red eyes
- Dark circles under eyes
- Blurry vision
- Earaches or ear infections
- Ringing in the ears
- Hearing loss
- Itching ears
- Ear drainage
- Stuffy nose
- Increased congestion
- Sinus problems
- Allergies
- Sneezing
- Coughing
- Clearing throat
- Sore throat
- Loss of voice
- Swollen tongue, gums, or lips
- Canker sores
- Rashes or hives
- Acne
- Hair loss or breakage
- Flushing
- Hot flashes
- Increased sweating
- Poor temperature regulation
- Irregular or skipped heartbeat
- Rapid heartbeat
- Chest pain
- Chest congestion
- Asthma
- Shortness of breath
- Difficulty breathing
- Nausea or vomiting
- Constipation
- Diarrhea
- Belching
- Increased gas
- Bloating
- Heartburn
- Stomach pains
- Frequent urination
- Frequent illness
- Genital itching
- Menstrual irregularity
- Spotting between cycles
- Painful periods
- Pain with intercourse
- Infertility

As you can see, many of the signs and symptoms of chronic inflammation are vague, and they are frequently dismissed by doctors. The most important takeaway is this: Chronic inflammation is not normal and disease is imminent. You should not be living like this. Your body is telling you that it is struggling. It is time to learn how to listen to what your body is telling you.

Why does chronic inflammation happen? What causes the immune system to be constantly turned on? Inflammation can result from infections and disease, but also, as we've been learning, from your daily life—what you eat, drink, and breathe, your stress and activity levels, sleep disruption, and exposure to toxins all contribute to your level of inflammation. Although we each have a different threshold of damage we can tolerate before our system is overwhelmed, our lifestyle contributes to our inflammatory burden often through increasing insulin resistance and a shift in our gut microbiome.

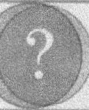 *Common Questions*

**If inflammation is bad, why can't I just take anti-inflammatory medication?**

The acute inflammatory response is responsible for cell healing and is an important part of menstruation, ovulation, implantation, and placental invasion. You can't just take anti-inflammatory medications and "treat" the inflammation, as this will also stop the helpful part of the inflammatory process. In fact, taking NSAIDs (nonsteroidal anti-inflammatory drugs), such as Motrin, Aleve, or ibuprofen, can prevent ovulation. Interestingly, in this scenario your cells still have hormonal changes associated with ovulation, but no egg is ever released, so you can't get pregnant.[20] Infertile women who chronically take NSAIDs may have ovulatory failure, which can be reversed by simply stopping the medication.[21]

Take-home message: Treating inflammation requires prevention. If you have pain before or around ovulation, don't take anti-inflammatory medication. Acetaminophen (Tylenol) is a better option.

## INSULIN RESISTANCE

Chronic inflammation and insulin resistance are tightly linked, leading to a cycle of hormone dysfunction. Insulin is an important hormone responsible for allowing glucose to move from the bloodstream into each cell, where it can be used to fuel cellular functions. When our body is working perfectly, insulin and glucose work in tandem every moment of the day. Insulin resistance is when our cells require a higher signal of insulin in order to allow glucose uptake. The net result is an elevation of blood glucose and insulin creating an inflammatory environment. Persistently elevated insulin levels also increase your visceral fat—worsening inflammation further.

Importantly, chronic inflammation can also lead to insulin resistance by interfering with both the insulin signaling pathway and the insulin receptor.[22] Since a healthy gut is an important contributor to your immune system and inflammatory burden, an abnormal gut microbiome increases chronic inflammation.[23] Inflammation and insulin resistance become a self-reinforcing cycle changing our cells on a metabolic level.

Insulin resistance harms your fertility in multiple ways—including impairing egg growth and maturation, decreasing egg quality and embryo growth, changing endometrial receptivity, and decreasing outcomes even with IVF, in addition to being a key component of polycystic ovary syndrome (PCOS).[24] To put it plainly, chronic inflammation and insulin resistance create a toxic environment for our fertility. Once we acknowledge that our lifestyle is pro-inflammatory and a contributing factor to insulin resistance, we begin to see the importance of breaking the cycle at its beginning.

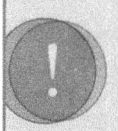

> ### *Important Study Findings:*
> ### Insulin Resistance and Pregnancy Loss
>
> "Increased Prevalence of Insulin Resistance in Women with a History of Recurrent Pregnancy Loss"[25]
>
> - **Study basics:** Rates of insulin resistance, defined as an elevated fasting insulin level or an abnormal glucose to insulin ratio, were evaluated in women with recurrent pregnancy loss compared to women without infertility.
>
> - **Results:** 27% of women with pregnancy loss had insulin resistance as compared to 9.5% of the control group. Fasting insulin levels were significantly higher in women with pregnancy loss.
>
> - **Conclusion:** Insulin resistance is an independent risk factor for pregnancy loss.

## AUTOIMMUNE DISEASE

At the far end of the inflammatory continuum is autoimmune disease. Autoimmune disease is a condition in which your immune system fails to distinguish "normal" from "abnormal" cells and begins to react to your own body, causing cellular damage and destruction. There are many different kinds of autoimmune disease, but they all share the common causal pathway of chronic inflammation. Most people will have symptoms of chronic inflammation before they are ever diagnosed with an autoimmune disease.

Autoimmune disease onset is believed to be caused by both a genetic predisposition (something you can't control) and an environmental exposure (many of which you can control).[26] Unfortunately, the diagnosis of autoimmunity does not happen until cellular damage is so extreme that blood tests for specific antibodies become positive. You may wait years for a diagnosis after symptoms start.

The time from disease initiation to cellular damage significant enough to warrant severe symptoms and a diagnosis is considered the "preclinical" time in autoimmunity. The preclinical disease state represents the opportunity for the biggest intervention and potential delay of true disease. If we know that you are at risk for an autoimmune disease but could change the trajectory of your course, imagine how that could change your life.

Interestingly, hormone changes increase autoimmune disease progression, so we are at higher risk of autoimmune disease during our reproductive years.[27] Autoimmune disease is associated with infertility, prolonged time to pregnancy, and an increase in pregnancy loss many years before actual diagnosis.[28,29] This means that infertility or pregnancy loss may be the first symptom of autoimmunity and represents the "preclinical" time where change can make the biggest impact.

Rates of autoimmune disease have increased 50 percent in thirty years, just as our lifestyle has become more inflammatory.[30] This is not a coincidence. Actively decreasing inflammation can make an impactful change in your long-term health and your fertility, and it is time we start to think about our fertility on a bigger scale.

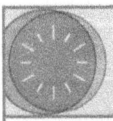 *Top Tip*

**How to get your doctor to take your inflammatory symptoms seriously**

I know how hard it is when your doctor dismisses your symptoms. I've been in that position myself, and it made me doubt my own body and my ability to know what was going on. You know your body best, and you deserve to have a doctor who not only believes you but wants to help you find an answer. As someone who has been on both sides of this situation, this is my best advice:

1. **Find the right care team:** Not every doctor will be a good fit. Although I know it can be easier said than done, if your doctor does not take your symptoms seriously, find another one.

2. **Pick the right visit:** Different visit types have a different amount of allotted time. If you are at an annual exam, it can be very difficult for your doctor to cover all the necessary health screenings and discuss new problems. Instead, schedule a specific problem-based appointment so the entire purpose of the visit will be to discuss the symptoms you are having.

3. **Know your story:** Take time to think about what is going on, how long you have been feeling this way, and if your symptoms are constant or if certain things make them come and go. The very first question your doctor will ask is "What is going on?" There is no reason to go into this visit unprepared. Write down your symptoms, timeline, and associated questions.

4. **Understand the next steps:** Don't leave this visit without knowing what needs to happen next. I always love it when a patient says, "I want to make sure I understand what to do next . . ." Also clarify how you will find out your lab results. How can you ask further questions? When should you schedule a follow-up visit to check in? You are the one in charge of your health, so make sure you know what to do next.

## FERTILITY IS A HEALTH MARKER

The World Health Organization defines infertility as a disease.[31] But I believe it can also be a sign of future illness. Infertility has been shown to put you at a greater risk for serious disease, chronic illness, and even earlier death than women who did not have infertility.[32,33] This risk persists regardless of whether you get pregnant or receive any fertility treatments.[34,35,36] It's not the infertility that causes these health risks, but the chronic inflammation—which contributes to both infertility and later disease development.

For instance, women with infertility have an 83 percent higher risk of a cardiovascular event, such as a heart attack, and a 79 percent increased chance of developing metabolic syndrome.[37] These huge percentages should be a wake-up call that infertility truly is a warning sign. As someone who had infertility, these numbers are scary!

**FUTURE HEALTH RISKS ASSOCIATED WITH INFERTILITY**

| | |
|---|---|
| High blood pressure | Kidney disease |
| Heart disease | Stroke |
| Myocardial infarction | Metabolic syndrome |
| Diabetes | Autoimmune disease |
| Liver disease | Cancer |

When we accept that our fertility is a health marker, the importance of optimizing our health becomes even more apparent. Our bodies are exposed to more inflammation in today's world than ever before. When your immune system is constantly working to fight external inflammation, your internal environment becomes toxic.

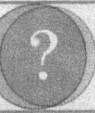 *Common Questions*

**Why do so many fertility doctors breeze over lifestyle interventions?**

It may be the case that by the time you get to the fertility clinic, you need more advanced treatment. I see patients who have been trying for years before coming to get help, and we may be in a race against the clock by the time I meet with them. Sometimes IVF is the answer. But if you have been through IVF, or know anyone who has, anything you can do to improve your chance of success is helpful when making such a huge emotional, physical, and financial investment. If you are in the midst of infertility and undergoing fertility treatments, please view this book as an adjunct to your care and not a replacement.

After our fourth pregnancy loss, I took matters into my own hands. I wasn't opposed to IVF; in fact, I was ready for that next step but had to wait due to my clinical schedule in fellowship. While waiting, I decided to do everything possible to improve our odds of success by decreasing the inflammation I was exposing my body to. My fellowship research supported this—even if my doctors told me there was nothing I could do. We changed our lifestyle, our diet, our kitchen, and our habits. We ended up getting pregnant in the months preceding IVF—and this time, we stayed pregnant.

In learning to listen to my body for inflammatory clues, I cut out gluten. It was one of many changes I made, but I wouldn't know the significance of this until over a decade later when I was ultimately diagnosed with celiac disease (an autoimmune disease resulting in a gluten sensitivity). Infertility and pregnancy loss were my body's warning sign that I was in the "preclinical" state of my autoimmune disease. Even though I didn't get a diagnosis at that point, the changes I made to my life had a huge impact on my fertility journey. After four pregnancy losses, pregnancies five and six became my children.

I'm not sure why healthcare providers sometimes tell their patients that there is nothing they can do to improve their fertility. This couldn't be further from the truth. You may not be able to "cure" your infertility by reducing inflammation, but you absolutely can make a difference in the outcome of your journey. We are conditioned to think about our bodies segmented off in different organ systems, but everything within you is connected. Of course the environment you subject your body to will make a difference on your fertility.

I know there are some things about your environment and your health that you absolutely cannot change. We can't rewind the clock or change our age. I can't go back and change how I treated my body in medical training. For both men and women, eggs and sperm are susceptible to the world around us. But the top causes of chronic inflammation are things you have control over. The lifestyle choices you make every single day directly determine the level of inflammation inside your body. It is clear that inflammation and fertility are tightly linked, and decreasing your inflammatory burden is the key to taking control of your reproductive future.

### Facts to Remember

- Your fertility matters long before you want to conceive.
- Infertility rates are increasing.
- Your fertility is a marker of your overall health.
- Infertility is both a symptom and a disease.
- Infertility is associated with a higher rate of future disease.
- Acute inflammation is an important part of reproduction, but chronic inflammation contributes to infertility and hormone dysfunction.
- Your lifestyle determines the level of inflammation inside your body.

# 2

# Decode Your Hormones and Menstrual Cycle

Maple, a thirty-six-year-old self-described "health freak," was trying to get pregnant. Her cycles were regular, she ate healthy, loved yoga, and didn't have any medical problems. But after about nine months with no success, she scheduled an appointment to check her hormones.

Maple favored natural approaches and routinely took essential oils or supplements instead of traditional medications. She didn't want to see a fertility doctor who would push invasive testing and treatments, so instead she scheduled an appointment with a holistic hormone specialist.

Her consultation was very detailed, and she had blood work done for a huge hormone panel. To her surprise, she had low progesterone, low testosterone, and high estrogen. The specialist recommended daily compounded progesterone and testosterone cream (sold by the clinic) and told her "estrogen dominance" was a hormone imbalance causing her infertility. Her husband was also seen and told his fatigue was due to low testosterone. He started on a daily injectable testosterone.

When Maple received a diagnosis and a treatment plan, she was happy that there was something she could do and hopeful for the future. What Maple didn't know was that the hormone specialist she saw had just prescribed both her and her husband birth control—without even knowing it!

This is why understanding your reproductive hormones is so important.

## HORMONES: YOUR BODY'S COMMUNICATION SYSTEM

Your hormones are your body's communication system, signaling the current state of affairs and providing instructions on what should happen next. Imagine best friends living in different states. They can't really "see" each other, but they rely on messages (hormones) being sent back and forth like texts letting the other know what they're doing.

Your hormones are responsible for coordinating all your bodily functions. They control growth, metabolism, digestion, blood pressure, water balance, mood, sexual function, ovulation, and reproduction. Your hormones are essential for life.

Unfortunately, there is a lot of misinformation about what hormones actually do, making them an easy scapegoat for any medical problem. *Less energy?* Must be your hormones. *Gaining weight?* You should get your hormones checked. *Low libido?* You need to take some hormones. At least once a week, I see a patient to discuss "balancing hormones." All these symptoms can absolutely be caused by a hormonal issue, but balancing hormones is a catchall phrase that doesn't really mean anything specific and is often used as a diagnosis without getting to the root cause. For our purposes, I define having balanced hormones as your hormone communication system working and responding correctly.

For instance, a regular and predictable period is one of the top signs that your hormones are working as they should. It is unlikely that you would have a major hormonal problem and still have a regular cycle, but many hormone issues present with subtle cycle changes, which can be hard to identify if you are not tracking your cycle. An understanding of the menstrual cycle is essential anytime we discuss your hormones (we'll go over this later in the chapter).

The hormone conversation is complex. Your hormones change all the time, based on time of day, what phase of your menstrual cycle you are in, and your environment. Some hormones are pulsatile, meaning they are released in bursts, while others have a constant release pattern. Hormone levels in urine, blood, and saliva can all be different, even if measured at the same time. In order to evaluate your hormones or interpret any testing, you must have a deep understanding of normal hormonal fluctuation and variation.

## HOW HORMONES WORK

There are multiple organ systems involved in hormone production: the thyroid gland; two adrenal glands (each sits on top of a kidney); your gonads (ovaries or testes); and your brain, specifically the hypothalamus and pituitary gland.

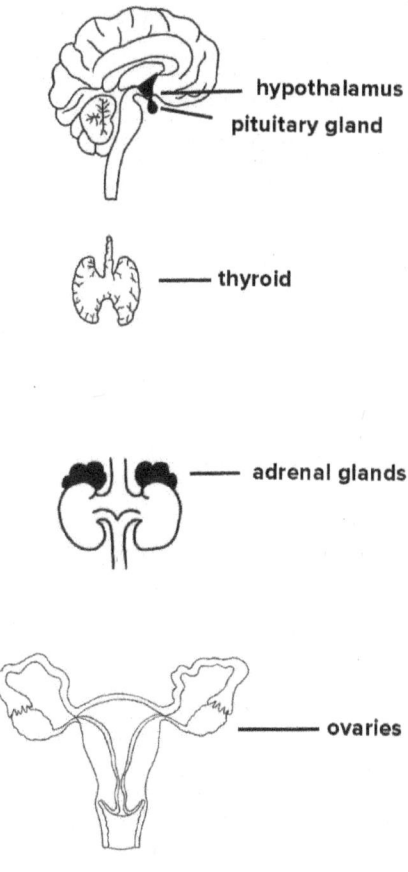

Hypothalamic-Pituitary-Ovarian (HPO) Axis

The brain is the primary hormone control center. Hormone signals from all over the body go through the brain, and the brain is responsible for responding accordingly. The hypothalamus is the central command station. It constantly interprets signals from other parts of the body—sent via hormones—and communicates to the pituitary gland with instructions to send out other hormones. But the pituitary gland is the real workhorse in the brain. It stores many of our hormones. Once signaled by the hypothalamus, the pea-sized gland sends out hormones to communicate with other organs in the body. This is your brain sending out the signal to *get to work!*

Pituitary hormones are essential for your body to function. Each is stored in a different section of the pituitary. This is something to keep in mind when treating infertility. For example, the pituitary hormones important in reproduction, FSH (follicle-stimulating hormone) and LH (luteinizing hormone), control ovulation and the production of estrogen and progesterone. The area of the pituitary gland that stores them is located the farthest from the blood supply. This means that if blood supply to the pituitary gland is decreased, reproductive functions are the first to go.

| Pituitary Gland Hormone | Target Organ | Function |
| --- | --- | --- |
| Growth Hormone (GH) | liver, muscle, bones, fat cells | cell growth |
| Follicle-Stimulating Hormone (FSH) | ovaries/testes | egg growth, estrogen production, sperm production |
| Luteinizing Hormone (LH) | ovaries/testes | ovulation, progesterone and testosterone production |
| Thyroid-Stimulating Hormone (TSH) | thyroid gland | makes thyroid hormones |
| Prolactin (PRL) | breasts | milk production |
| Adrenocorticotropic Hormone (ACTH) | adrenal gland | makes cortisol and other steroids |

| Pituitary Gland Hormone | Target Organ | Function |
| --- | --- | --- |
| Melanocyte-Stimulating Hormone (MSH) | skin | melanin production, skin protection |
| Oxytocin | brain, breasts, uterus | pleasure, decrease stress, milk production, contractions |
| Antidiuretic Hormone (ADH) | kidneys | control water/salt balance |
| Endorphins | brain | decrease pain |

The pituitary gland and hypothalamus work in tandem to interpret and balance your hormones to the best of their ability. The pituitary gland only interprets hormone signals from the hypothalamus.

But—and this is one of the most important concepts to understand about hormones—the hypothalamus signals the pituitary gland based solely on *your brain's interpretation of your hormone status*. Your hypothalamus decides if the signal it sees from the rest of the body is sufficient or deficient—meaning that the hormone level *you* may need and the level I may need might be very different. Your brain is truly personalized for you.

Your immune system and hormone production are tightly linked. If you have acute inflammation and are trying to heal, your body is going to want energy readily available to use. This results in a shift in hormone production, which is helpful in the short term but harmful long term. Chronic inflammation interferes with hypothalamic-pituitary communication, resulting in abnormal hormone release.[1] Decreasing inflammation is the key to balancing your hormones.

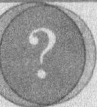 **Common Questions**

**Can I balance my hormones?**

Your hormones change throughout the day, making it hard to check one hormone level and detect an imbalance or confirm normalcy. However, when you have a disconnect between the brain-organ communication system, it will result in an abnormal hormone response. We don't initially know where the issue is, and it is important to think about potential sources of disruption. These can include the following:

1. Your brain is not interpreting signals correctly.
2. Your brain is not responding to signals appropriately.
3. Your target organs are not interpreting signals correctly.
4. Your target organs are not responding to signals appropriately.
5. The communication system has interference.

"Balanced hormones" mean your body is functioning correctly and "unbalanced hormones" indicate a failure of your hormone system to interpret or respond appropriately to a signal. As you can see, one lab test can mean many different things and can even be "normal" if something is wrong. Hormone testing is dependent on which hormone was checked at what time *and* the knowledge of the person interpreting the results. You are now on your journey to understanding how to interpret your hormones yourself.

## YOUR REPRODUCTIVE HORMONES

Estrogen and progesterone are the two reproductive hormones primarily responsible for much of how your body and menstrual cycle function, and they are essential determinants of your health and wellness. How we feel on any given day throughout a normal menstrual cycle is directly related to these hormones. When our hormones are off, the symptoms that we recognize as abnormal—from fatigue, bloating, and mood changes to low libido—are due to abnormal levels of estrogen and progesterone. Both estrogen and progesterone are also important modifiers of your immune system—influencing inflammation and insulin sensitivity.[2]

## Estrogen

Estrogen can be made by fat cells and the adrenal glands, but the main form of circulating estrogen in your reproductive years is made by your ovaries. The brain sends out FSH, which stimulates an egg to grow. As the egg is maturing, you make higher levels of estrogen, peaking at ovulation.

There are three main types of estrogen that can be made in your body:

- Estrone (E1)—made by fat cells, main form of estrogen after menopause
- Estradiol (E2)—made by developing follicles in the ovary, main form of estrogen in reproductive years
- Estriol (E3)—made by the placenta in pregnancy

Estrogen receptors are located in many types of tissue throughout your body, making estrogen important to numerous important bodily functions, including regulating metabolism, blood sugar, cholesterol, bone and muscle mass, collagen production, brain function, and your immune system. Estrogen has anti-inflammatory properties, with inflammation markers decreasing significantly as estrogen levels rise during a normal menstrual cycle.[3] In fact, most premenopausal heart attacks in women occur in the early follicular phase, when estrogen is the lowest.[4]

Since ovulation is the primary driver of estrogen production, regular cycles help keep inflammation low. However, chronic inflammation can interfere with the HPO axis, resulting in delayed or absent ovulation and longer menstrual cycle length.[5] The cycle of inflammation can continuously worsen unless you break the pattern.

Irregular or absent periods can occur with both abnormally elevated or decreased estrogen levels. Consistently elevated estrogen levels can lead to irregular or absent cycles, as the brain cannot interpret the need to grow a follicle. Estrogen levels are often elevated due to increased production, decreased ability to metabolize estrogen, or external sources. Conditions that can lead to elevated baseline estrogen include PCOS, obesity, excess alcohol intake, liver problems, ovarian tumors, stress, toxins, and supplements.

Low estrogen can occur when the ovaries are not functioning or are removed. Understanding the cause for low estrogen is important in determining appropriate treatment options. Common causes of low estrogen include irregular or absent ovulation, perimenopause, ovarian failure (menopause), stress, and surgical removal of the ovaries.

Your brain and body love estrogen. Abnormal estrogen levels can significantly impact your quality of life, as seen in the table below.

**SYMPTOMS OF ABNORMAL ESTROGEN**

| Low Estrogen | High Estrogen |
| --- | --- |
| Hot flashes | Acne |
| Night sweats | Difficulty sleeping |
| Brain fog | Fatigue |
| Vaginal dryness | Mood changes |
| Decreased libido | Headaches |
| Mood changes | Breast changes |

## Progesterone

After ovulation, LH from the brain stimulates progesterone production from the ovaries. Progesterone prepares the body for a potential pregnancy, often resulting in many undesired side effects, and it is only made after you ovulate. It opens and closes the implantation window, meaning the uterus can only allow an embryo to implant during a set number of days. To do this, progesterone thickens the cervical mucus to prevent bacteria from ascending into the uterus and decreases the immune system, permitting implantation.

Since inflammation is important for ovulation and implantation, higher inflammatory markers are often seen when progesterone levels are higher.[6] However, progesterone is immunosuppressive at high levels, as seen during pregnancy.[7] Many autoimmune disease symptoms actually improve during pregnancy due to this immune suppression. The truth is that progesterone is a potent immune modulator—activating some parts of the immune system and suppressing others.[8]

**SYMPTOMS OF HIGH PROGESTERONE**

| | |
|---|---|
| Decrease in energy | Nausea |
| Increase in appetite | Increased sense of smell |
| Sleepiness | Food sensitivity |
| Tender breasts | Acne |
| Bloating | |

Progesterone elevation is not problematic or attributed to any medical diagnosis. On the other hand, low progesterone is more common and is almost exclusively due to problems with ovulation. If your brain is not properly interpreting or sending out LH, or your ovaries are not properly responding to LH, you will have difficulty ovulating and making progesterone.

Progesterone is made by the ovary in pulses, directly stimulated from LH pulses from the brain. After ovulation, progesterone levels can range anywhere from 3 ng/mL to 40 ng/mL, depending on when blood was drawn in response to an LH surge.[9] Checking progesterone can only confirm that ovulation occurred, not whether your body is making enough progesterone. This means there is no set level of progesterone that confirms a "good" luteal phase.

However, progesterone production should significantly increase with pregnancy because hCG (human chorionic gonadotropin), the pregnancy hormone, binds to the same receptor as LH. Once pregnant, the ovary now has a constant stimulus to make progesterone, unlike when it was relying on LH pulses from the brain, and progesterone production should now increase and stay elevated.

Until the placenta becomes functional, around nine to ten weeks of pregnancy, all progesterone production comes from the ovary. The link between progesterone, infertility, and miscarriage is complex, but without a doubt, progesterone is essential in implantation, and poor progesterone production is the first stage of ovulatory dysfunction.

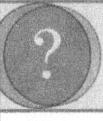

## *Common Questions*

**What is estrogen dominance?**

Estrogen dominance is not a true medical diagnosis but instead a sign that something else is happening inside your body. Some people will say it is an abnormal "estrogen-to-progesterone ratio," which is also false. When people are diagnosed with estrogen dominance it means that lab results show an elevated estrogen and a low progesterone. This occurs in two circumstances: (1) everything is normal and blood was drawn in the follicular phase, or (2) you are not ovulating and by definition are "stuck" in the follicular phase (an example of this is PCOS). If we think back to Maple's case, she was diagnosed with "estrogen dominance" in the follicular phase of her cycle, which is a normal time to be estrogen dominant. Since ovulation had not occurred, there was no progesterone. By definition, the follicular phase is estrogen dominant. Drawing a random hormone panel, seeing a high estrogen and low progesterone, and falsely diagnosing estrogen dominance can lead to prescribing progesterone when not needed. This daily progesterone acts like birth control and prevents pregnancy.

## OTHER IMPORTANT HORMONES IN REPRODUCTION

Other hormones play an important role in your fertility. Abnormalities in these hormones may directly cause infertility or be a symptom of an underlying issue. Many of these will be discussed more in chapter 4, but for now, here's a quick overview.

## Prolactin

Prolactin is made by the pituitary gland and is important in controlling breast growth and lactation. Outside of these specific situations, prolactin levels are usually low but will fluctuate throughout the day and in response to food, exercise, and sex. Elevated prolactin levels impair the ability of the pituitary gland to release FSH and LH, resulting in lack of ovulation and a low estrogen state.

## Thyroid Hormones

The thyroid gland is important in metabolism and energy regulation and is a butterfly-shaped gland in the neck. The pituitary gland sends out thyroid-stimulating hormone (TSH), which directs the thyroid gland to send out the thyroid hormones, triiodothyronine (T3) and thyroxine (T4). Abnormal thyroid hormone levels impair the pituitary gland's ability to send out FSH/LH, resulting in abnormal ovulation.

## Testosterone

Testosterone is made by both the ovaries and the adrenal glands in women. Testosterone can play an important role in libido, bone density, and muscle mass. Testosterone is converted to estrogen, and levels are generally low but vary throughout the menstrual cycle just as estrogen does.[10] High levels of testosterone can be seen with PCOS, ovarian tumors, and androgen resistance syndrome. When the ovaries stop making estrogen in menopause, they continue to make testosterone, and testosterone becomes more impactful in your body after menopause.

## Dehydroepiandrosterone (DHEA)

DHEA is made by the adrenal glands and is measured by checking the sulfated version, named DHEAS. DHEA is converted in the bloodstream to testosterone and is the main source of circulating androgens in premenopausal females. An increased level of DHEAS can be seen with adrenal gland tumors or PCOS, often causing irregular periods.

## Cortisol

Your adrenal glands make cortisol, also known as the stress hormone. The hypothalamus is constantly interpreting how much cortisol you have in your body, so it knows if it needs to direct the pituitary gland to send out ACTH. The adrenal glands control our "fight-or-flight" response, so cortisol is meant to increase when your body needs to direct resources elsewhere in a time of stress. Cortisol is an inflammatory hormone, meaning that in chronic stress, continually elevated cortisol contributes to chronic inflammation.[11]

## Insulin

Insulin is released by the pancreas in response to food. It allows your cells to utilize glucose for energy, store glucose for later use, and regulate your blood sugar. Insulin resistance is when your cells stop responding to insulin, leading to high circulating insulin levels and chronic inflammation. High insulin acts directly on the ovary, stimulating increased androgen production, and the endometrium, impacting endometrial receptivity and implantation.[12] Insulin resistance is often seen with PCOS, but it is also associated with infertility and pregnancy loss even when PCOS is not present.[13]

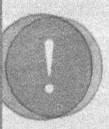

## *Important Study Findings:*
## Biotin Supplements and Hormone Levels

"Association of Biotin Ingestion with Performance of Hormone and Nonhormone Assays in Healthy Adults"[14]

- **Study basics:** Biotin is a B vitamin (B7) which helps the body metabolize carbohydrates, fats, and proteins into usable amino acids. It is important in hair, skin, and nail growth and proper nervous system functioning. Biotin can bind to the assay that we use in the lab to test some of your hormone levels. In this study, healthy adults were given 10 mg of biotin a day for seven days, and hormone levels were tested before and after dosing.

- **Results:** Biotin interference was seen in many of the hormone levels, resulting in both falsely high and falsely low results.

- **Conclusion:** Biotin is found in many multivitamins and prenatal vitamins. At the daily recommended dose of 300 mcg a day, biotin does not interfere with lab tests. However, many over-the-counter products will contain extremely high doses of biotin (ten to thirty times the daily average). This megadose of biotin can result in abnormal lab results and misdiagnosis. Look carefully at products marketed for fertility, hormone health, beauty, greens powders, or collagen to make sure you are not taking too much biotin.

## YOUR MENSTRUAL CYCLE

As mentioned, a normal and predictable menstrual cycle is one of the biggest indicators that your hormones are working as they should. Chronic inflammation interferes with the brain's ability to interpret and send out correct hormone signals, and one clear sign of this is a change in your menstrual cycle pattern. In order to know what is abnormal, you must first know what is normal.

Of course, what's normal looks different for everyone. But in general, here's what should happen.

The menstrual cycle is divided into four phases: (1) menses, (2) follicular phase, (3) ovulation, (4) luteal phase. Then the cycle starts over again with menses. Communication is required between the brain, ovaries, and uterus to regulate ovulation and production of estrogen and progesterone, which dictate the beginning and end of each phase. The hypothalamus sends out gonadotropin-releasing hormone (GnRH) in pulses, based on the interpretation of estrogen and progesterone. The frequency and amplitude of the

GnRH pulses control the pituitary gland release of FSH and LH (think of it like Morse code). FSH and LH work throughout your cycle to control estrogen, ovulation, progesterone, and menses, also known as your period.

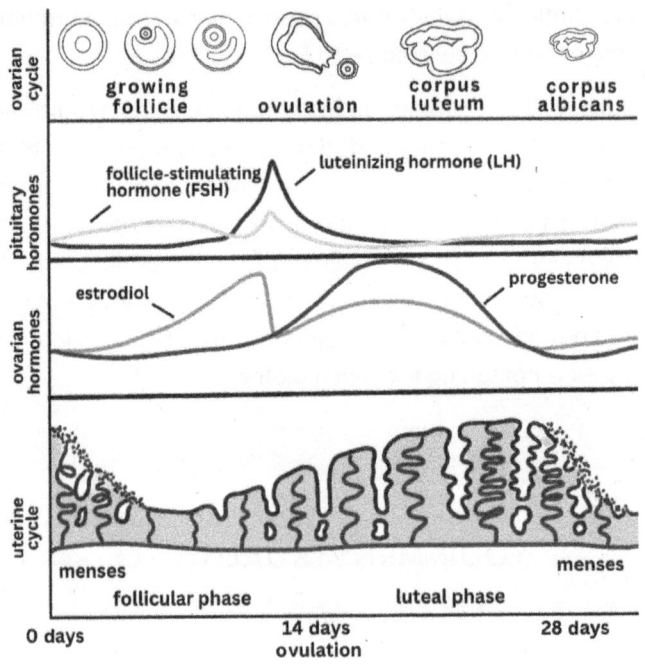

Menstrual Cycle

## Menses

The menstrual cycle begins with the first day of menses, or when your period begins. Menses is the shedding of the uterine lining, or endometrium, since pregnancy did not occur. The signal for your body to begin menses is a drop in progesterone at the end of the luteal phase. Your ovary is healing from the prior cycle. You have small follicles, each with an egg inside, ready to respond, but no follicle has yet been selected to ovulate. The pituitary gland begins to send out FSH in order to select a new follicle.

During menses, you will have bleeding and uterine cramping. Your estrogen and progesterone levels are both low, which can result in some symptoms commonly seen with low hormone levels, including mood changes, irritability, increased appetite.

The menstrual phase is actually a phase within the follicular phase, as the ovary is starting to grow the follicle for the next month while you are bleeding. In fact, the estrogen made by the new follicle is what stops your menstrual bleeding. For simplicity, we will consider menses and the follicular phase different cycles. Your menstrual phase is as long as your period, with the average menses lasting four to six days.

## Follicular Phase

The follicular phase is the first half of your menstrual cycle, when an egg is growing in preparation for ovulation. Each egg grows inside a follicle. In the follicular phase, your pituitary gland sends out just enough FSH to stimulate one follicle to grow. I like to think of FSH as the food for the eggs. As that follicle is growing, the egg inside is maturing, and estrogen is made at increasing levels.

Estrogen communicates back to the brain, telling it that a follicle is growing. Since your body does not want to have every egg mature and ovulate (after all, humans cannot carry twenty babies at one time), FSH decreases once estrogen is being made. This FSH-estradiol feedback loop is essential in order to ovulate only one egg at a time.

The follicular phase is an estrogen-dominant phase, with high estrogen levels and low progesterone levels. This results in increased focus, energy, and sexuality. The length of the follicular phase can vary cycle to cycle and throughout different phases of reproductive life. As we age, the FSH signal from our brain increases, resulting in earlier ovulation and a shorter follicular phase.

## Ovulation

Ovulation is when the follicle containing the egg ruptures, releasing the egg into the body to be captured by the fallopian tube. As the egg matures and gets closer to ovulation, estrogen levels exponentially increase, peaking around 200 pg/mL. Once estrogen has reached this peak for fifty hours, the brain will then send out a surge of LH (luteinizing hormone).[15] This LH surge begins the process of ovulation, with egg release occurring on average twenty-four to thirty-six hours after the LH surge is detected.

Immediately prior to ovulation, peak estrogen levels increase your cervical mucus and sex drive. Some people may have ovulatory spotting, which can occur from a transient decrease in estrogen production as the follicle ruptures and the cells that make estrogen are disrupted for a short period of time.

An interesting fact: Your body typically has a hard time interpreting pain signals from the pelvis, and many people do not feel their ovaries at all. However, you may have one-sided cramping from the follicle rupturing at ovulation, and this is called mittelschmerz, German for "middle pain," as it occurs in the middle of the cycle.

## Luteal Phase

The luteal phase is the second half of your cycle, from ovulation to your next period. After ovulation, the follicle that grew the egg re-forms into a new cyst, called a corpus luteum. This corpus luteum becomes a progesterone production factory. Progesterone is secreted from the corpus luteum in pulses, stimulated directly from brain pulses of LH. Progesterone stabilizes the uterine lining, prepares it for pregnancy, and opens and closes the implantation window. Typical symptoms from this high-progesterone state are all meant to conserve energy and include an increase in appetite, decrease in energy, and decrease in focus.

The corpus luteum cannot live forever, and without a pregnancy it typically lasts only twelve to fourteen days. At this time, the corpus luteum dies, progesterone production drops, and your body will begin a period, entering back into the menses stage of the menstrual cycle. The time when progesterone drops *prior* to bleeding can lead to what many people know as PMS, premenstrual syndrome, associated with mood changes and irritability due to the hormone changes of the late luteal phase.

If you do happen to conceive, a pregnancy will begin to implant about seven to nine days after ovulation, and hCG will be made from the pregnancy. Since hCG and LH are similar in structure, they share a receptor and hCG can "rescue" the corpus luteum. The rising hCG levels constantly stimulate progesterone production, leading to a progesterone increase after implantation.

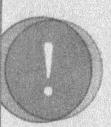

### Important Study Findings: Inflammation and the Menstrual Cycle

"Systemic Inflammation and Menstrual Cycle Length in a Prospective Cohort Study"[16]

- **Study basics:** This study evaluated menstrual cycle length in a prospective cohort of women trying to conceive. Researchers evaluated 1,409 cycles from 414 women. Systemic inflammation was defined as a blood test for C-reactive protein >10 mg/L (normal levels are <1 mg/L).

- **Results:** Women with systemic inflammation had over three times the odds of long cycles (more than thirty-five days) and two times the odds of a long follicular phase.

- **Conclusion:** Long cycles have been associated with decreased pregnancy rates and infertility. These results suggest that chronic inflammation may result in delayed ovulation and impaired fertility.

## IS YOUR CYCLE NORMAL?

Everyone will have their own different version of a normal cycle, but there are certain characteristics that differentiate what's normal from what's abnormal. When I am evaluating if someone has a normal cycle, I always ask these three questions: (1) Is your cycle regular? (2) Is your bleeding normal? (3) Is your cycle painful? We'll delve into this in chapter 4, but for now, consider whether this is you.

## Is Your Cycle Regular?

Your period should be regular and predictable, meaning it should arrive around the same time every month, without skipping a month. Although many textbooks use a twenty-eight-day average menstrual cycle length for simplicity, only 13 percent of women have a twenty-eight-day cycle. A normal cycle for an individual can span between twenty-four and thirty-five days, with most cycles between twenty-seven and thirty-two days.[17]

To determine the average length of your cycle, the first day of bleeding is considered the first day of your menstrual cycle. The last day before the next period begins is the last day of your cycle. Cycle length is the number of days from day one until the last day before your next period. Menses length is the number of days you typically bleed.

## Is Your Bleeding Normal?

Although it often feels like you lose a lot of blood during your period, the average blood loss is only about two ounces—approximately the volume of an egg! Since most people don't measure their menstrual blood, a normal rate of flow equals filling a tampon or soaking a pad every four hours.

Remember, spotting with ovulation or implantation can be normal. Ovulatory spotting is typically seen along with sticky, egg-white cervical mucus and can be pink, red, or brown and is due to a transient drop in estrogen after the follicle is ruptured. Implantation spotting begins about a week after ovulation and is seen as an embryo begins to invade the uterine lining. However, irregular or constant spotting may be a sign of a bigger problem.

## Is Your Cycle Painful?

Menstruation is the process of shedding the lining of the uterus, and during this time, the uterus contracts, causing cramping as you bleed. Menstrual cramps are normal, but they should not interfere with your daily life, keep you home from school or work, or require narcotic pain medication. Passing out or throwing up from your menstrual pain is not normal. Normal cramping typically lasts one to two days and is relieved with heat and anti-inflammatory pain meds. Although it is bothersome, it should not cause you to miss out on your life.

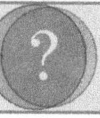 **Common Questions**

### Am I having a period on birth control pills?

Hormonal birth control works to stop the menstrual cycle by suppressing the brain and the uterine lining. Birth control often refers to the birth control pill, which is made of ethinyl estradiol and a type of progestin, synthetic versions of estrogen and progesterone. The ethinyl estradiol acts as estrogen and prevents your brain from sending out any FSH, preventing ovulation. Since you are taking ethinyl estradiol, you will not have low estrogen symptoms. The daily progestin in the birth control pill keeps the uterine lining thin, decreasing menstrual blood loss and cramping. When you take the placebo or take a pill break, you will have a drop in progesterone and will subsequently have what is known as a withdrawal bleed (since progesterone has been withdrawn).

Maple was so upset to learn that the daily progesterone she was taking was preventing pregnancy and that her husband's testosterone had made his sperm count almost zero. Testosterone and sperm are made together, and the testosterone he was taking was telling his brain that there was plenty of sperm and testosterone, thus shutting down the hormones making sperm. This is exactly how the birth control pill works with ovulation in women.

Maple couldn't believe that someone who claimed to be a fertility specialist and sold compounded hormones in their office could give such bad medical advice. We stopped the progesterone and had to give Maple a month of estrogen to help her lining thicken. Her husband stopped the testosterone and started on a medication to improve both his sperm count and natural testosterone production. After four months of treatment, his sperm count improved, and they conceived with intrauterine insemination (IUI). Maple learned the importance of understanding how her hormones really work.

Your reproductive hormones are important in immune regulation, largely driven by the anti-inflammatory properties of estrogen. The net result of the hormonal impact on the immune system is that anything causing delayed, infrequent, or absent ovulation will by default result in fewer estrogen days and will increase inflammation. In addition, chronic inflammation interferes with the HPO axis, resulting in delayed or absent ovulation and a change to your menstrual cycle. This all means that your hormones and menstrual cycle are influenced by your inflammatory burden.

Remember, the best sign that your reproductive hormones are balanced is a regular and predictable period. I always tell my patients that any change from what is normal *for you* should be evaluated. Learning to track your cycle (as we will in chapter 5) will also help you detect small, subtle hormonal changes before they become bigger problems.

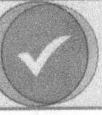

### Facts to Remember

- Your menstrual cycle is a sign of your hormonal health.
- Your hormones fluctuate in response to the world around you.
- Chronic inflammation interferes with normal hormone production.
- Balanced hormones are not determined by lab values but by a properly functioning hormone system.
- Your menstrual cycle is a tightly controlled system of hormone communication and production between the brain, ovaries, and uterus.
- The first half of the cycle is the follicular phase, characterized by estrogen production.
- The second half of the cycle is the luteal phase, characterized by progesterone production.
- A normal cycle is regular, predictable, and occurs at an interval of twenty-four to thirty-five days.

# 3

# Your Biological Clock

Six years ago, I sat across from Holly, a thirty-year-old physician in her last year of a surgical residency program. Holly had had an IUD for the past seven years. One common side effect of an IUD is not having a period, and Holly didn't mind this at all. But recently, she had started to feel like something was off. She was experiencing extreme fatigue, low energy, and having a hard time concentrating. A friend mentioned that maybe her symptoms were due to her IUD, so Holly had it removed.

Without the IUD, her symptoms actually worsened, and her period did not return. Concerned, Holly went to see her primary care doctor, who said it was probably stress from residency and advised her to try to sleep more. Yes, surgery residency is very stressful, but she had a gut feeling something else was going on.

When Holly came to see me, we reviewed her symptoms and decided to check her blood work. It turned out that Holly had a very low egg count, but she was not yet in ovarian failure (which would mean no eggs remaining). In Holly's case, her low egg count meant she was no longer ovulating regularly. Even though she was only thirty, her biological clock was ticking.

Holly's plan had been to finish surgical residency, get settled in her first job, and then start a family. She had a partner, wanted to have two kids, and was planning to conceive in four to five years. But Holly was now faced with the fact that her old plan no longer made sense. Knowing that she was running out of eggs changed her entire strategy. Luckily, Holly still had the opportunity to intervene.

Age is a hard subject to talk about when it comes to fertility. We cannot rewind the clock. If we are lucky, we will all live to an old age—but our fertility is finite. Even with advancements in reproductive technology, fertility is limited and it is harder to conceive as we age due to the following factors:

1. We are born with all the eggs we will ever have.

2. Our eggs are fragile and sensitive to the environment around them.

3. Our egg quality decreases the longer our eggs are inside our body.

4. We will eventually run out of eggs and go into menopause.

I learned this myself the hard way. Like many career paths, medical training overlaps with your most fertile years. I started my OB-GYN residency at age twenty-seven and completed my REI fellowship at thirty-four. These were the busiest and hardest years of my life, but also my "prime" reproductive years. The question that kept me up at night was: "When is the right time to have kids?"

The truth is that for each of us there is no perfect time. You will never be truly ready, and only you can balance the contrasting needs of pursuing one goal to the potential detriment of another. I knew that waiting would make it harder to get pregnant, but I didn't truly understand why or what it meant.

The studies on when you should start your family are eye-opening and can be overwhelming, but you can't make decisions on data you don't know. Choosing to ignore your fertility or hormones just because you have other goals at the moment doesn't make having a family one day any easier. In fact, if having kids is a life goal of yours, does it ever make sense to completely ignore that goal?

Sadly, many of us are not taught about the natural decline in our fertility and vastly overestimate our chance of success from fertility treatments like IVF. In fact, most physicians have limited knowledge of the success of these treatments.[1] Adding to this is how common it now is to see celebrities getting pregnant at older ages, without always being transparent about the means through which they conceived, leaving many of us without any real facts around which to base one of our biggest life decisions.

That is what this chapter is about.

## WHAT IS THE BIOLOGICAL CLOCK?

The number one question I get asked as a fertility doctor is, "When should I have kids?" I know that decision is complex and often feels like an impossible choice to make. Do you focus on your career goals and put family planning to the side? Or do you start a family knowing it might affect the trajectory of your career? And then there are the factors out of your control, such as the economy and your partner status.

To make the best and most informed decision, you first must understand how your biological clock really works. Your "biological clock" refers to more than just running out of eggs. Your biological clock is determined by both your egg *number* and egg *quality*. What many people don't realize is that egg quality starts to decline well before you are out of eggs. In fact, fertility is often capped approximately ten years before you enter menopause due to the change in quality of your eggs, not just how many are left.

Yes, fertility and age are tightly connected. The odds of getting pregnant decrease with each year older you get when you start trying. One in four women will have infertility at age thirty-five, and over half of all women over forty will have infertility.[2] You also have a higher rate of miscarriage as you age.[3]

But again, age is only one factor affecting our egg quality. I always like to say that all our cells age together. We get wrinkles and back pain, just as our eggs get older. This means the same factors that keep you healthy can also help improve your egg quality. The opposite is also true: The same factors that cause inflammation can lead to an increased rate of cellular damage inside your eggs.

## OVARIAN RESERVE: YOUR EGG COUNT

Most women don't realize that we have been running out of eggs since before we were born.[4] Unlike men, who make millions of sperm every single day, women are born with all the eggs they will have. Your ovarian reserve is an estimation of the number of eggs you have remaining.

You have the most eggs—approximately six to seven million—when you are a fetus and your mom is five months pregnant with you. After this, your egg number continually decreases. You will have one to two million eggs at birth, and only three hundred thousand to five hundred thousand eggs remain by the time you start puberty.[5] You lose the majority of your eggs before you ever have your first menstrual cycle![6] In fact, women only ovulate around four hundred eggs over the course of their reproductive life.

I often get asked, "What happens to all the other eggs if we're born with one to two million eggs but we only ovulate four hundred eggs?" Here's the analogy I created to explain.

Imagine that all your eggs are inside a vault within the ovaries. Nobody can see inside the vault, so there is no way to definitively count how many eggs you have left. At the start of each month, a group of eggs is released from the vault and comes to the surface of the ovary. Each egg is microscopic and grows inside a small, fluid-filled cyst known as a follicle. The small follicles outside the vault each month (each follicle contains an egg) can be seen on ultrasound and are known as antral follicles. The brain will send out just enough FSH to stimulate one antral follicle to grow; as the follicle grows the egg matures and makes estrogen, eventually ovulating.

In other words, out of all the eggs released from the vault, only one egg will be chosen to ovulate. All the other eggs outside the vault that were not chosen to ovulate will die, and the process will start over again.

When the vault has more eggs inside (more total eggs remaining), you have an increased number of eggs released from the vault each month. When the vault has fewer eggs remaining, there is a decrease in the number of eggs sent out each month. This means the number of eggs outside the vault—the ones we can see—give us an idea of how many eggs you may have remaining. The more eggs outside the vault, the more inside the vault.

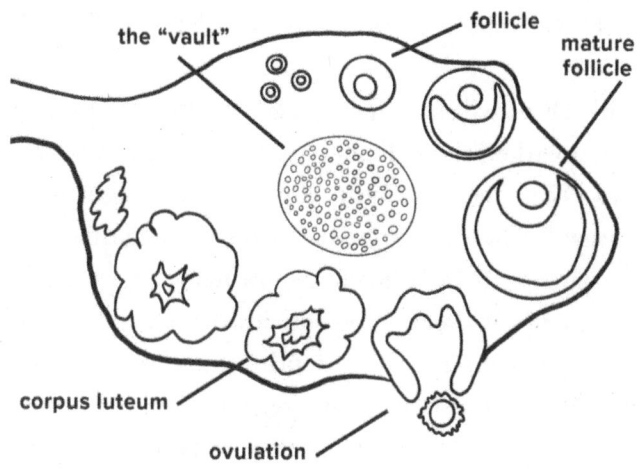

**Natalie's Ovarian Vault Analogy**

Eggs come out of the vault every month—before puberty, when you are on birth control, with irregular cycles, when you are pregnant, and when you breastfeed. Once eggs have been released from the vault, they are on a pathway to either ovulate or die. Even if you are not constantly ovulating, you are constantly losing eggs as they are constantly released from the vault.

Fertility treatments like IVF and egg freezing attempt to get all the eggs outside the vault to grow instead of letting all the eggs that did not ovulate die, as seen naturally. When you have a lower egg count, all fertility treatments become harder because you are limited by the number of eggs you have in a given month. Fertility medications can only get the eggs outside the vault to grow; we cannot tap into the vault or stimulate eggs that are not available in that month. This is why women with a low egg count often need to go through multiple cycles of egg freezing or IVF in order to get eggs from multiple months and have a cumulatively higher total number of eggs to work with.

Having a low number of eggs for your age, like Holly, is called diminished ovarian reserve (DOR). Running out of eggs early—before age forty—is premature ovarian insufficiency (POI), or premature menopause.

## DIMINISHED OVARIAN RESERVE (DOR)

A woman with DOR will have fewer eggs remaining than her peers, will enter menopause earlier, and will not have as many eggs available for fertility treatments. This does not mean you can't get pregnant now. Think about it this way: If you and your bestie are the same age and have different egg counts, what is actually different is how many eggs are released from the vault each month. As long as you both are ovulating, you have a similar chance of being pregnant in a given month because you are both ovulating one egg. The difference is how many eggs will die in that month, which determines how long you have to complete your family.

DOR should always be evaluated, especially if your egg count is considerably low for your age. A diagnosis of DOR may completely change your plan. When Holly discovered her DOR, she reevaluated her fertility plan. Although she did not meet the definition of infertility, she had the opportunity to intervene and change her future.

Even though we cannot always get to the root cause of DOR, potential causes include endometriosis, genetic conditions, chemotherapy, toxic exposures, and inflammation. Chronic inflammation is clearly associated with lower ovarian reserve.[7] This is just further evidence that your lifestyle choices do impact your current and future fertility. Although we can't reverse the egg loss that has occurred, knowing the cause can help mitigate future damage.

Low ovarian reserve can also occur when you are a fetus inside your mom, meaning an exposure your mother had when she was pregnant with you—such as testosterone exposure, high weight gain, smoking, and other toxin exposure—may be contributing to your lower egg count.[8] In mice, poor dietary choices (such as increased sugar) and chronic inflammation have been associated with low ovarian reserve in offspring.[9]

**POTENTIAL CAUSES OF DOR**

| | |
|---|---|
| Genetics | Ovarian surgery |
| Autoimmune disease | Chemotherapy |
| Endometriosis | Chronic inflammation |
| Environmental toxins | |
| Smoking | Maternal exposure |

One of the first and only clinical signs that your egg count is dropping may be a change in your menstrual cycle length. The ovary gets more stubborn as your egg count drops—it doesn't want to run out of eggs. When you have fewer eggs released from the vault, you need a stronger FSH signal to get one to grow. Since FSH is the hormone responsible for selecting an egg to ovulate, increased FSH results in earlier egg selection, earlier ovulation, and a shorter cycle length than before.

As your egg count continues to drop, your cycle will eventually become longer, irregular, and spaced out; it will eventually stop completely as you transition from DOR to perimenopause to menopause. You may even have signs and symptoms of low estrogen before you truly notice cycle changes.

It's important to know that there is a genetic link to age of menopause. If you have a first-degree relative—meaning your mom or sibling—go through menopause before age forty-six, your risk for early menopause is six times higher.[10] Ask your family members the age they went through menopause. For many, the topics of fertility and menopause are still taboo, but you can be the one to start that conversation simply by asking. Important note: If your family member had a hysterectomy, they may or may not have had their ovaries removed too; this can make it difficult to determine when menopause truly occurred.

## OVARIAN RESERVE TESTING

Ovarian reserve tests are an estimation of your "egg count" by evaluating the eggs outside the vault. We don't actually know the exact number of eggs you have remaining, but we try to estimate by quantifying the eggs outside the vault. They are imperfect measurements, but they help to approximate where you are in your reproductive lifespan.

Ovarian reserve tests are helpful in planning your future, understanding your proximity to menopause, and predicting response to fertility treatments.[11] Although no test of ovarian reserve can precisely predict menopause, low values for your age are highly concerning and warrant further evaluation, as they indicate you are at risk of POI.[12] However, there is some controversy around checking ovarian reserve in women who are not trying to conceive.

The American College of Obstetricians and Gynecologists (ACOG) released a committee opinion in March 2019 titled "The Use of Antimüllerian Hormone in Women Not Seeking Fertility Care."[13] In this document, ACOG presents the case that anti-müllerian hormone (AMH) should not be used as a screening test for women to gauge their fertility potential. ACOG's argument is that ovarian reserve tests in a young population may cause undue stress or anxiety and lead women to seek more aggressive treatments than needed.

I have been outspoken in my disagreement with this statement and perspective. Honestly, I think it is sexist and the perfect representation of everything that is wrong with medicine. We have a data point that might help you make decisions in your life, but instead you are being told that a professional organization doesn't think you are smart enough to understand what it does and does not mean. This is wild—and it is exactly why this book exists.

Although ovarian reserve is just one piece of the puzzle, testing your egg count now can give you the opportunity to evaluate your reproductive life and weigh the options that may be best for you. Normal testing does not mean you will be fertile later in life, just as low testing does not mean you will be infertile. Ultimately, testing your ovarian reserve lets you be the one making decisions about your future instead of just assuming everything will be fine. Would this information change your entire reproductive plan, just like it did for Holly?

Holly could have learned about her very low egg count and chosen not to change her plan, but at least she would have known and could have viewed her future differently. Your fertility is time sensitive. Simply being able to make the choice, as opposed to having a decision forced by the passage of time, is very powerful. Knowledge is essential. You are the one who must advocate for your own health.

I believe fertility should be discussed at every annual visit. Just as your OB-GYN may ask, "What would you like for birth control?" they should also ask, "Do you want to have kids someday?" If the answer is yes, a discussion about age, fertility, and ovarian reserve should follow. Since this is not how many doctors are trained or taught, it is up to you to ask the question and advocate for testing if having kids is a future goal.

Current options for ovarian reserve testing include:

- Antral follicle count (AFC)
- Follicle-stimulating hormone (FSH) and estradiol (E2)
- Anti-müllerian hormone (AMH)

## Antral Follicle Count (AFC)

The antral follicle count is the number of all the small follicles "outside the vault" in one month—which correlates with the total number of remaining eggs.[14] Your AFC can be determined at any point in the monthly cycle, and it is often tested with your initial fertility evaluation. Important note: If you have an ultrasound ordered by your OB-GYN, they usually do not measure your AFC. Typically, an AFC is only measured at a fertility clinic.

As your total follicle count declines with age, your average AFC will also decrease.[15] A low AFC for your age has been associated with decreased success in achieving pregnancy following IVF and a closer proximity to menopause.[16,17]

**AVERAGE AFC BY AGE**

| Age (Years) | AFC |
| --- | --- |
| 25–30 | 20 |
| 31–35 | 15 |
| 36–40 | 12 |
| 41–45 | 7 |

Women with infertility are more likely to have a low AFC than age-matched fertile women.[18] This further suggests that the ability to conceive is about more than just ovulating, and that women who have a lower follicle count may have an underlying mechanism that also impairs fertility.

## Follicle-Stimulating Hormone (FSH) and Estradiol (E2)

Remember, FSH is the signal from the brain that stimulates one follicle to grow and the egg to mature and make estradiol, the type of estrogen made by the ovary from the growing follicle. The brain relies on feedback from the ovary to determine how much FSH to send out. As your egg count drops, the brain sends out a stronger signal of FSH.

Importantly, FSH needs to be checked on cycle day two or three (cycle day one is the day you start bleeding). This can sometimes be difficult to schedule. Normal FSH levels are usually between 5 and 10 IU/L, and FSH levels rise as the number of remaining eggs decreases.[19] FSH levels of >40 IU/L indicate menopause.[20] The following table helps identify your reproductive stage based on your FSH and E2 levels.

## AVERAGE FSH AND E2 LEVELS BY REPRODUCTIVE STAGE

| Reproductive Stage | FSH (IU/L) | E2 (pg/mL) |
| --- | --- | --- |
| Not ovulating | <5 | <20 |
| Normal | 5–10 | <60 |
| DOR | 5–10 | >60 |
|  | 10–25 | <60 |
| Perimenopause | 25–40 | variable |
| Menopause | >40 | <20 |

Each small follicle makes a small amount of E2. As the egg matures, E2 levels rise to around 200 pg/mL with a mature egg. E2 alone has limited utility in determining ovarian reserve. However, cycle day two or three levels can help interpret normal FSH values.

In early stages of reproductive aging (before the ovary becomes stubborn), FSH from the brain will be a stronger signal to each egg (less dilution). This means a dominant follicle will be chosen earlier, and E2 levels will start to rise early in the cycle. Elevated estradiol levels (>60 pg/mL) with normal FSH values are suggestive of a low egg count.

Since FSH and E2 require blood work on a set cycle day, these tests have largely been replaced by AMH for testing ovarian reserve. That said, FSH and E2 are still important in the evaluation of absent or irregular periods and are discussed more in chapter 4.

## Anti-Müllerian Hormone (AMH)

AMH is made by the cells that surround each follicle. When you have more follicles outside the vault, you have a higher AMH. When you have fewer follicles outside the vault, your AMH will be lower. AMH is relatively unaffected by cycle day, making it an easy screening test for how many eggs are outside the vault at a specific moment.[21]

The vault is not perfect and will not release the exact same number of eggs every single month, meaning AMH will vary slightly month to month. Studies testing AMH in multiple menstrual cycles in the same women have shown up to a 28 percent variation month to month.[22] One single measurement of AMH is only an estimation of the number of follicles that were recently sent out of the vault.

Normal AMH levels depend on age, but estimates for the low end of normal values are shown in the table below.[23] Essentially, if your AMH value is below the level for your age, you may have diminished ovarian reserve.

**MINIMUM AMH LEVEL BY AGE**

| Age (Years) | AMH (ng/mL) |
| --- | --- |
| 25 | 3.0 |
| 30 | 2.5 |
| 35 | 1.5 |
| 40 | 1.0 |
| 45 | 0.5 |

AMH is clearly a marker for how many eggs you can get with IVF or egg freezing and your reproductive lifespan.[24] It is important to note that a single value only tells us about a single moment—we do not know the rate of decline. AMH helps us guide fertility planning and fertility treatments. How aggressive should we be? How much medication do you need to get the ovary to respond? What type of protocol will be best? How many eggs do we expect?

Just like your egg count, your AMH may not reflect your ability to get pregnant, as long as you are still ovulating.[25,26] However, a low AMH is a reflection of your fertility and is associated with a longer time to pregnancy.[27] AMH is important in your family planning. I always ask the question, "Why do you have a low AMH?" Some potential causes of low ovarian reserve can absolutely also cause infertility, such as endometriosis, autoimmune disease, and smoking. For people to universally say that a low AMH has "no impact" on your natural fertility without trying to figure out *why* your AMH is low is simply wrong.

## Common Questions

**Does birth control decrease your ovarian reserve?**

Hormonal contraception can temporarily decrease ovarian reserve. When you are not ovulating for a prolonged time, such as when you are using birth control or during pregnancy and breastfeeding, the ovaries become suppressed and go into a quiet state. You are still losing eggs each of these months—it's just that none of them are ovulating. You may have very small antral follicles, which can be difficult to see on ultrasound, and overall less AMH is being produced. The temporary decrease in AMH is dependent on which form of contraceptive you are using. With the birth control pill, AMH may be up to 24 percent lower; the ring, 22 percent lower; and the progesterone arm implant, 23 percent lower. Hormonal IUDs have a much lower impact on AMH levels, with only a 7 percent decrease, and the copper IUD (which is nonhormonal) does not change AMH at all.[28] Stopping hormonal contraception results in a return to baseline AMH values after two months.[29] I still advocate for testing your ovarian reserve without stopping your birth control if you aren't ready to be pregnant. Most of the time your testing will be normal and you never risked an unplanned pregnancy. If your results do come back low, you can then stop your hormonal contraception and retest in a couple months.

## EGG QUALITY: MORE THAN JUST GENETICS

Egg quality is both the genetic normalcy of your eggs and the metabolic competency for maturation and development. It is well established that as we age, our eggs become increasingly abnormal, because the longer your eggs are in your body, the more they accumulate damage from the wear and tear of your life, including inflammation. Unfortunately, there is no test for egg quality. Age is the best marker we have to estimate egg quality.

The chromosomes inside your eggs are held in a stage of cell division called meiosis until you ovulate. For example, when you are twenty-five, your egg has been held in this stage for twenty-five years; likewise, when you are forty, your egg has been holding this position for forty years. The longer we ask our eggs to remain in this holding pattern, the more the egg accumulates cellular damage and chromosomal issues.

Imagine a line of kindergarteners in alphabetical order. The longer I ask them to wait in line, the greater the odds that someone is going to get out of place. Now, imagine asking them to stand in line for forty years. We all know that somebody will definitely be out of line! Not only have we asked our chromosomes to wait in line, but we have subjected them to inflammation and toxins, which cause further chaos. Inflammation is similar to bringing in a puppy. How many kindergarteners will stay in their place if there is a puppy to distract them?

It should be no surprise that by the time we are forty, most of our chromosomes will have moved out of line, and the vast majority of our eggs will be chromosomally abnormal.[30] Most chromosomally abnormal eggs will not fertilize, develop correctly, or implant, or they will miscarry early.

But genetics is just one piece of the egg quality picture. Once you ovulate, the egg resumes meiosis and has to have the metabolic competency to finalize maturation and permit fertilization. The mitochondria inside your eggs, the powerhouse of the cell, require energy in the form of glucose to properly function. Anything that increases inflammation—such as obesity, insulin resistance, and aging—affects mitochondrial function and egg quality.[31] Even with IVF, insulin resistance (in women with and without PCOS) results in a lower number of mature eggs and decreased embryo quality.[32,33]

In other words, embryo development is dependent on the mitochondrial function and metabolic health of our eggs, reinforcing the importance of decreasing inflammation to help our eggs function properly.[34]

Age impacts more than just the genetics of our eggs. Women over age thirty-five have been shown to have different metabolic by-products inside their eggs than younger women.[35] Even more startling is the fact that women who are thirty-eight and older have a significantly higher number of abnormally shaped and poorly functioning mitochondria than women under age thirty-eight.[36]

This is why the probability of pregnancy per cycle, called our fecundability, drops significantly with age. At age thirty, your fecundability is about 20 percent per month. For every year that passes, your fecundability decreases. If you are trying to conceive for the first time at age thirty-eight, your fecundability is 5 percent.[37] The rate of miscarriage at age forty is over 40 percent.[38] The decline in fertility with age is not due to running out of eggs, but to the change in egg quality.

I know this can be shocking to learn. If you are starting your family at age thirty-five, more than half your eggs are already genetically abnormal.[39] This doesn't mean that getting pregnant is impossible after age thirty-five, but it explains why thirty-five is an important age marker for fertility.

I want you to see this as information you can use rather than as information to fear. If part of the change seen with aging is a metabolic issue within your eggs, you can start to change *now*. No, you can't rewind the clock or mitigate all chromosomal change seen with age. But you can control the inflammatory burden inside your body and work to improve the metabolic competency of your eggs.

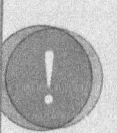

## *Important Study Findings:* What Are Your Odds of Getting Pregnant?

"Impact of Female Age and Nulligravidity on Fecundity in an Older Reproductive Age Cohort"[40]

- **Study basics:** This prospective study looked at women age thirty to forty-four who had just started trying to conceive and were tracking cycles. Fecundability rates were determined by age groups and prior pregnancy.

- **Results:** Your monthly odds of conception decrease as your age increases. Women who'd already given birth to a prior child (gravid) had higher fecundability rates than women who had not had a child (nulligravid).

MONTHLY FECUNDABILITY BY AGE AND PARITY

| Age (Years) | Nulligravid | Gravid |
|---|---|---|
| 30–33 | 17–19% | 22–23% |
| 34–37 | 11–12% | 16–22% |
| 38–41 | 3–5% | 10–17% |
| 42–44 | 3% | 9% |

- **Conclusion:** Natural fertility declines with age, more significantly for women attempting to have their first child. In both groups, the impact of age and fertility is most pronounced after thirty-seven years old.

## THE RELATIONSHIP BETWEEN EGG QUANTITY AND QUALITY

Low ovarian reserve does not always mean you have poor egg quality—it depends on why you have DOR. If you ever get diagnosed with DOR, it is important to determine why your egg count is low to understand if this will also impact your egg quality. There are certainly some factors, like smoking and endometriosis, that can cause both a low egg count and decreased egg quality. And there are others, like genetics, that may cause a low egg count but can have no impact on egg quality. Most studies show limited correlation between low ovarian reserve and low egg quality.

If you are young, even if you don't have as many eggs, your egg quality should still be relatively consistent with your age. Since the top driver of genetic abnormalities is age, even young women with severe DOR should be given the opportunity to proceed with fertility treatments. Reproductive outcomes and planning options will differ based on the reason you have DOR, so I recommend that all women with DOR have a complete fertility evaluation to understand all the variables impacting your ability to conceive.

Any woman under the age of thirty-five who is told she will not be able to get pregnant with her own eggs but is still ovulating should absolutely seek a second opinion. Some IVF clinics have AMH cutoff levels, which exclude DOR patients from pursuing IVF in order to protect the clinic's IVF success rates. I think this is wrong and completely unfair—and it's a huge reason it's important to choose a fertility clinic you trust.

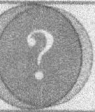

## Common Questions

**When should I start trying to have kids?**

In order to have a 90 percent chance of having kids (without needing IVF), you should start trying to get pregnant at age thirty-two if you want one child, twenty-seven if you want two children, and twenty-three if you want three children.[41] If you are OK with possibly needing IVF, you need to start trying at age thirty-five for one child, thirty-one for two children, and twenty-eight for three children. It is important to note that IVF does not always work, and IVF success is largely dependent on age (younger is better). This means that if you are waiting to start a family in the later age ranges, you need to know when to seek a fertility evaluation and how to optimize your chances of conceiving. To be honest, these ages are all much younger than most people think! I know I wasn't ready to start trying at age twenty-three, or even twenty-seven, but I wish I had understood what I could do at a younger age and how to improve my odds of success once I did want a pregnancy.

## WORKING WITH YOUR BIOLOGICAL CLOCK

It can be very upsetting to find out that your egg count is low or that you have poor egg quality. I know it can feel like you are being blamed for your infertility—though that is never the case. Every single person's body will respond differently to the exact same exposure. As both egg count and quality are tied to age, and you can't change your age, it is up to you to understand what to do to support your egg health.

Even though time itself is a huge variable in your fertility, I like to think about the eggs in the vault and trying to support them in holding that perfect position while supporting your mitochondria. We want to decrease inflammation and increase healthy nutrients. Although a single egg is in your body for your entire life, it takes 290 days for full follicular development, with 60 days to become a full antral follicle.[42] This means the few months preceding ovulation are when this egg is most sensitive and susceptible to damage. We want to support the proper metabolic function of your eggs. I like to imagine that the eggs that will come out of the vault next are already selected and starting to line up in position. This is why the sooner you make lifestyle changes to decrease inflammation, the greater the improvement you can see in your egg quality and fertility.

You can control what your eggs are exposed to now. You can also focus to improve the environment inside your body and give yourself the tools you need to repair cellular damage and fight oxidative stress.[43] If you smoked since your early twenties, you can't go back and undo the past, but you can stop smoking today. Inflammation has been shown to negatively impact egg quality, so if you have a low egg count, you should absolutely control all the other factors you can to optimize your fertility (reviewed in detail in part III).

In short, what's good for your body is good for your eggs—and what's bad for your body is bad for your eggs.

## INFLUENCE OF LIFESTYLE FACTORS ON EGG QUALITY

| Beneficial | Harmful |
| --- | --- |
| Vitamins | Environmental toxins |
| Antioxidants | Inflammation |
| Sleep | Smoking |
| Exercise | Marijuana |
| Normal weight | Alcohol |
| Increased blood flow | Stress |
| Fiber | Obesity |
| Fruits and vegetables | Chronic illness |
| Whole grains | Processed food, processed meats |

What should you do if you find out you have poor egg quality or low ovarian reserve? My recommendations:

1. **Learn about your body.** We cannot change our age, and sometimes things happen on a timeline we don't plan. This doesn't mean you shouldn't understand what happens as you age.

2. **Review any inflammatory symptoms with your doctor.** Make sure you are not missing an underlying diagnosis that may change your treatment plan (reviewed in chapter 1).

3. **Be honest with yourself about lifestyle changes you can make to try to reduce inflammation.** (This will be discussed further in part III.) Just as there was not one thing that caused you to have infertility, there is no single change or pill that makes everything "better."

4. **Consider testing your ovarian reserve.** These tests are not perfect but can help you understand your reproductive timeline.

5. **Consider seeing a fertility doctor to learn about egg freezing.** This is especially worth considering if you know you do not want to begin having children until after age thirty-two. If your starting age is

closer to thirty-five to thirty-seven years old and you potentially want more than one child, then you should seriously consider this option.

6. **Understand how to optimize your natural fertility and track your cycles.** When you are ready to conceive, make sure you are making your best effort with each cycle. (This will be discussed further in chapter 5.)

## EGG FREEZING

Egg freezing allows you to potentially delay conception and maintain an opportunity for successful pregnancy at a later age. I like to describe egg freezing as trying to get all the eggs outside the vault to grow, instead of just the one your body would have chosen to ovulate. We are saving eggs instead of letting the majority of them die. Egg freezing does not deplete your future egg count or harm your future fertility because the eggs were going to be lost no matter what.

Freezing your eggs when you are younger directly correlates with improved odds of success when you are ready to use them. The current freezing technique, called oocyte vitrification, has drastically improved egg survival and has increased access to egg freezing. Everyone asks if egg freezing is just a trend, but the truth is that the ability to freeze your eggs is a relatively new technology that was considered experimental until 2014! It isn't trendy, but it is now available at almost all fertility clinics.

Surprisingly, egg freezing is a relatively quick process and is usually completed within two weeks. Gonadotropin hormone injections, mostly synthetic FSH, stimulate the growth of many eggs at one time. This process is called "controlled ovarian hyperstimulation" and takes around eight to twelve days. During ovarian stimulation, you will be monitored with ultrasounds to measure follicular growth and blood work to check estradiol levels.

Once the eggs reach maturity, they will be removed in a procedure called an egg retrieval. While you are sedated, a needle is attached to a vaginal ultrasound and enters each follicle. The fluid is drained, and the eggs are aspirated into test tubes and identified. All mature eggs undergo vitrification, where the central liquid of the egg is removed and the egg is collapsed and then frozen in liquid nitrogen. In vitro fertilization (IVF) will be required when you want to use your eggs. Although some loss is expected in the freeze/thaw process, egg freezing has expanded reproductive options for women.

The average live birth rate per frozen egg is approximately 4 to 5 percent, indicating that most women will need a substantial number of eggs frozen in order to have at least one child, let alone complete their entire family.[44] The success of egg freezing, no matter when you want to use your eggs, will always be linked to the age you were when you froze your eggs. The take-home message as it is related to your eggs is the sooner the better.

If you are considering freezing your eggs, now is the time to look into it and learn more about the process. Egg freezing will not be right for everyone, but any eggs you put in the freezer now will create an opportunity that otherwise might be lost by waiting.

I've had patients freeze "fewer" eggs than the math would recommend, and they still end up with a child that might otherwise not have been possible. Based on modeling, the highest probability of live birth from one round of egg freezing is observed when you freeze your eggs between thirty-one and thirty-four years old, but there was still an improvement in live birth as compared to no action up to age thirty-seven.[45] Personal goals and beliefs influence the chance of success, and there is not one right answer for each person. Seeing a fertility doctor, testing your ovarian reserve, and learning about your own odds of success can help you make this decision. In short, there is no perfect time, but freezing your eggs when you are younger will make things easier when you are older and ready for a family.

Some women who freeze their eggs will get pregnant naturally without a problem. Some women may never use these eggs, but many will use them later to grow their family and add future children. Regardless, they were proactive in preserving their fertility, have decreased anxiety about family building, and granted themselves a slight reprieve from the biological clock.

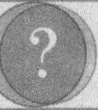 **Common Questions**

**Is egg freezing an insurance policy for my fertility?**

As a fertility doctor, I often see patients who are concerned about their fertility because they desire a family but are not yet ready for motherhood or are not in a relationship. I believe that egg freezing is a game changer. Allowing yourself the freedom for reproductive flexibility is a beautiful thing. It is important to remember that there are no guarantees. Egg freezing is not an insurance policy for your fertility but an investment in your future. Just like investing in the stock market, the return on your investment depends on factors we cannot control and often do not know until the future (such as sperm quality). But overall, investing is a smart strategy to plan for your future. With egg freezing, you are giving yourself the best available option to have the family you want and on the timeline you desire.

---

Holly thought surgical residency was the least ideal time to start a family, but she also knew that she wanted to have kids. When faced with her DOR, we discussed her options: (1) try to get pregnant now, (2) freeze her eggs or embryos, or (3) don't do anything now but know she may need donor eggs to get pregnant later.

After a long discussion, Holly knew that the only way to guarantee she would have kids would be to try to have them now. She started IVF. Holly had a great response considering her low ovarian reserve. She decided to do multiple IVF cycles to get more eggs, and she is now pregnant and has three frozen embryos remaining for her second child. Although there are no guarantees, Holly is thankful that she was able to learn the truth in time to take action.

You can't roll back the clock and change your age, but you deserve to understand where your biological clock stands and how to work with it. If having children is a life goal for you, I want you to be the one who makes the decisions about your future. You can decide to test your own ovarian reserve now. You can decide to prevent further chromosome damage and improve the metabolic function of your eggs by decreasing inflammation.

There is no one right answer, but giving yourself the opportunity to make these fertility decisions is important. Time should not be what makes them for you.

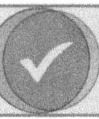

### Facts to Remember

- You are born with all the eggs you will ever have.
- Each month you lose a group of eggs, and eventually you will be out of eggs.
- Both egg quantity and egg quality decrease with age.
- Ovarian reserve tests estimate the number of eggs you have remaining, but they do not predict future fertility or infertility.
- Your eggs are susceptible to wear and tear from the world around you; chronic inflammation decreases egg quality and quantity.
- The percentage of genetically abnormal eggs increases with age.
- Egg quality consists of both genetic normalcy and metabolic competency.
- Freezing your eggs can be an option to help preserve your fertility.

# PART II

# PREPARING FOR CONCEPTION

# 4

# Getting to the Root Cause of Abnormal Cycles

As we've learned, a regular and predictable menstrual cycle is the best indication that your hormones are functioning properly. Your period is a vital sign telling you a lot about your body, ovulation, and fertility. If you don't have a normal cycle, it is important to get to the root cause before you start trying to get pregnant.

Unfortunately, I see patients every week who were told that their period symptoms were normal. Women are dismissed by doctors, confused by the internet, and ultimately gaslit into thinking they just don't "handle" their period symptoms as well as everyone else.

Hazel had terrible acne and irregular periods as a teenager. It was embarrassing, and she tried everything she could, but nothing really helped. Her acne continued to worsen, her cycle got longer, and her period got so heavy that she bled through her clothes at school. At age sixteen, she started taking a birth control pill. Hazel felt great on the pill. Her acne subsided, and her heavy bleeding stopped—she never bled through her clothes again. Her cycles also became regular and predictable, and she continued the birth control pill until she was ready to get pregnant at age thirty-two.

After sixteen years, Hazel didn't know what to expect when she stopped the pill. The first month was fine, but each subsequent month her cycle started to get longer, and each period was further apart. She gained weight and felt terrible. Hazel searched online and found people talking about "post–birth control pill syndrome." Maybe her problems were all due to the birth control pill?

Hazel followed all the online advice about how to cure her post–birth control pill syndrome. She bought expensive online cleanses to rid her body of the birth control pill, but as more time passed her cycle only got worse, and she was gaining weight. She started restricting calories and getting up early for a HIIT workout to try to lose a few pounds. When her acne started to return, she found herself crying in frustration.

Hazel came to see me and was diagnosed with polycystic ovary syndrome (PCOS), not "post–birth control pill syndrome." PCOS is an inflammatory disease that affects hormone function and ovulation, so Hazel's acne and irregular cycles (symptoms of PCOS) returned once she stopped the pill. The birth control pill prevents ovulation and decreases circulating levels of testosterone—often improving the symptoms of PCOS. Once you stop the pill, the symptoms of PCOS return, including cycle and hormone changes.

Why was Hazel not diagnosed with PCOS at age sixteen? The short answer is that the pill was a good enough treatment for her problems. It was easier for her doctors to say, "Take this," than evaluate what was really going on. Ultimately, the pill was a Band-Aid solution. Unknowingly, Hazel had made her symptoms worse by getting less sleep, exercising too much, and restricting calories—all of which contribute to inflammation.

Since PCOS impacts ovulation and hormone production, women with PCOS often have infertility. Without addressing her PCOS, Hazel would likely have a difficult time getting pregnant.

Just like Hazel, many women use the pill not for birth control but rather to mitigate abnormal menstrual cycles and other related symptoms. We now have a generation of women who were started on the pill without ever knowing their underlying diagnosis. Like so many aspects of women's health, the birth control pill has been used without proper education for decades—and women are paying the price. At sixteen, Hazel should have had the opportunity to know what was happening with her body and how to make things better. Understanding her true diagnosis would have saved her time and money later in life.

Abnormal cycles can be hard to diagnose because our cycles are unique and different. Here are the top questions I ask my patients when considering whether their cycle is normal:

1. Is your cycle regular?
2. Is your bleeding normal?
3. Is your cycle painful?

Many hormone imbalances present with irregular cycles, while many structural abnormalities present with pain or abnormal bleeding. For simplicity, in this chapter I've categorized each disease based on the top presenting symptom I see in my patients, although some etiologies fit into multiple categories.

## IRREGULAR CYCLES AND OVULATION

All absent or irregular periods warrant an evaluation. It doesn't matter if you have been trying to get pregnant or not. Your body is meant to have regular, predictable periods, and when you don't, something is wrong. Regular, predictable cycles are a sign that you are ovulating. Not ovulating, known as anovulation, will make it hard to get pregnant and may significantly impact your long-term health.

Irregular cycles are the result of some deviation from the normal menstrual cycle. But the menstrual cycle can have gradients of dysfunction, ranging from cycles that are too short (luteal phase defect) or too long (long follicular phase) to cycles that are unpredictable, all the way to amenorrhea, the absence of a period.

Regular Cycles | Luteal Phase Defect | Long Follicular Phase | Irregular Cycles | Amenorrhea

**Cycle Length Progression**

## STAGES OF OVULATORY DYSFUNCTION AND CYCLE PATTERN

| Luteal Phase Defect (LPD) | • Luteal phase less than 11 days in length<br>• LH pulses not strong enough to maintain the corpus luteum and make progesterone |
|---|---|
| Long Follicular Phase | • Cycle length longer than 35 days<br>• FSH signal not strong enough, resulting in delayed ovulation |
| Irregular Cycles | • Cycles not regular or predictable<br>• Skipping months |
| Amenorrhea | • Absence of a period for 6 months<br>• Primary amenorrhea: no period by age 16<br>• Secondary amenorrhea: prior periods that have stopped |

There are several reasons a cycle may be irregular, and they all have to do with hormone dysfunction. Dysfunction can happen at the level of the hypothalamus, pituitary gland, thyroid, ovaries, or the adrenal glands. Each location presents in different symptoms, as outlined in the table below. That said, the first step in an evaluation should always be a pregnancy test, as irregular and absent bleeding are both signs of pregnancy.

## TOP CAUSES OF IRREGULAR CYCLES

| Hypothalamus | Hypothalamic amenorrhea (HA)<br>Hypothalamic dysfunction |
|---|---|
| Pituitary | Hyperprolactinemia<br>Sheehan syndrome |
| Thyroid | Hypothyroidism<br>Hyperthyroidism |
| Ovary | Ovarian failure<br>Polycystic ovary syndrome (PCOS) |
| Adrenal Glands | Congenital adrenal hyperplasia (CAH) |

Remember, inflammation affects our hormones, so it should come as no surprise that irregular cycles are worsened by the world around us. Chronic inflammation is associated with longer cycle lengths and impairment of the HPO axis.[1] Women who have premature ovarian failure have higher levels of inflammatory markers than women who do not.[2] And as we've learned, inflammation and insulin resistance are hallmarks of PCOS.[3]

You can improve your ovulatory pattern by decreasing your inflammatory exposures.[4] I always tell my patients that they owe it to themselves to control the factors they can. Sometimes you will not be able to reverse your ovulatory dysfunction with lifestyle changes alone, but decreasing chronic inflammation will help you have the best response to treatment.

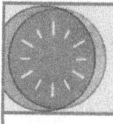

## Top Tip

**What to expect for the evaluation of an irregular cycle**

1. **History:** The first key is to make sure *you* have a clear idea of the timeline of your symptoms. When was your last normal period? Have they been irregular or absent before this? Do you have any other symptoms? When were you last on any type of hormones or contraception? Have you taken a pregnancy test?
2. **Blood work:** A typical lab panel starts with FSH, LH, E2, TSH, PRL, AMH, and hCG.
3. **Imaging:** Imaging typically includes a vaginal ultrasound or MRI.

## Hypothalamic Causes of Anovulation

As we learned in chapter 1, the hypothalamus interprets signals from your body and sends out gonadotropin-releasing hormone (GnRH) telling the pituitary gland to release gonadotropins (FSH and LH). Failure at the level of the hypothalamus is known as "hypo-hypo," or more accurately, hypogonadotropic (low FSH) hypogonadism (low estrogen).

## POTENTIAL CAUSES OF HYPOTHALAMIC ANOVULATION

| | |
|---|---|
| Stress | Autoimmune disease |
| Calorie restriction | Malabsorption |
| Eating disorder | Chronic illness |
| Weight loss | Brain mass |
| Excess exercise | Pituitary damage |

As the hypothalamus is the control center for all hormones, it should be no surprise that chronic inflammation and stress play a role in hypothalamic function.[5] Think of the hypothalamus as a dimmer switch, not an on-off switch. When the switch is off, you will not ovulate, resulting in amenorrhea. Stages of dimming can result in more subtle changes of ovulatory dysfunction. The most common hypothalamic causes of irregular cycles are hypothalamic amenorrhea (HA) and hypothalamic dysfunction.

### Hypothalamic Amenorrhea

Hypothalamic amenorrhea is characterized by low FSH and low estrogen, resulting in an absence of a period. HA is often caused by energy deficiency, such as low calorie intake for your metabolic requirements, known as functional hypothalamic amenorrhea (FHA). I describe FHA as being in a state where your brain has decided that your body cannot support a pregnancy. Your brain has interpreted some stressor as too much and shuts off the ovulatory pathway by no longer sending out GnRH. Remember that our bodies all have different responses to having an energy deficit, and not everyone will be classically "thin."

Symptoms of HA are caused by low estrogen levels. Treatment for HA depends on the underlying cause, but replacing estrogen is key. If you have FHA, focusing on improving energy availability is crucial. The goal will be to decrease stress and inflammation, improve healthy calories, get sleep, and engage in low-intensity exercise.

One frustrating aspect of HA is that it may take years after returning to an energy balance for your body to resume a normal ovulatory pattern.

This doesn't mean that your lifestyle changes are not working, but it does mean they are not a quick fix. If you want to get pregnant while you have HA, you will likely need fertility treatments with either ovulation induction with gonadotropins or IVF, as we will learn about in chapter 7.

### HYPOTHALAMIC AMENORRHEA

| | |
|---|---|
| **Symptoms** | Amenorrhea |
| | Fatigue |
| | Headache |
| | Low libido |
| | Vaginal dryness |
| | Weight gain/loss |
| | Infertility |
| **Diagnosis** | Low FSH/LH, low E2 |
| **Treatment** | Lifestyle modifications |
| | Estrogen replacement |
| | Ovulation induction or IVF |

## Hypothalamic Dysfunction

With hypothalamic dysfunction, the GnRH signal is decreased, resulting in less FSH and LH release. This can present as a long follicular phase with delayed ovulation (a longer duration of FSH release was needed because the FSH signal was not as high as normal), or a short luteal phase (poor LH pulses resulting in less progesterone production). These subtle hormonal changes are distinctly different from a normal cycle.

Hypothalamic dysfunction is an underdiagnosed cause of cycle abnormalities. Symptoms are similar to HA but often less pronounced, since some estrogen is made and ovulation occurs. If you track your ovulation, you will be able to detect ovulatory issues. Treatment can include lifestyle optimization and ovulation induction if you are trying to conceive.

## HYPOTHALAMIC DYSFUNCTION

| Symptoms | Short luteal phase |
| --- | --- |
| | Long follicular phase |
| | Fatigue |
| | Infertility |
| Diagnosis | Low/normal FSH, low E2 |
| Treatment | Lifestyle modifications |
| | Ovulation induction |

### Common Questions

**Why do I need to get a brain MRI if my doctor said my HA is from not eating enough?**

Everyone will have a different set point for what their brain interprets as an appropriate energy need for their body. We should never assume someone has FHA based on their history without testing other treatable causes, such as thyroid, prolactin, and brain masses. The treatment options and clinical implications are different, as a brain mass cannot be fixed by eating more calories.

## Pituitary Causes of Anovulation

Prolactin is a major pituitary hormone, and abnormal secretion can result in anovulation. Although prolactin levels are usually low, they vary throughout the day and are higher in response to certain stimuli (see the following table).

## POTENTIAL CAUSES OF ABNORMAL PROLACTIN

| | |
|---|---|
| Brain mass | Exercise |
| Pituitary damage | Intercourse |
| Medications | Eating |
| Nipple stimulation | Lack of sleep |

The most common pituitary causes of anovulation include hyperprolactinemia and Sheehan syndrome.

### Hyperprolactinemia

Elevated prolactin, known as hyperprolactinemia, impairs the ability of the pituitary gland to release FSH. This results in anovulation and low estrogen, causing a spectrum of menstrual irregularity, including luteal phase defect at mildly elevated levels and amenorrhea at high levels. Because the pituitary gland makes prolactin to control breast growth and lactation, the classic symptom of hyperprolactinemia is spontaneous milk production, known as galactorrhea.

Prolactin can, and should, always be checked with cycle changes or amenorrhea. Three causes of elevated prolactin that should always be ruled out include:

1. Pregnancy

2. Medications (especially antidepressants or seizure medications)

3. Pituitary tumor

Since prolactin can be influenced by time of day and phase of your cycle, an elevated prolactin level should be repeated in your follicular phase while you are fasting. If you are on any medications or using any recreational drugs, please make sure your doctor is aware so they can review medication causes of an elevated prolactin. All women with hyperprolactinemia should have a brain MRI to evaluate for a pituitary mass.

Elevated prolactin is usually treated with dopamine agonists, a medication to stop prolactin production. Once prolactin levels are normalized, ovulation should resume. Dopamine agonists should be stopped with a positive pregnancy test, since prolactin is important in pregnancy.

**HYPERPROLACTINEMIA**

| | |
|---|---|
| **Symptoms** | Irregular or absent periods |
| | Galactorrhea |
| | Low libido |
| | Breast growth |
| | Headache, vision changes |
| | Infertility |
| **Diagnosis** | Labs: high PRL, low FSH, low E2 |
| | Brain MRI: may have pituitary mass |
| **Treatment** | Dopamine agonists |
| | Ovulation induction |

## Sheehan Syndrome

Prolactin levels are usually low, so it is rare to have an underproduction of prolactin, but one notable cause is Sheehan syndrome. This is when you have extreme blood loss after delivery, resulting in lack of blood flow to the pituitary gland. It is often discovered with failure to make milk postpartum.[6] Treatment involves hormone replacement therapy.

**SHEEHAN SYNDROME**

| | |
|---|---|
| **Symptoms** | Absent periods |
| | No milk production |
| | Fatigue, low energy |
| **Diagnosis** | Labs: low PRL, low FSH, low E2 |
| **Treatment** | Hormone replacement |

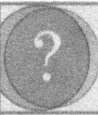 **Common Questions**

### Can you get pregnant while breastfeeding?

High prolactin while breastfeeding is considered "nature's birth control" and known as lactational amenorrhea. If you are exclusively breastfeeding every four hours during the day and every six hours at night, breastfeeding is 98 percent effective at preventing ovulation and pregnancy during the first six months.[7] Once your baby begins to eat other foods or has formula, ovulation generally resumes. Although you can get pregnant while breastfeeding, it may be more difficult. It is important to note that exclusive breastfeeding during pregnancy is associated with a three times greater risk of miscarriage.[8] If you have infertility or are going through fertility treatments, you will want to discuss with your doctor the best plan for breastfeeding.

## Thyroid Causes of Anovulation

Your thyroid is important in metabolism. The pituitary gland sends out thyroid stimulating hormone (TSH), which directs the thyroid gland to make the thyroid hormones T3 (triiodothyronine) and T4 (thyroxine). These hormones affect every cell in your body to control your metabolism—including your weight, temperature, and energy levels. When you brain is not getting the right amount of thyroid hormones, the hypothalamus and pituitary have to work together to release more or less TSH, and when this occurs, it can interfere with the ability of the pituitary gland to regulate normal FSH and LH release, resulting in ovulatory dysfunction.

Every person needs a different amount of T3 and T4 for your body to function best. This is why TSH is the best *screening* test for your thyroid. If I check your TSH, I can see if *your* brain thinks *you* have enough thyroid hormone.[9] Of note, a screening test is just that, and if you have symptoms of thyroid dysfunction, checking your thyroid hormone levels, in addition to TSH, is helpful to get to a diagnosis.

Sadly, thyroid disease is one of the most common endocrine disorders in women.[10] Many women with thyroid disease will have irregular cycles, as thyroid disease is associated with an increase in infertility and miscarriage.[11] Everyone with an irregular menstrual cycle should be screened for thyroid disorders.[12]

The two most common types of thyroid disorder that affect ovulation are hypothyroidism and hyperthyroidism.

### Hypothyroidism

In hypothyroidism, your thyroid gland is not making enough thyroid hormones, so your metabolism slows; this is known as an "underactive thyroid." To compensate, your brain sends out more TSH in an attempt to stimulate more thyroid hormone production. Not having enough circulating thyroid hormones will result in weight gain, fatigue, irregular or heavy periods, and the symptoms common with hypothyroidism. Even if your T3/T4 are in the normal range, an elevated TSH is a sign that *your* brain is not getting enough thyroid hormones.[13]

The most common cause of hypothyroidism is an autoimmune disease called Hashimoto's disease, where your body makes antibodies that attack, damage, and prevent the thyroid gland from making enough (or any) thyroid hormones.[14] You can measure the Hashimoto's antibodies, called TPO (thyroid peroxidase) antibodies, in the blood.

Treatment of hypothyroidism involves thyroid hormone replacement, most commonly with levothyroxine, a synthetic T4. Ninety-six percent of the thyroid hormone produced is T4, which is converted into T3 (the more active form of thyroid hormone).[15] Since T4 can be converted into T3, many people do not need T3 replacement, but hypothyroidism is complex and sometimes T3 is needed—always listen to what your doctor recommends. Importantly, during pregnancy only T4 crosses the placenta (T3 does not), so it is important to make sure anyone with hypothyroidism has sufficient levels of T4 replacement.[16] This typically means changing over to T4-only medication (instead of both T4 and T3). That said, occasionally continuing T3 replacement *in addition* to T4 is the right option, as long as thyroid hormone levels are checked and followed closely by a professional.

When we are replacing your thyroid hormones prior to pregnancy, it is my goal to get you on medication that appropriately replaces what you need, makes you feel better, and helps you conceive. I follow first trimester thyroid hormone recommendations (goal TSH < 2.5 mIU/L) and want my patients on a treatment plan we can continue in pregnancy, as thyroid hormone requirements increase by 30 percent once pregnant.[17]

**HYPOTHYROIDISM**

| | |
|---|---|
| **Symptoms** | Weight gain |
| | Fatigue |
| | Irregular or heavy periods |
| | Feeling cold |
| | Having dry skin and hair |
| | Hair loss |
| | Slow heart rate |
| | Constipation |
| | Depression |
| **Diagnosis** | Labs: high TSH, low T3/T4 |
| **Treatment** | Thyroid hormone replacement |

## Hyperthyroidism

In hyperthyroidism, you have high levels of the thyroid hormones (high T3/T4) and an overactive metabolism, resulting in weight loss, hair loss, insomnia, and irregular or absent periods, among other symptoms.[18] The brain responds by decreasing the amount of TSH released (low TSH), but often the thyroid gland is not listening.

The most common cause of hyperthyroidism is an autoimmune disease known as Graves' disease, where the thyroid gland is attacked by antibodies that stimulate the production of thyroid hormones while causing pain, swelling, and inflammation of the thyroid gland. Inflammation is a huge part of what makes autoimmune thyroid disease so problematic for the body.

Treatment for hyperthyroidism is more complicated and can include medications, surgery, or radioactive destruction of the thyroid gland. If a patient has definitive treatment with surgery or radiation, they will then be hypothyroid and need thyroid hormone replacement. Some treatment options for hyperthyroidism will delay your timeline to conceive.

**HYPERTHYROIDISM**

| | |
|---|---|
| **Symptoms** | Weight loss |
| | Insomnia |
| | Irregular or absent periods |
| | Feeling hot |
| | Warm and sweaty skin |
| | Hair loss |
| | Rapid heart rate |
| | Diarrhea |
| | Anxiety |
| **Diagnosis** | Labs: low TSH, high T3/T4 |
| **Treatment** | Medications |
| | Surgery |
| | Radioactive ablation |

## Ovarian Causes of Anovulation

The ovary is a hormone-producing factory, making estrogen and progesterone in response to FSH and LH from the pituitary gland. Remember that the ovary makes a small amount of estrogen from each antral follicle and only makes high levels of estrogen as an egg matures. When you are not ovulating, you are not making as much estrogen as your body needs.

The most common ovarian causes of anovulation include ovarian failure and PCOS.

### Ovarian Failure

Ovarian failure, also known as menopause, is when the ovary is out of eggs and no longer able to make estrogen (since estrogen is made as eggs mature and ovulate). Before you are completely out of eggs, your egg supply will get to such a low level that you'll often see a change in your ovulatory pattern. As your egg count drops, the ovaries become more stubborn, not wanting to run out of eggs. The brain must send out a stronger signal of FSH to get the ovary to respond, resulting in faster follicular growth due to the elevated FSH. Ovarian failure is diagnosed with low estrogen and FSH levels over 40 mIU/mL.

As your egg count declines, the classic cycle pattern evolves from shorter cycles with earlier ovulation, to longer cycles with later ovulation, to irregular cycles, skipping months, and then amenorrhea. This period of menstrual irregularity associated with a declining egg count is known as perimenopause and can last anywhere from two to ten years. Initial cycle changes may be bothersome but not detrimental, but once your cycles start to lengthen and ovulation is delayed or irregular, you will start to experience more days with low estrogen symptoms. It is important to note that hormone change and symptoms begin while you are still having a cycle, and ovulation tracking (reviewed in chapter 5) will alert you to subtle cycle changes and present the opportunity for earlier intervention.

The average age of menopause, or ovarian failure, is fifty-one to fifty-two years. Ovarian failure prior to age forty-five is considered early menopause. Premature ovarian insufficiency (POI) is ovarian failure before the age of forty. POI is diagnosed after four months of absent cycles and two FSH levels >25 mIU/mL.[19] POI is distinct from diminished ovarian reserve (DOR), as women with DOR are presumed to still be ovulating while those with POI no longer have responsive ovaries. Women with DOR are at risk for POI, but they have a different reproductive potential.

POI is associated with future health risks such as osteoporosis, heart disease, and dementia.[20] All patients with POI should have a complete evaluation to determine the nature of ovarian failure. Almost half of patients with a normal genetic evaluation will have a positive antibody for an autoimmune disease when an expanded panel is completed.[21] Even when an autoimmune cause is not identified, an increase in pro-inflammatory factors have been found in women with POI—suggesting that inflammation contributes to the early loss of ovarian function.[22]

Estrogen replacement is recommended for women with POI to improve long-term health and quality of life. I'm a big believer in estrogen replacement. Your body and brain love estrogen, and I want you to feel your best. I often titrate levels of E2 in women with POI to replicate a more physiologic state.

Hormone replacement should always be done with a healthcare provider. There are two important truths about estrogen treatment:

1. Estrogen is not birth control.
2. If you have a uterus, you also need to take progesterone, either daily or at minimum every three months.

POI does not mean you are 100 percent out of eggs (though you are very close), but it does mean you will no longer respond to fertility treatments. Although the most successful treatment for women with POI is egg donation, 3 to 4 percent of women with POI can achieve a spontaneous pregnancy once estrogen treatment has been started.[23] If you desire a pregnancy and have POI, I recommend having unprotected intercourse and using progesterone every one to three months if not pregnant. I had a patient who had POI in her twenties and had her first child via egg donation. She then spontaneously conceived her second child while on estrogen replacement.

### OVARIAN FAILURE

| | |
|---|---|
| **Symptoms** | Amenorrhea |
| | Fatigue |
| | Headache |
| | Low libido |
| | Vaginal dryness |
| | Weight gain or loss |
| | Infertility |
| **Diagnosis** | Labs: high FSH, low E2 |
| **Treatment** | Estrogen replacement |
| | Donor eggs |

## Polycystic Ovary Syndrome (PCOS)

PCOS is the most common endocrine disease in reproductive-age women.[24] As we saw with Hazel, in PCOS, the communication between the brain and the ovary is broken, resulting in hormone abnormalities and anovulation.

Remember the ovarian vault? With PCOS, you are born with too many eggs and have a higher number of eggs inside the vault, which means more eggs are released each month. The brain sends out a normal amount of FSH, but this FSH signal gets diluted among the high number of follicles. The FSH signal from the brain is not strong enough to get one follicle to grow, resulting in delayed or no ovulation. In addition, each small antral follicle makes a tiny amount of estrogen. If you have more follicles, you will have a higher baseline estrogen. Your brain assumes that estrogen is from a growing follicle instead of many small ones, thus the brain does not release a stronger FSH signal. Since the ovary can't make high levels of estrogen without ovulation, the brain begins to send out LH, stimulating androgen production (such as testosterone). This becomes the preferred pathway, as testosterone is made at a higher rate than normal.

The majority of women with PCOS will have insulin resistance.[25] Insulin is extremely important; it helps your body use and store glucose, the fuel for cells. Without insulin, your cells cannot utilize glucose. Low intracellular glucose levels result in the liver breaking down stored glucose, which increases blood glucose levels. In response to the elevated glucose, your pancreas starts to make even more insulin. Since your cells have become resistant to insulin, this process creates a vicious cycle. High insulin levels are harmful throughout the body—causing inflammation and a change in cellular function, especially the ovaries and uterus. Insulin resistance results in an increase in ovarian androgen production, impaired egg maturation, and changes endometrial receptivity.[26] In addition, high insulin levels result in increased fat accumulation, which further exacerbates inflammation and hormonal changes.

High androgen levels manifest as acne, increased face and body hair, and male pattern baldness. If you have PCOS, you are also at risk for an increase in breakthrough bleeding. The low, but slightly elevated, estrogen level from all the small follicles continually stimulates growth of the uterine lining. Without ovulation or progesterone, the lining never stabilizes or sheds.

I compare bleeding in PCOS like placing a cup under a faucet on constant drip. Imagine the water is estrogen. After ovulation, progesterone is meant to turn off the faucet, and the drop in progesterone tells your body to pour out the water from the cup, representing your period. If your faucet is constantly on drip and never turns off, the cup will overflow, and you will bleed even though it is not a "real" period.

PCOS is diagnosed when you present two of the three factors listed below, known as the Rotterdam criteria:[27]

1. High androgens (testosterone, androstenedione, and DHEAS), determined through blood tests or symptoms (facial hair, acne, or losing hair).

2. Irregular or absent periods.

3. Polycystic ovaries on ultrasound, defined as >20 antral follicles on at least one ovary or an ovarian volume of >10 mL. This ultrasound appearance is described as a "string of pearls" as the small follicles are pushed to the external surface.

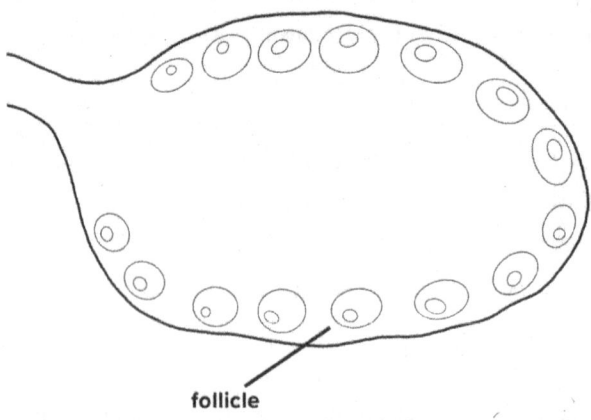

**PCOS "String of Pearls" Appearance**

PCOS is a complex disease, so there is no one-size-fits-all treatment recommendation. The important components in treatment include:

1. Improving insulin resistance
2. Weight optimization
3. Endometrial protection
4. Ovulation induction (if trying to conceive)

Let's go through these one by one.

### IMPROVING INSULIN RESISTANCE

Insulin resistance results in high blood glucose and insulin levels—creating inflammation and further hormone disruption. In order to fully treat PCOS, we cannot ignore the metabolic changes seen with high insulin levels. Insulin resistance is reversible, and it is important to not just treat (with medication) but to also change behaviors that worsen your glucose metabolism.

The lifestyle recommendations to reverse insulin resistance will be reviewed at length in part III, but I recommend starting by removing any factors that are worsening your metabolic status. This approach includes: getting more high-quality sleep, decreasing chronic stress, building skeletal muscle, and shifting dietary habits to fight inflammation. Often the greatest opportunity for improvement of insulin resistance includes a high-fiber diet full of fruits and vegetables while avoiding ultra-processed foods and added sugars.[28]

In addition to lifestyle changes, sometimes medical options are needed to improve insulin sensitivity, such as metformin or myo-inositol. Metformin is an insulin sensitizing medication, which works to help your cells respond to lower levels of insulin—resulting in a lowering of your blood glucose and insulin levels. Metformin can cause side effects such as nausea and diarrhea, and often needs to be titrated up in dose slowly to avoid these. Around 30 percent of women with PCOS will ovulate in response to metformin treatment alone.[29] Metformin treatment improves live birth rates in women with PCOS over placebo, and although it may not restore ovulation in all women with PCOS, it should be considered as a potential first-line treatment option or an adjunct to treatment due to the benefit of improving insulin resistance.[30] Myo-inositol is important in glucose uptake into the ovary, and supplementing with myo-inositol can improve insulin sensitivity and ovarian response to FSH.[31]

### WEIGHT OPTIMIZATION

Women with PCOS can have any body type. However, obesity worsens PCOS in multiple ways: (1) fat cells make a form of estrogen called estrone; (2) obesity is associated with a decrease in the liver's production of sex hormone binding globulin (SHBG); and (3) obesity is linked with insulin resistance and inflammation. An increase in estrone makes the brain believe an egg is growing, preventing sufficient FSH release, and estrone can be converted into testosterone. SHBG floats around your blood and binds to your free hormones like testosterone. Your body can't use hormones that are bound to SHBG, but when SHBG levels are low, you have more "active" circulating testosterone, worsening hormone imbalance and high androgen symptoms. If you are overweight, losing weight can decrease estrone, increase SHBG, and improve your metabolic parameters, potentially restoring ovulation.

### ENDOMETRIAL PROTECTION

Another component of treating PCOS is what we call endometrial protection. If you are not ovulating, as is often the case with PCOS, you are not fully shedding the uterine lining. This can result in endometrial changes that can lead to endometrial cancer. Treatment includes exposure to progesterone, either by inducing ovulation, giving a daily progesterone or birth control pill, or cyclic progesterone for one to two weeks every one to three months. If you have not had a regular cycle for an extended amount of time, and especially if your endometrial lining is thick on ultrasound, you may need an endometrial biopsy to confirm there are no cancerous or precancerous cells present. If you are not ready for pregnancy, the birth control pill can have advantages for women with PCOS. The birth control pill can provide endometrial protection, contraception, and improvement of hormonal symptoms by increasing SHBG and lowering testosterone. The birth control pill has side effects and is not the only option. A full discussion with your doctor should always take place before starting the pill.

## OVULATION INDUCTION

Many women with PCOS will have infertility and need ovulation induction in order to conceive. Ovulation induction is reviewed in chapter 7 in detail, but often includes metformin, oral medications—such as clomid or letrozole—and/or gonadotropins. The decision on which to use will depend on your scenario, but you should review what to expect with treatment and the goals of each cycle. Importantly, women with PCOS have a higher risk of pregnancy complications, including miscarriage, gestational diabetes, and preeclampsia, especially in the setting of insulin resistance.[32] Managing chronic inflammation and insulin resistance is important for your fertility and pregnancy outcomes. Some women with PCOS will not respond to ovulation induction medications and may need IVF to conceive.

### POLYCYSTIC OVARY SYNDROME (PCOS)

| | |
|---|---|
| Symptoms | Irregular cycles |
| | Weight gain |
| | Acne |
| | Hair growth (facial hair) |
| | Hair loss (male pattern baldness) |
| | Fatigue |
| | Insulin resistance |
| | Depression |
| | Infertility |
| Diagnosis | Rotterdam criteria (2 out of 3): <br> • Irregular cycles <br> • High androgen labs or symptoms <br> • Ultrasound appearance of ovaries |
| Treatment | Lifestyle modifications |
| | Weight loss |
| | Improve insulin resistance |
| | Endometrial protection |
| | Ovulation induction, IVF |

## Adrenal Causes of Anovulation

Your adrenal glands are important in the production of many hormones, including aldosterone, cortisol, and testosterone. Since the adrenal glands make cortisol and are involved in the stress pathway, they are poorly understood and often blamed when getting to a diagnosis is difficult.

*Adrenal fatigue* is the term coined for the group of symptoms including fatigue, body aches, insomnia, anxiety, GI upset, and abnormal cycles. However, adrenal fatigue is not a recognized medical diagnosis. *This does not mean your symptoms are not real.* But accepting a fake diagnosis will prevent you from getting to the real source of your symptoms. For many people, the symptoms to which "adrenal fatigue" refers may be the first presentation of an autoimmune disease or hypothalamic dysfunction.

The most common adrenal disease that impacts your cycle is known as congenital adrenal hyperplasia (CAH).

### Congenital Adrenal Hyperplasia (CAH)

CAH is an inherited genetic disease resulting in mutation of an enzyme important in adrenal gland hormonal production, most commonly 21-hydroxylase. One form of CAH is severe and diagnosed at birth, but the more common version, known as non-classic CAH, will present after puberty. In CAH, the adrenal glands' hormone production encounters a block where the enzyme defect is present, resulting in a shift of adrenal gland hormone production toward increased androgens, often mimicking PCOS with irregular cycles and hyperandrogenism. Diagnosis is made with high levels of 17-hydroxyprogesterone (17-OHP), a hormone that builds up due to the enzyme mutation, or genetic testing. Treatment usually includes steroids and ovulation induction.

## CONGENITAL ADRENAL HYPERPLASIA (CAH)

| | |
|---|---|
| **Symptoms** | Early puberty |
| | Irregular cycles |
| | Weight gain |
| | Acne |
| | Hair growth (facial hair) |
| | Hair loss (male pattern baldness) |
| | Infertility |
| **Diagnosis** | Labs: high 17-OHP, genetic testing |
| **Treatment** | Steroids |
| | Ovulation induction |

 *Common Questions*

**Should I take adrenal support supplements?**

Some patients are told to take adrenal hormone supplements to help their adrenal glands function, but this can be harmful and is not recommended. Adrenal support supplements are usually cow or pig adrenal glands plus a variety of other hormones, including progesterone, cortisone, cortisol, aldosterone, and thyroid hormones. The FDA does not regulate supplements, and each pill can be different. The hormones in the adrenal supplement also tell your brain to stop sending out ACTH and can cause adrenal insufficiency, a serious medical problem.

## ABNORMAL BLEEDING AND STRUCTURAL ABNORMALITIES

The amount of bleeding that is considered normal varies from person to person, but on the whole, spotting, light bleeding, and heavy bleeding are all abnormal. Most abnormal uterine bleeding is a result of structural issues, as compared with hormonal issues, which more typically present with cycle irregularity.

**TOP CAUSES OF ABNORMAL BLEEDING**

| | |
|---|---|
| **Spotting** | Uterine polyps |
| | Cervical stenosis |
| | Endometritis |
| | Cancer |
| | Infections |
| | Vaginal atrophy |
| | Retained pregnancy tissue |
| | Pregnancy |
| | Luteal phase defect |
| **Light Bleeding** | Hormone suppression |
| | Asherman syndrome |
| | Low ovarian reserve |
| **Heavy Bleeding** | Fibroids |
| | Adenomyosis |
| | Uterine polyps |
| | Cancer |
| | Anovulation |
| | Retained pregnancy tissue |

Many of the causes on the list represent much more than just an ability to get pregnant, emphasizing the importance of using your period as a vital sign. As you can see, this list is diverse, and some causes can create more than one type of bleeding abnormality, depending on size and location. That said, any change in bleeding should be evaluated.

The structural abnormalities that contribute to abnormal bleeding often disrupt normal anatomy. The following diagram represents your normal anatomy, and we will review the structural changes in each section.

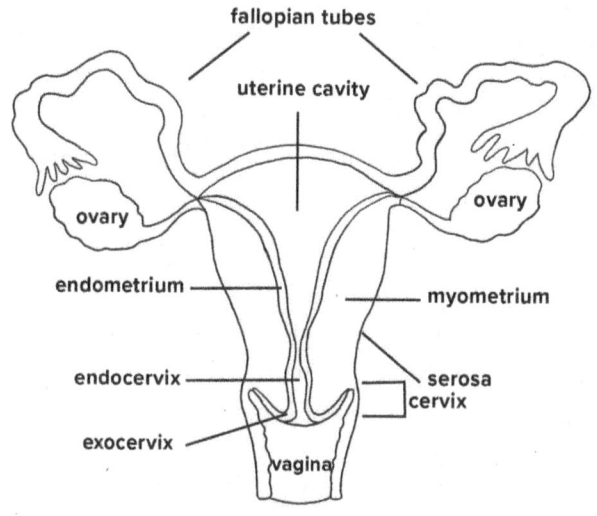

Normal Reproductive Anatomy

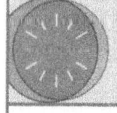 *Top Tip*

**What to expect for the evaluation of abnormal bleeding**

1. **History:** You need to be able to describe how long your bleeding lasts, how heavy your bleeding is, and if there is any change from a prior bleeding pattern. Any spotting should be described as either always occurring at a set point in your cycle or random.

> 2. **Blood work:** The first step is usually an updated Pap smear and a negative pregnancy test. Blood work may be ordered if your bleeding could be due to abnormal ovulation.
>
> 3. **Imaging:** The first step is often a physical exam prior to imaging. Ultrasound is the simplest and most accessible first-line option.

## Top Causes of Spotting

Although typically not painful, spotting more than a couple days before or after your period is abnormal. The timeline of spotting can help aid in diagnosis. Think about when you are spotting and track your bleeding level along with your cycle.

The most common structural causes of spotting are uterine polyps and endometritis.

### Uterine Polyps

A uterine polyp is a projection of endometrial glands and stroma into the uterine cavity. Around 8 percent of women have polyps—and the top symptom is spotting.[33] I want to rule out a polyp anytime a patient has spotting.

Polyps are typically painless and do not impact ovulation, but they are associated with infertility.[34] Polyps may interfere with sperm getting through the uterus, cause uterine inflammation, and impair implantation. Up to 45 percent of women undergoing IVF will be diagnosed with uterine polyps.[35] Although you can get pregnant with a polyp, removal of polyps is associated with an improvement in pregnancy rates.[36]

Most polyps are benign, but they can be malignant, especially if your cycles are infrequent. I had one patient who had a cancerous polyp without abnormal bleeding. That was one case too many, and it is why I think even asymptomatic polyps should be removed.

Polyps are not always seen on transvaginal ultrasound because the inside of the uterine cavity is not well visualized. Instead, for diagnosis, a saline infusion sonogram (SIS) or hysterosalpingogram (HSG), where water or dye is inserted into the uterine cavity, allows visualization inside the uterine

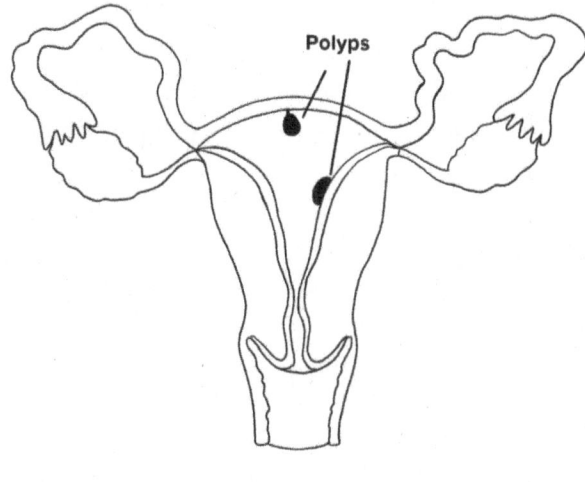

Uterine Polyps

cavity. Hysteroscopy is another method for diagnosis that also allows immediate removal. Polypectomy is a simple surgical procedure that can be done in an outpatient setting with minimal risks.

**UTERINE POLYPS**

| Symptoms | Spotting |
| --- | --- |
| | Heavy bleeding |
| | Painless |
| Diagnosis | Imaging: SIS or HSG |
| Treatment | Hysteroscopic polypectomy |

## Endometritis

Endometritis is an inflammation of the endometrium that can occur after procedures, infections, or from intrauterine structures (like polyps or fibroids). Although endometritis can present with spotting, it is sometimes asymptomatic. Endometritis is diagnosed with uterine biopsy.

Up to 50 percent of women with unexplained infertility will have uterine inflammation on biopsy.[37] I often empirically treat my patients for endometritis without putting them through an endometrial biopsy. The standard treatment for endometritis is the antibiotic doxycycline, which also has anti-inflammatory properties. In the case of a polyp or fibroid, surgical removal resolves the endometritis.[38]

**ENDOMETRITIS**

| | |
|---|---|
| **Symptoms** | Spotting |
| | Vaginal discharge |
| **Diagnosis** | Uterine biopsy |
| | Imaging: SIS or HSG (to rule out polyp/fibroid) |
| **Treatment** | Antibiotics |

## Top Causes of Light Bleeding

Light bleeding may be a sign that your endometrial lining is not able to grow as thick as before. The endometrium has two layers, a basal layer that regenerates and a functional layer that is hormonally responsive and sheds each month during your menses. Light bleeding results from either:

1. Suppression of the functional layer (from progesterone exposure)
2. Damage to the basal layer (from trauma or uterine procedures), known as Asherman syndrome.

If you were recently on hormonal contraception and have lighter cycles since stopping, it may be due to prolonged exposure to progesterone. This will typically resolve with further ovulatory cycles, but sometimes profound suppression (more likely if you had no cycles at all on your contraceptive) will need evaluation and possible treatment with estrogen.

The top structural cause of light bleeding is Asherman syndrome.

## Asherman Syndrome

Asherman syndrome is adhesions inside the uterus caused by the destruction of the basal layer of the endometrium. In Asherman syndrome, ovulation still occurs, but scar tissue has replaced the functional endometrium, resulting in less tissue to bleed.

Concerning history that might point to Asherman syndrome includes heavy blood loss, uterine infection, retained placenta, dilation and curettage (D&C), or significant damage to the uterus during a procedure. Although less common, prior uterine surgery, IUD placement, or uterine infections pose a risk of traumatizing the basal layer of the endometrium, resulting in adhesions.

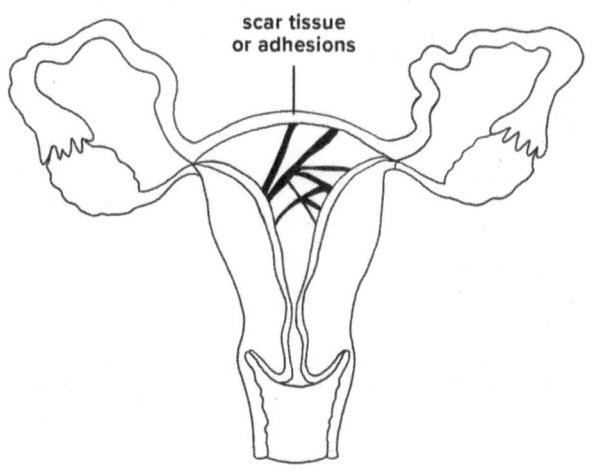

**Asherman Syndrome**

Uterine adhesions can present with light bleeding or amenorrhea. Surgical resection of the adhesions is standard treatment, but 27 to 50 percent of adhesions return.[39] Postoperatively, I often recommend treatment to prevent recurrence with both placement of an intrauterine balloon and high-dose estrogen. Since adhesion recurrence is high, it is important to confirm normal uterine cavity with repeat imaging.

After surgical treatment, an important discussion with your doctor should focus on your family goals and timeline. I always prioritize preventing further uterine damage to the best of our ability and expediting pregnancy.

Sometimes this means accelerating to IVF to genetically test embryos (decreasing the risk of pregnancy loss) and optimizing endometrial growth in a frozen embryo transfer.

**ASHERMAN SYNDROME**

| | |
|---|---|
| Symptoms | Amenorrhea |
| | Light bleeding |
| | Cyclic pain |
| | Ovulatory symptoms |
| Diagnosis | Imaging: SIS or HSG |
| Treatment | Hysteroscopic polypectomy |

## Top Causes of Heavy Bleeding

Approximately 10 percent of women have heavy bleeding.[40] Passing blood clots, bleeding through clothes, changing your pad or tampon every hour, and feeling short of breath, lightheaded, dizzy, or passing out are all signs that your bleeding may be too heavy. Heavy bleeding is known as menorrhagia.

The top causes of heavy bleeding include uterine fibroids and adenomyosis.

### Uterine Fibroids

Fibroids are benign growths of myometrial tissue in the uterus and occur in 70 percent of reproductive-age women.[41] Fibroids can be located inside the uterus (submucosal), in the myometrium itself (intramural), on the outside of the uterus cavity (subserosal), and even connected to the uterus with a stalk (pedunculated). The symptoms and reproductive impact of your fibroids will depend on where they are located.

Fibroids can cause heavy bleeding and painful periods, significantly impacting quality of life. You should not bleed through your clothes, pass out, or need a blood transfusion when you are on your period. Depending on

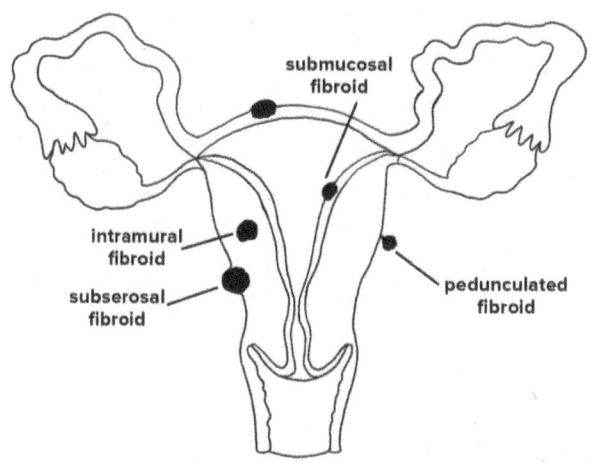

Uterine Fibroid Locations

the size of the fibroid, you may have "bulk symptoms," where the uterus is so large that it presses on your organs, causing frequent urination and pain with bowel movements. I once saw a seventy-year-old woman present to the emergency room convinced she was pregnant because her uterus was so large—due to fibroids!

Not all fibroids impact your fertility or need to be removed. I recommend only removing fibroids that may impact implantation. To improve pregnancy rates, surgical removal of fibroids that are inside the uterine cavity or distort the uterine cavity should be considered in women who desire pregnancy.[42]

**UTERINE FIBROIDS**

| | |
|---|---|
| Symptoms | Heavy bleeding |
| | Painful, regular periods |
| | Bulk symptoms |
| Diagnosis | Imaging: transvaginal ultrasound |
| Treatment | Myomectomy |

## Adenomyosis

Adenomyosis is an inflammatory disease where endometrial-like tissue migrates into the myometrium, the muscle of the uterus, presenting as lesions. Adenomyosis rarely occurs without a prior pregnancy or surgical procedure on the uterus, as those situations represent a potential pathway for the tissue to invade the myometrium. Due to the increased size of the myometrium, periods are often longer, heavier, and painful.

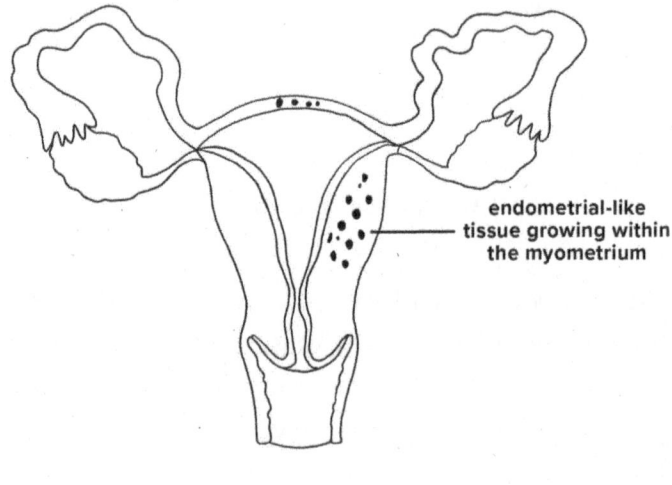

Adenomyosis

Adenomyosis lesions can typically be seen on ultrasound or MRI. On a physical exam, the uterus is often enlarged and soft, called "boggy." Adenomyosis is not inside the uterine cavity, which means uterine biopsy is not helpful in diagnosis.

Adenomyosis causes lower pregnancy rates and higher miscarriage rates due to increased inflammation.[43] Medical management includes hormone suppression and decreasing inflammation. Since these lesions are responsive to estrogen (like the endometrium), the only way to fully decrease local inflammation is to stop ovulating. Women treated with hormone suppression have about half the rate of disease progression as women who were not suppressed.[44]

To treat adenomyosis, I also often recommend a multifaceted approach of decreasing inflammatory lifestyle behaviors through diet, movement, sleep, stress reduction, and more, as well as IVF with hormonal suppression prior to embryo transfer.[45] I rarely recommend surgery, as removing adenomyosis tissue from the myometrium poses a risk of damage to the uterus and can harm your fertility.[46] In fact, I have seen women who were no longer able to carry a pregnancy after extensive adenomyosis resections.

### ADENOMYOSIS

| | |
|---|---|
| **Symptoms** | Painful, regular cycles |
| | Heavy bleeding |
| **Diagnosis** | Transvaginal ultrasound |
| | MRI |
| **Treatment** | Ovulation suppression |
| | Surgery |
| | IVF and hormone suppression |

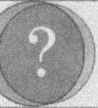

## Common Questions

**How do I know if my abnormal bleeding is from endometrial cancer?**

The most concerning cause of abnormal bleeding is always cancer. Endometrial cancer can present with painless, heavy bleeding. Anovulation and obesity are risk factors for uterine cancer as the increased estrogen without regular bleeding predisposes endometrial cells to cancerous changes. Taking unopposed estrogen (without progesterone) also increases the risk of cancer. Endometrial cancer is typically diagnosed with a uterine biopsy. Treatment can include hormonal suppression and/or uterine surgery, and prognosis is good if diagnosed early. Although endometrial cancer is not common, the risk of it is real if you are not ovulating—further supporting the need for a prompt evaluation.

## DYSMENORRHEA: PAINFUL MENSTRUAL CYCLES

Painful periods are known as dysmenorrhea. It can be difficult to understand what constitutes normal period pain because we all have cramps when the uterus contracts and we bleed. But how much pain is too much?

A good medical history is key to expediting a diagnosis for dysmenorrhea. This means you must know your cycle. Many causes of dysmenorrhea will also present with abnormal bleeding. But the top cause of dysmenorrhea seen without any bleeding change is endometriosis.

### TOP CAUSES OF DYSMENORRHEA

| | |
|---|---|
| Endometriosis | Uterine scar tissue |
| Adenomyosis | Infections |
| Uterine fibroids | Cervical stenosis |

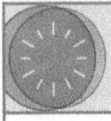

### Top Tip

**What to expect for the evaluation of a painful cycle**

1. **History:** You need to be able to describe your pain, symptoms, and timeline. Consider keeping a symptom log. Each day, mark your symptoms on your calendar, in a planner, or in an app. Important questions include:
    i. Do you have pain only with your menses or at other times?
    ii. Do you have any associated symptoms, like bleeding changes or GI symptoms?
    iii. How long have you had the pain?
    iv. Does the pain interfere with your quality of life?
2. **Blood work:** Blood work is not typically helpful with painful cycles unless your bleeding is also irregular.

> 3. **Imaging:** Imaging is typically the next step to evaluate pain. Ultrasound is the simplest and most accessible option.

## Endometriosis

Endometriosis occurs when endometrial-like tissue grows outside of the uterus, most commonly on the ovaries, fallopian tubes, and the pelvic sidewall. The endometrial implants respond to estrogen with each cycle and trigger a large immune response, leading to chronic inflammation, scarring, adhesions, and distortion of the normal pelvic anatomy.

Endometriosis pain typically occurs with menstrual bleeding. Associated symptoms are due to the huge inflammatory burden and include GI symptoms, fatigue, bloating, and pain with intercourse or bowel movements.

The severity of endometriosis is categorized into four stages:

- Stage I: minimal
- Stage II: mild
- Stage III: moderate
- Stage IV: severe

The early stages of endometriosis are characterized by inflammation, while the later stages involve more extensive scarring and anatomical distortion. Although the stage of endometriosis reflects the burden of disease, it does not correlate with symptoms.

One of the biggest challenges with endometriosis is the significant delay in diagnosis—on average, it takes seven to nine years for women to receive a diagnosis.[47] This delay is due to both the dismissal of women's pain and the limited options available for diagnosis. Endometriosis is formally diagnosed with surgery, as it is not always seen on ultrasound or detected on physical exam.

Up to 50 percent of women with infertility have endometriosis.[48] Endometriosis can reduce fertility through several mechanisms, largely chronic inflammation that impacts egg quality, embryo development, and implantation.[49]

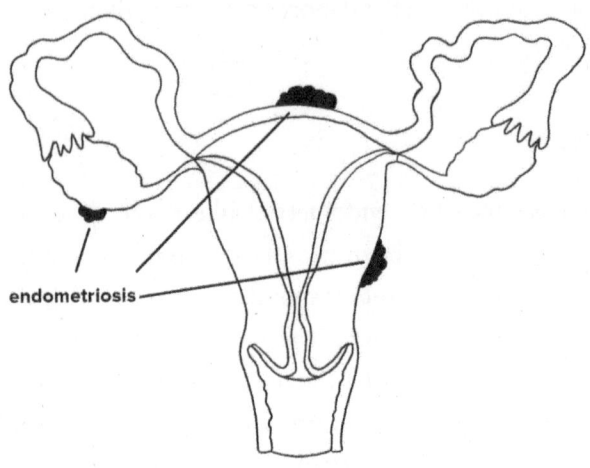

**Endometriosis Lesions**

Scarring and adhesions can distort the normal pelvic anatomy, preventing the egg from being released or traveling properly. The prognosis worsens as the stage of endometriosis increases—fewer than 25 percent of women with moderate to severe disease will conceive naturally.[50] Additionally, endometriosis is associated with a decline in ovarian reserve due to chronic inflammation, so women with endometriosis have less time to complete their family.[51,52]

The right treatment plan for endometriosis will depend on the stage of your disease, your age, and your fertility goals. I encourage my endometriosis patients to always start with lifestyle factors that can help reduce inflammation. Medical treatments will suppress ovulation and decrease estrogen production. These include birth control pills, progestin-only treatment, aromatase inhibitors, and GnRH agonists. Medications may help control the growth and spread of endometriosis but will not get rid of any existing disease. Since these medications suppress ovulation, you cannot conceive while using them, so fertility treatments are often needed.

Surgical options to treat endometriosis include excision or destruction of endometriosis lesions. However, surgery is not straightforward, as some women have increased pain or scar tissue after surgery. Surgical resection of endometriosis implants results in a transient decrease in inflammatory markers, which begin to rise again after three months.[53] The decision to proceed with surgical resection should be personalized after a full fertility evaluation and based on treatment goals. While surgery can significantly improve pain, it appears to have a limited utility to improve pregnancy rates, especially in higher-stage disease, and may not be the right decision for everyone.[54]

Endometriosis is a real, treatable condition that deserves to be taken seriously. The sooner you can get an accurate diagnosis and begin appropriate treatment, the better your chances of preserving your fertility. Remember, you are your own best advocate. If you suspect you may have endometriosis, be persistent in getting answers. If you decide to pursue a surgical approach, make sure you are in the hands of an experienced surgeon trained in minimally invasive gynecology who frequently treats women with endometriosis.

**ENDOMETRIOSIS**

| | |
|---|---|
| **Symptoms** | Painful, regular cycles |
| | Bloating |
| | Nausea |
| | Vomiting |
| | Diarrhea |
| | Constipation |
| | Gas |
| | Fatigue |
| **Diagnosis** | Laparoscopic surgery |
| **Treatment** | Ovulation suppression |
| | Surgery |
| | IVF |

> 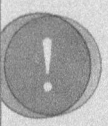 ***Important Study Findings:***
> **Endometriomas**
>
> "Prospective Assessment of the Impact of Endometriomas and Their Removal on Ovarian Reserve and Determinants of the Rate of Decline in Ovarian Reserve"[55]
>
> - **Study basics:** Women with endometriomas (ovarian endometriosis cysts) >2cm had AMH and AFC levels checked before and six months after removal and compared to controls without endometriomas.
>
> - **Results:** At baseline, women with endometriomas had lower AMH and AFC levels. AMH decreased even further after removal.
>
> - **Conclusion:** The presence of an endometrioma is associated with a decrease in ovarian reserve, which is accelerated after surgical removal. Delaying or avoiding surgery may need to be considered if future fertility is desired.

After learning about her PCOS, Hazel started to understand how sensitive her HPO axis is to outside factors and decided to make changes. Hazel revamped her life to decrease inflammation. She ate more whole foods, decreased toxin exposure, and changed her behaviors—prioritizing sleep, outdoor walks, and weight training. After a full fertility evaluation, she started ovulation induction with letrozole. Hazel began to feel more like her old self, and she got pregnant after only a few ovulatory cycles.

Getting to the root cause of your abnormal cycle is an essential step in preventing future fertility problems. And because all stages of abnormal cycles are worsened by external inflammation, decreasing inflammation is a key aspect of treatment.

Your cycle reveals a lot about your hormones and your body, if you know what you are looking for. As you can see, many causes of abnormal cycles can have a lot of overlap. This means being able to give a good menstrual history is the first step in getting to a diagnosis. But to give a good history, you must know how to track your cycle. That's the topic of the next chapter.

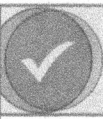

### Facts to Remember

- Your period is a vital sign.
- Your period should be regular and predictable.
- Your bleeding should not soak through clothes.
- Your pain should not interfere with your activities.
- Your ability to describe the timeline of your symptoms will aid in diagnosis.
- Many hormonal imbalances can present with irregular or absent periods.
- Many structural abnormalities can present with pain and abnormal bleeding.
- Treatment of abnormal cycles is important for your future fertility.

# 5

# Mastering Cycle Tracking

Fertility awareness methods (FAM) and cycle tracking are more than just knowing when your next period will start. Understanding your cycle allows you to detect early changes in cycle pattern, which can impact your current and future fertility. In addition, FAM can decrease time to pregnancy as well as help prevent pregnancy, also known as natural family planning.

Unfortunately, medical professionals are often dismissive about cycle tracking, even if they don't mean to be. This is usually because they (1) were not taught (only 6 percent of physicians know how to properly evaluate fertility awareness methods to prevent pregnancy or aid in conception),[1] (2) do not have time to explain, or (3) believe patients are coming to see them for more advanced medical treatments. This has left FAM to be considered a "granola" approach to reproductive medicine and ultimately puts holistic care and advanced reproductive technology at odds, leading to a knowledge gap and lack of trust between patients and medical professionals.

Cycle tracking and FAM were not a part of my initial training either. It wasn't until I had my own pregnancy losses that I started to truly understand the importance of cycle tracking and was able to research FAM and natural fertility and apply this knowledge to work with my own patients.

Dawn had been trying to get pregnant for over a year. She was tracking her cycle and felt like she had done everything in her power to conceive before coming to see me. When reviewing her medical history, I asked about menstrual history. Dawn relied on her cycle-tracking app to tell her when her fertile window would be and said everything was normal. But when she shared her app's tracking data with me, it became very obvious that she was actually missing her fertile window. Since having frequent intercourse had become stressful (which is common), Dawn and her partner were only having intercourse when the app recommended. But her app was not calculating her fertile window correctly, and they were completely missing their opportunity to get pregnant.

Imagine the frustration! Unfortunately, Dawn's story is not uncommon. Today, more than ever, it is essential that we take ownership of our menstrual cycles and not rely on technology or assumptions to tell us how we're doing.

App technology is fascinating. I have used many of the app-based cycle-tracking options myself (for science, of course). There are so many high-tech options. Some are calendar based. Others combine calendar tracking with other methods, such as temperature or measurement of urinary hormone metabolites. But I have been shocked to see that the app's determination of my "peak fertility" has sometimes been completely off, even missing my fertile window—just like what happened to Dawn.

One of the most important skills we can learn for our fertility is how to track our menstrual cycle and pinpoint ovulation. For this reason, this chapter will focus primarily on how to do so without apps or web-based tech. Understanding how to use different types of fertility awareness methods will allow you to decide if wearable or app-based tracking is a good solution for you.

## THE INS AND OUTS OF CYCLE TRACKING

All cycle tracking begins with an understanding of what happens in a normal menstrual cycle. We learned this in chapter 2, but to recap: Your menstrual cycle is divided into two phases—the follicular phase and the luteal phase. The follicular phase begins on the first day of your period and ends with ovulation, when a mature egg is released from the ovary. During the follicular phase, an egg is growing and estrogen is rising. After ovulation, the luteal phase begins, lasting until your next period starts. In the luteal phase, the follicle that grew the egg becomes a cyst known as a corpus luteum, making progesterone. Unless pregnancy occurs, the corpus luteum will die after two weeks, progesterone will drop, and you will have a period, starting the cycle again.

Determining your fertile window, or the only period of time in which conception is possible, is key to cycle tracking. An egg can only be fertilized for twenty-four hours after it is ovulated. Meaning the more precisely you can detect the day of ovulation, the better you will be able to define your fertile window. On the other hand, sperm can survive for up to five days in the female reproductive tract. This means that the only possible days in which conception can occur are the five days before and the day of ovulation. This is the fertile window.

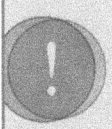

## *Important Study Finding:* Ovulation and the Fertile Window

"Timing of Sexual Intercourse in Relation to Ovulation—Effects on the Probability of Conception, Survival of the Pregnancy, and Sex of the Baby"[2]

- **Study basics:** 221 women trying to conceive collected daily urine specimens to check estrogen and progesterone and kept daily records of whether they had intercourse.

- **Results:** The chance of conception ranged from 10 percent when intercourse occurred five days before ovulation to 33 percent when intercourse occurred on ovulation day. The chance of conception was 0 percent on each day outside this six-day window, including intercourse on the day after ovulation.

- **Conclusion:** Conception occurred only when intercourse took place during a six-day period that ended on the estimated day of ovulation.

## THE CALENDAR METHOD

One of the most common methods for cycle tracking is the calendar method, based on the idea that the corpus luteum has a relatively set lifespan. This means that of the two phases of the cycle, the follicular length varies, while the luteal length is a standard length of fourteen days. According to this method, if you subtract fourteen days from the length of your average cycle, you'll find your expected day of ovulation. Again, your fertile window is the five days before and ending on ovulation day.

However, there are many flaws with this method. For one, the idea that everyone ovulates on cycle day fourteen is actually faulty and taken from a simplified four-week menstrual cycle. In a study looking at hormone levels and ovulation, only 10 percent of women with a twenty-eight-day cycle ovulated on day fourteen. The majority of women actually ovulated prior to this, representing a longer luteal phase and an earlier fertile window than the simple calendar method would predict.[3]

Additionally, the calendar method doesn't account for or detect early stages of ovulatory dysfunction (luteal phase defect), and is only accurate if your cycles are always extremely regular. Despite these limitations, the simple calendar method is the formula on which many apps base their entire fertile window calculation.

Although the simple calendar method is easy to use and is better than no tracking, it only provides limited information. By combining calendar tracking with a fertility awareness method, you will be able to determine if your calendar tracking is accurate.

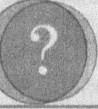 *Common Questions*

**Should I use an app to track my cycle?**

Many app-based methods use the simple calendar method for cycle tracking, which is based on a typical twenty-eight-day cycle, but only 13 percent of women truly have a twenty-eight-day cycle.[4] In fact, only 21 percent of mobile apps that rely on the calendar method alone to determine ovulation day are actually accurate.[5] Emerging tech options combine various methods of calendar tracking and fertility awareness, which improves reliability and accuracy. However, use of any technology includes a risk of data and privacy breach. Some tracking and pregnancy apps recently asked users to update the country and state they live in, which is highly concerning! Why does your app need to know where you live in order to predict your ovulation? As reproductive health is starting to be regulated, it is essential that you have access to accurate health information. If you like using an app, I recommend also co-tracking with another method(s) of fertility awareness to see if the app's determined fertile window and ovulation day appear correct for you.

## FERTILITY AWARENESS METHODS

Unlike the simple calendar method, methods for fertility awareness use physical signs and symptoms to more accurately detect ovulation. Types of FAM include temperature tracking, cervical mucus and position detection, and urinary hormone tracking.

All methods of fertility awareness can help you get pregnant faster than using no method of FAM. Some studies show more than twice the chance of getting pregnant per month when using any FAM and timing intercourse versus random intercourse.[6] Ultimately, no single method has been proven to be superior—and in my opinion, this is good news. The best option for you is going to be the method you can consistently stick with and know how to interpret.

### Basal Body Temperature (BBT)

Your basal body temperature (BBT) is your body's lowest temperature during a twenty-four-hour period, typically first thing in the morning before you even get out of bed. Your temperature fluctuates throughout your cycle in a very predictable pattern. In the follicular phase, your temperature will be relatively low, between 96°F and 98°F. Starting the day after ovulation, your temperature will rise by at least 0.4°F (0.2°C) and stay elevated for the rest of your cycle due to the increase in progesterone.[7] If you are not pregnant, when the corpus luteum dies and progesterone drops, your temperature will drop also.

Basal body temperature tracking requires taking your temperature every morning and watching for a temperature shift as your cycle progresses. Determining an exact ovulation day with BBT can be difficult, because BBT only confirms ovulation once your temperature increases at least 0.4°F (0.2°C), lasting for three consecutive days. Some experts even have a hard time identifying the exact day of ovulation with BBT tracking.[8] Therefore, this method is most effective when used to first establish your pattern of ovulation; then you use that information to estimate your fertility window.

In a perfect cycle, your temperature will be lowest at the time of the LH surge, approximately twenty-four hours before ovulation. Temperature then begins to sharply rise after ovulation. In theory this sounds easy, but it can be difficult to interpret as temperatures are not consistent every day. It is much easier—and more effective—to look back at your cycle to determine patterns when you are first starting to track BBT.

In addition, ovulation is a dynamic process, and every woman is different. The speed of follicle rupture, formation of the corpus luteum, and progesterone production differs for everyone. In clinical practice, progesterone levels are low at the time of ovulation, but in reality, there is a lot of variability among women. The lowest temperature point can occur anywhere from three days before ovulation up to the day of ovulation, but in 95 percent of cycles, the BBT nadir (lowest point) occurs in the sixty-six hours before ovulation.[9] To put this another way, your lowest temperature is likely anywhere from one to three days before ovulation. Once your temperature rises, by definition, ovulation has already occurred.[10]

Only 30 percent of women using BBT were able to predict their exact day of ovulation, but 94 percent could predict within a four-day range.[11] To me this means that BBT is *very* good at determining the fertile window, even if it is less accurate at detecting the precise day of ovulation.

To simplify BBT tracking, use the coverline method. With this technique, you are trying to detect what temperature rise you are looking for to make BBT tracking a more predictive method. Take your temperature every morning starting on day one of your cycle. After cycle day ten, look at your chart and determine when your highest follicular phase temperature occurred. Draw a line, known as the coverline, at 0.1°F above this value. Ovulation will occur between the day of the nadir and the day that your temperature crosses the coverline.[12]

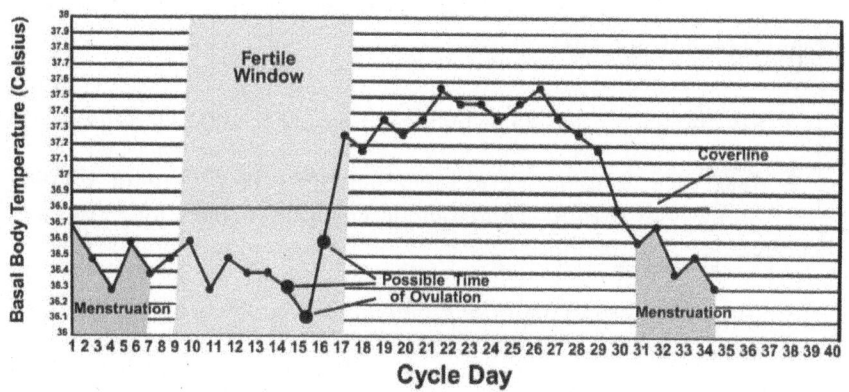

**Example of BBT Chart with Biphasic Shift**

Once your temperature is above the coverline for three days, your BBT is biphasic, or has progressed from a phase of lower temps (the follicular phase) to a phase of higher temps (the luteal phase), confirming ovulation has occurred. BBT does not proactively tell you when to have intercourse, because your temperature rises only after ovulation has occurred. Once you are familiar with identification of your temperature nadir and the coverline, you will be able to take a more proactive approach to determining your fertile window.

This can be tricky, especially for those with irregular sleep schedules, shift work, or busy mornings. Your core temperature will vary based on your lifestyle and the world around you, and it may not be accurate in times of illness, changing wake-up time, changing room temperature, or even after drinking alcohol the night before.

BBT tracking provides insights into your overall reproductive health. Irregularities in your temperature pattern, such as a short luteal phase or erratic fluctuations, can be a sign of hormone imbalance that may require medical attention. By closely monitoring your BBT, you can identify potential issues early and get the support you need.

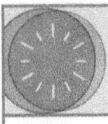

### Top Tip

**The steps to track BBT**

1. You need a thermometer that can measure to 1/10 of a degree.
2. Take your temperature at the same time every morning, before getting out of bed or engaging in any other activity (even before checking your cell phone).
3. Get BBT charting paper or create your own. Record your temperature.
4. After ten days of tracking, mark your coverline 0.1°F above the highest value.
5. Ovulation occurs between the day of the nadir and the day your temperature crosses the coverline.
6. Confirm ovulation by checking BBT and confirming three days above the coverline.

## Cervical Mucus Monitoring (CMM)

Your cervical mucus changes as estrogen rises in the days leading up to ovulation, becoming more stretchy, like egg whites. This peak fertile cervical mucus signals that ovulation is imminent. CMM predicts ovulation within one day for most women.[13] The only tricky part is learning to accurately identify different types of cervical fluid.

The best way to monitor your cervical mucus is to evaluate your vulvar secretions throughout your cycle. You do not have to insert your fingers into your vagina for this. You can detect the mucus at the vulva itself by wiping with toilet paper prior to using the restroom and then inspecting the paper. Some women will want to separate their labial lips before wiping in order to capture the mucus on the toilet paper (everyone has different anatomy).

You should evaluate the following:

1. How does your vulva feel? (dry, damp, wet)
2. How does the toilet paper feel as you wipe? (rough, smooth, slippery)
3. How does the mucus look? (no secretions, thick and creamy, stretchy and elastic)

Note that Type 4 cervical mucus, the wettest and most slippery, may fall immediately into the toilet if you do not wipe first, or it may be absorbed into a panty liner if you routinely wear one.

Once you see the external secretions, classify the type of cervical fluid you have based on both sensation at the vulva and the properties of the cervical mucus itself.

| Mucus Type | Sensation | Mucus Properties |
| --- | --- | --- |
| Type 1 | dry, rough | no secretions |
| Type 2 | damp, smooth | no secretions |
| Type 3 | damp, smooth | thick, creamy, and whitish; sticky |
| Type 4 | wet, slippery | transparent, stretchy, elastic, and like egg-whites *ovulation day* |

With a maturing egg, your estrogen levels increase in preparation for ovulation. This increase in estrogen changes the cervical mucus; it progresses from no secretions (Type 1 and Type 2) to thicker/sticky secretions (Type 3), then to transparent and stretchy mucus (Type 4). Type 4 mucus is similar to raw egg white and can be stretched at least one inch between your fingers.[14] It is seen the day before ovulation and/or on ovulation day and helps sperm swim through the cervix. If you have multiple days of Type 4 mucus, the last day is considered ovulation day. After ovulation, the cervical mucus disappears as it thickens around the cervix to prevent infections.

I love CMM because you get immediate feedback. When you see Type 4 cervical mucus, you know ovulation is imminent, and you should have intercourse if you are trying to conceive. There is a 29 percent chance of pregnancy when you have intercourse on a day with Type 4 cervical mucus, as compared to 0 percent on a day with no cervical secretions.[15] Checking your cervical mucus is also safe, free, and requires no technology. It is one of the easiest FAM available.

Cervical mucus can be affected by external factors, including recent intercourse, lube, douching, and vaginal infections. Hormone changes—including breastfeeding, recent hormonal contraception, and perimenopause—can also affect your mucus patterns. Prior cervical surgery, such as excisional procedures for precancer treatment, can permanently change your cervical mucus, and you should use other fertility awareness methods in this instance.

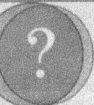

## Common Questions

**Can Mucinex help me get pregnant?**

Mucinex is an over-the-counter expectorant, known as guaifenesin, commonly used to thin out respiratory secretions. One study evaluated cervical mucus in a group of women before and after guaifenesin treatment (200 mg of guaifenesin three times a day from day five of their cycle until a confirmed temperature rise). After Mucinex, 75 percent of women showed an improvement in mucus quality, with a cumulative pregnancy rate of 70 percent.[16] The mechanism of action in the cervix is likely similar to that of the respiratory tract, pulling water into the cervical mucus and thinning it out, making it easier for sperm to swim through. This study was limited, lacking a control group, but if you feel like your cervical mucus might be low, adding Mucinex may be an option.

## Cervical Position

Your cervical position can indicate peak fertility, but it is a more difficult sign to track. As estrogen rises, your cervix changes from firm (like the tip of your nose) and closed to softer (like your lips) and open by the time of ovulation. In addition, the cervix actually moves position based on the amount of estrogen and progesterone present. Within twenty-four hours of progesterone production after ovulation, the cervix will return back to a low and firm position.

| Cycle Phase | Cervical Position | Cervical Texture | Cervical Opening |
|---|---|---|---|
| Not fertile | low | firm | closed |
| Fertile window | midway | medium | partial opening |
| Peak fertility | high | soft | open |

To check your cervical position, insert a finger into your vagina and feel for your cervix. To make it easier, keep your nails short, insert your middle finger (it is longer), and try to check at the same time every day. It is easiest to check your cervical position by elevating one leg on the side of the tub when you are in the shower.

I've looked at thousands of cervixes over my career, and I can tell you every woman has a different "normal" position, size, and opening. Prior C-sections, severe endometriosis, or pelvic scarring will change the position and orientation of your cervix. Previous vaginal birth will also change the cervical opening. Cervical procedures for abnormal Pap smears can remove a portion of your cervix and will change the length, feel, and responsiveness of your cervix. Focus on what is normal for *you*.

## Ovulation Predictor Kit (OPK)

One of my favorite ways to track ovulation if you are trying to conceive is with an ovulation predictor kit. Once estrogen reaches a threshold of at least 200 pg/mL for fifty hours (seen with a mature egg), the brain sends out a surge of luteinizing hormone (LH), triggering ovulation twelve to thirty-six hours later.[17] OPKs detect this LH surge in your urine. The great thing about these tests is that they provide very clear, objective data. You get either a positive or a negative result.

You should start using OPKs five days before you expect to ovulate. If you are not sure when this would be, take your average or estimated cycle length and subtract twenty days. So cycle day six for a twenty-six-day cycle, cycle day eight for a twenty-eight-day cycle, and cycle day ten for a thirty-day cycle. Once you have tracked for a few cycles, or if you use OPK testing and another fertility awareness method, you can likely shorten this interval, but remember to start testing before the earliest ovulation could potentially occur. The day you get a positive LH surge is the day *before* ovulation.

Many OPKs say to test your first morning urine, but I do not recommend this. In 85 percent of cycles the LH surge is released before 8 a.m., so checking first thing in the morning may not give LH enough time to actually be present in your urine.[18] You could completely miss your surge. Instead, take an OPK once per day, sometime between 10 a.m. and 2 p.m. If that time interval is hard for you, then I recommend checking twice a day.

If you want to get pregnant, you should target intercourse for the day of the positive result and the next day. Once you see an LH surge, you no longer need to keep testing because you already know that LH is going to be released from the brain in pulses throughout the luteal phase.

OPK tests come in simple versions with control and test lines, and digital versions, much like pregnancy tests. With simple testing, a positive OPK is a test line that is as dark or darker than the control line. Digital tests can be more expensive but can alleviate some of the stress of interpreting the darkness of the lines. Some ovulation tests now measure more than just LH; they also detect rising estradiol levels in an attempt to accurately define the fertile window based on high estrogen levels. In these tests, "high" fertility is an estrogen measurement, while "peak" fertility is your actual LH surge.

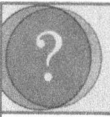

### Common Questions

**What causes a false positive OPK?**

False positive LH levels occur in about 7 percent of cycles.[19] Some women have a higher baseline LH, especially those with PCOS or low ovarian reserve, which can lead to false positive tests. Women with PCOS may have many "peak" days with LH testing that are not true peaks. Women with DOR (perimenopause) will have higher LH levels at baseline and may have false positive tests when taken early in their cycle. Many fertility medications can cause a false positive OPK due to their mechanism of action. For example, Clomid and letrozole are medications used to improve ovulation, and both cause an increase in LH and FSH from the brain. Also, since hCG and LH share a receptor, pregnancy (or an hCG trigger shot) can result in a positive LH test as well.

## Mid-Luteal Progesterone Levels

Although progesterone levels have limited utility in predicting ovulation, a blood progesterone test can confirm that ovulation did occur. Remember, progesterone is made in pulses in response to LH from the brain. Just like LH levels can fluctuate in the luteal phase, progesterone levels can range anywhere from 3 to 40 ng/mL after ovulation. Any serum progesterone level of 3 ng/mL or greater is confirmation of ovulation.

That said, progesterone testing has not proven to be an accurate or effective method for determining one's fertile window.[20] Progesterone production is not immediate upon ovulation, so progesterone should only be checked a week after suspected ovulation, known as a mid-luteal progesterone. This is often called a "day twenty-one progesterone," because one week after ovulation in a twenty-eight-day cycle would likely be day twenty-one, based on the simple calendar method. However, everyone's cycle is different, so many people are not mid-luteal on cycle day twenty-one.

The urinary metabolite for progesterone is pregnanediol 3-glucuronide (PdG), which can provide an easier alternative for confirming ovulation.

An elevated urinary PdG of over 5 μg/mL for three consecutive days is confirmation that ovulation did occur.[21] Some urinary hormone–tracking options incorporate progesterone metabolites, which, if utilized consistently, can help you understand your cycle and detect subtle abnormalities. Although these tests have limited utility in predicting ovulation, they can be helpful in cycle tracking.

## Other Fertility Signs

As estrogen rises and your cycle moves closer to ovulation, there are other physical changes you may notice. Peak estrogen levels around ovulation increase libido to encourage intercourse and promote sperm survival. You may also experience a heightened sense of smell and taste, breast sensitivity, light spotting, and a fuller labia. After ovulation, your body will change again in order to protect and support a potential pregnancy. The chart below reviews common changes that confirm ovulation.

**UNDERSTANDING FERTILITY SIGNS**

| Fertility Sign | Physiologic Reason |
| --- | --- |
| Ovulatory spotting | Drop in estrogen with follicle rupture at time of ovulation can cause temporary spotting |
| Ovulation pain (mittelschmerz, German for *middle pain*) | The follicle ruptures in order to allow the egg to be released, and free fluid enters the abdomen, causing pain |
| Labial fullness | Increased blood flow with increase in estrogen, specifically on the side you ovulated |
| Pelvic lymph nodes | Palpable groin lymph node on the side you ovulated |
| Increased libido | Increase in estrogen at time of ovulation increases sex drive |
| Increased sense of smell and taste | Increase in progesterone after ovulation, so you are less likely to eat potentially dangerous food |
| Breast sensitivity and tenderness | Increase in progesterone after ovulation changes breast tissue |

## NATURAL FAMILY PLANNING

Every woman deserves the opportunity to control when she wants to start a family. Many of us are familiar with the most common methods of contraception: barrier methods (condoms, diaphragms), hormonal options (the pill, IUD, patch, shot, ring), and surgical options (tubal ligation, vasectomy). But understanding your cycle and utilizing the tracking methods we just learned to *avoid pregnancy* is also an option. This is called natural family planning (NFP).

Not all of us have access to hormonal contraception or are good candidates, for various reasons, such as history of stroke, clotting disorder, migraines with aura, or hormonally sensitive cancer. Hormonal contraception is also not without side effects—notable ones include mood changes, headache, nausea, and decreased libido. Many women may opt to avoid hormonal contraception in order to not mask their cycle characteristics or to avoid potential side effects of contraceptives. For those who want to avoid hormonal contraception, NFP can be an option to still feel protected against an undesired pregnancy. It is important to understand your cycle in order to truly take charge of your reproductive health.

However, just as no one treatment will guarantee pregnancy, no method of natural family planning will completely prevent pregnancy. The stakes are still high. This means that some methods with less accurate or personalized detection might recommend a period of abstinence during your fertile window. Although some people may opt to use barrier methods like condoms on potentially fertile days, they are not perfect at preventing pregnancy. You can decrease the rate of failure with NFP by combining multiple methods. But you should be the one deciding what makes the most sense for you, including the risk of failure, expense, ease of use, and potential side effects for each option.

The natural family planning methods we'll discuss include:

- Rhythm method
- Standard days method

- Basal body temperature
- Two-day method
- Billings method
- Symptothermal method

## Rhythm Method

The rhythm method is an antiquated option of NFP where you avoid intercourse during any possible fertile days based on your cycle length. Due to inaccuracy, I do not recommend this method but think it is important to review the rhythm method since it is well known. You need to observe the length of six menstrual cycles prior to starting. Looking at these cycles, take the shortest cycle length and subtract eighteen days. This is your first fertile day. Then, take the longest cycle length and subtract eleven days. This is your last fertile day. Your fertile window falls between these two days: (shortest cycle length −18) to (longest cycle length −11).

A disadvantage of the rhythm method is that it does not track ovulation day itself, has a long abstinence interval, and is ultimately unreliable. For example, if your shortest cycle length was twenty-six days and your longest was thirty-one days, you would calculate your abstinence interval as follows: 26–18 = day 8, and 31–11 = day 20. Your fertile days would be estimated between days eight and twenty, so you would avoid intercourse at this time.

## Standard Days Method

The standard days (or fixed formula) method defines the fertile window as days eight to nineteen of the menstrual cycle, for cycles that are regular and last twenty-six to thirty-two days. If your cycle is irregular, or the length of your cycles falls outside of that range, the standard days method will not be accurate for you.

If you are using the standard days formula, you do not need to make any calculations to determine your fertile window. You simply consider days one to seven not fertile, days eight to nineteen fertile, and days twenty and on not fertile. You would time or avoid intercourse during the fertile days.

One of the method's downfalls is that it requires a relatively long abstinence interval. On the other hand, not having to calculate fertile days may decrease stress and simplify cycle tracking for you.

## Basal Body Temperature

If you're trying to avoid pregnancy, you can use the temperature shifts seen with BBT to identify that ovulation has occurred and that you are no longer in your fertile window. For the most effective contraception, you should not have sex from cycle day one until you have confirmed ovulation, which means three consecutive days of a BBT rise. This would mean using barrier methods or not having intercourse for around two and a half weeks of your cycle, which may not be realistic for many people.

## Two-Day Method

The two-day method requires you to check your cervical mucus twice a day (morning and night) to determine your fertile window. Ask yourself:

1. Did I have any cervical secretions yesterday?
2. Do I have any cervical secretions today?

If the answer to either of these is yes, then it is considered a potentially fertile day. Once you answer no to both questions, ovulation has already occurred and you are safe to have intercourse.

An easier way to think about the two-day method:

- Non-fertile day = no cervical mucus that day or the day before (checking twice a day)
- Fertile day = any day with cervical mucus yesterday or today (checking twice a day)

The two-day method has proven to be an effective way to prevent pregnancy in that it allows for cycle-to-cycle variation and is easy to use.

The key is to remember that once you have two consecutive days in a row without cervical mucus, conception is unlikely and you should feel confident proceeding with unprotected intercourse.[22]

## Billings Method

The Billings method, named after its originators, Drs. Evelyn and John Billings, uses cervical mucus monitoring to time intercourse around your fertile window. With perfect use, it has a low failure rate and high satisfaction.[23]

There are four protocols, called Early Day Rules, you must follow to practice this method:

1. Early Day Rule 1: No intercourse on your period.
2. Early Day Rule 2: After your period, you can alternate intercourse in the evening of days with no cervical mucus.
3. Early Day Rule 3: When you notice any cervical mucus, stop having intercourse and wait for peak fertility. If your cervical secretions disappear for three days in a row, you can go back to Rule 2 until secretions return.
4. Peak Rule: After peak cervical mucus (last day of Type 4 cervical mucus), you can resume intercourse on the fourth day after cervical mucus has disappeared.

Although the Billings method might seem complex, essentially you are avoiding intercourse on any potentially fertile days. Think about it this way: After your period has finished, you can have intercourse every other night when you have Type 1 or Type 2 cervical mucus. Once you have Type 3 or 4 cervical mucus, avoid intercourse. After your last day of Type 4 cervical mucus, wait for three more days, then resume intercourse on the fourth day.

## Symptothermal Method

The symptothermal method uses two different methods of FAM to determine when you should avoid intercourse, most often cervical mucus monitoring and basal body temperature, which I like because it provides insight into when ovulation is occurring (CMM), then confirms that ovulation did in fact occur (BBT). When tracking with both CMM and BBT, the symptothermal method is more effective at preventing pregnancy than either method alone.[24]

## CHOOSING THE RIGHT METHOD FOR YOU

You deserve to have *all* the data when deciding which natural family planning method is right for you. My goal is to highlight options you may not have been aware existed and educate you on how to use them correctly. If you want to learn more about NFP, I recommend you read *Taking Charge of Your Fertility* by Toni Weschler.

To help you evaluate your options, the table below includes the effectiveness of both natural family planning and traditional birth control methods.[25,26] Perfect use rates have higher effectiveness than typical use, reflecting the importance of understanding and following your method of choice.

**EFFECTIVENESS OF CONTRACEPTIVE OPTIONS**

|  | Contraceptive Method | Perfect Use | Typical Use |
|---|---|---|---|
| Natural family planning options | Rhythm method | 85% | 85% |
|  | Standard days method | 95% | 87% |
|  | Basal body temperature | 98% | 93% |
|  | Two-day method | 96% | 86% |
|  | Billings method | 97% | 77% |
|  | Symptothermal method | 99% | 98% |

|  | Contraceptive Method | Perfect Use | Typical Use |
|---|---|---|---|
| Other contraceptive choices | Combined birth control pill | 99% | 93% |
|  | Birth control patch | 99% | 93% |
|  | Birth control ring | 99% | 93% |
|  | Progesterone-only pill | 98% | 93% |
|  | Depo-Provera shot | 99% | 96% |
|  | Progesterone IUD | 99% | 99% |
|  | Copper IUD | 99% | 99% |
|  | Implant | 99% | 99% |
|  | Spermicide prescription | 93% | 86% |
|  | Spermicide over the counter | 84% | 79% |
|  | Diaphragm | 84% | 83% |
|  | Withdrawal | 96% | 80% |
|  | Condoms | 98% | 87% |
|  | Sterilization | >99% | >99% |

Dawn was frustrated to learn that the fertile window her app had been giving her was completely wrong. Before delving into the various fertility awareness methods, we decided to proceed with a complete fertility evaluation to make sure we weren't missing any underlying diagnoses or issues. All testing was normal. Since Dawn only wanted one child, we reviewed cycle tracking and decided to give it a few months before starting fertility treatments. Dawn conceived after three months with CMM and BBT tracking, and now she has the added skill of knowing how to interpret her cycle moving forward.

I want you to know what Dawn didn't know. There are so many different ways you can utilize the data your body is giving you to understand not only your natural fertility but also your hormones and overall health. This information is invaluable whether you're trying to conceive or simply want to be more in tune with your hormonal health. There is no one way to track your cycle, but consistency is the key to having reliable results. In today's world, access to accurate information about your body without being dependent on technology is more important than ever.

### Facts to Remember

- The fertile window is the six days ending on the day of ovulation.
- An egg can live for twenty-four hours.
- Sperm can live in the female reproductive tract for up to five days.
- Fertility awareness methods use your body's symptoms to detect ovulation.
- Using two FAM together can improve the accuracy of detecting the fertile window.
- Natural family planning allows you to utilize cycle tracking to prevent a pregnancy.

# 6

# Trying to Conceive

At twenty-six, Violet was the first of her friends to get married, and she was the first to try to have kids. She was OK being the first, as it suited her goal-oriented nature, but it also meant that she had nobody to talk to about how to get pregnant. Her friends were all at a different stage of life. But Violet was young, healthy, and never had any medical issues. She thought it would be pretty easy to conceive.

The first few months of trying, Violet decided not to stress about it. She stopped the pill, and she and her husband started having intercourse when they felt like it. She got pregnant after only a few months of trying, but sadly, Violet miscarried before her first doctor's appointment. They kept trying, and two months later, Violet had a faintly positive pregnancy test. Her period started the next day.

After a few months, Violet asked her OB-GYN about infertility at her annual appointment. She was concerned because she and her husband had been trying for nine months, resulting in two losses. She was young, so wasn't it even more worrying that she hadn't gotten and stayed pregnant?

However, her doctor said the exact opposite. "You are young! Stop worrying about it. It will just happen." Violet was told the losses were just bad luck. She left that appointment feeling defeated. She was expecting a referral to a fertility doctor, or at least testing to make sure everything was OK, but instead she was sent away and told to come back if she wasn't pregnant in six months.

Violet didn't know what to do next. Was her doctor right? Should she just keep trying? Was it bad luck? Was she timing intercourse wrong? Or was something else going on? She felt more confused than ever.

Sadly, Violet's confusion is a common experience. Isn't it ironic that we spend so many years trying to prevent pregnancy but then don't know what to expect when we are ready to conceive? Violet already felt behind and was even more frustrated to be brushed off by her doctor. Surely there was something she could be doing to improve her chances of getting pregnant?

In this chapter, I'm answering the top questions I hear from women who are ready to conceive:

1. Where do I start?
2. How do I improve my chances?
3. I'm pregnant—now what?

## BEFORE YOU START TRYING

The moment you decide to get pregnant, it feels like everything changes—and it does. Suddenly, you have questions you've never thought about. You may be rethinking old habits—like your afternoon coffee and your nightly cannabis—or trying to decide next steps—what vitamins should you take and what testing do you need? Growing another human is a really big deal.

Step back and think about it for a moment. Egg and sperm will combine, an embryo will implant, and your body will nourish and support a new life. The metabolic demands, the strain on your body, and everything you do now potentially have a much bigger impact than before.

In a perfect world, your pregnancy plan begins long before you are trying to conceive. The first step is to reduce inflammation by making proactive lifestyle adjustments that help set the stage for a healthy pregnancy. You should:

1. Eat a nutrient-dense diet high in fruits and vegetables.
2. Limit caffeine.
3. Eliminate toxin exposure, including smoking, marijuana, and excessive alcohol.

We'll delve into all of this in greater detail in part III of the book. But if you know you're ready to conceive, this is my "where to start" list (I love a good to-do list):

- Wait between pregnancies.
- Stop birth control.
- Schedule a preconception visit.
- Start taking prenatal vitamins.

## WAIT BETWEEN PREGNANCIES

The changes to your body and your uterus with pregnancy are incredible. If you have recently given birth, you need time to recover prior to conceiving again. The time between pregnancies is known as the interpregnancy interval. This interval allows your uterus to heal from where the placenta implanted and for your cycles and ovulation to return. Short interpregnancy intervals have been associated with subsequent pregnancy complications, including preterm birth, growth restriction, and stillbirth.[1]

Most professional organizations recommend waiting eighteen months from delivery until your next pregnancy, but a large study recently suggested that most negative outcomes occur with intervals shorter than twelve months.[2] I know that balancing advancing age with waiting between pregnancies can be hard. If you are thirty-five or older, I would recommend waiting a minimum of six months and concluding breastfeeding before trying again. Individual delivery characteristics may impact this recommendation, with longer intervals potentially recommended after large blood loss, cesarean section, or prior uterine surgery.

In patients undergoing IVF with frozen embryos, we want to transfer an embryo when you will have the highest chance of success, so I recommend waiting at least twelve months. Your doctor may have different recommendations, but studies show the optimal timing for a transfer is twelve to eighteen months after delivery.[3]

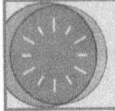 **Top Tip**

### How to try again after a miscarriage

First and foremost, I have been there, and I know the desire to get the show on the road ASAP. That said, there are no universal recommendations, because each pregnancy loss is different. You should think about your situation and make a plan with your doctor. Remember, your doctor knows your personal case best and may recommend something specific for you.

In general, for a chemical pregnancy loss where you had a positive pregnancy test but lost the pregnancy prior to ultrasound, I allow my patients to try again immediately as the pregnancy did not fully implant. For clinical losses, where you had a pregnancy seen on ultrasound, the amount of recommended wait time will depend on the treatment needed and gestational age of pregnancy loss. While the World Health Organization recommends waiting six months after any loss, a large review study showed no benefit of a mandatory interval of waiting.[4] In general, make sure your body is ready for the next pregnancy. I typically make the following recommendations to my patients:

1. Follow hCG to zero or a negative pregnancy test to confirm no residual retained placenta fragments.

2. Wait until you get your next period after your loss to allow your uterus to recover.

3. If you had a D&C or required medication to induce a pregnancy loss, consider asking for a uterine evaluation prior to trying again. This is even more important if it took more than six weeks for your hCG to become negative.

### Stop Birth Control

Depending on the type of birth control you are using, you will need a plan for stopping it. You want to give your body enough time to reveal your cycle pattern and alert you to any ovulatory issues before getting pregnant.

Sometimes you will find that your period is not regular and predictable after stopping birth control. It can take months of cycle tracking to determine your cycle pattern, and then more time for an evaluation to reveal the root cause (as discussed in chapter 4).

What follows is not an exhaustive review of birth control options, a discussion of side effects, or an endorsement for one option over another. As I've mentioned, contraception is a personal decision. You should choose what is best for you. My goal is to help you come off birth control in preparation to conceive. Each type of birth control requires a different kind of plan.

## Combined Birth Control Pill ("The Pill")

The birth control pill, which is a combination of ethinyl estradiol (a type of estrogen) and a progestin (a type of synthetic progesterone), works by telling the brain to stop sending out FSH and LH. Without FSH and LH, you won't ovulate. There are multiple different uses for the birth control pill, as well as different doses/combinations of ethinyl estradiol and progestins.

The pill can be used monthly or continuously. With monthly cyclic use, you either take placebo pills or have four to seven pill-free days a month, allowing your body to bleed every cycle. This bleed is known as a "withdrawal bleed" since progesterone levels drop when you stop taking active pills, signaling to the uterus it is time to bleed. Continuous use is taking an active pill every single day without breaks for bleeding. A combined option is a three-month cycle, where you continuously use the pill for three months then take a break to bleed. All options are excellent for contraception, but cyclic use decreases the incidence of breakthrough bleeding, which is when you have bleeding while you are taking the active pills and between withdrawal bleeds, and is overall less suppressive to the ovaries than continuous use.

The birth control pill does *not* last in your body for weeks or months. The pill has a half-life of twenty-eight hours, which means half the medication is out of your system in one day.[5] There is no need to be "cleansed" with any expensive alternative treatment.

However, with continuous pill use, your uterus is constantly exposed to progesterone, which can thin the uterine lining. Depending on the length of time you take the pill, you may not get a period when you first stop. Even if ovulation resumes immediately, you may need time to grow the lining before having a bleed. If you are continuously using the pill and want to conceive soon, switch to cyclic use six months before you want to get pregnant. If you start bleeding every month, it is a sign that your lining is growing back and getting thicker. It may take a few months to track your cycles and get to see your cycle pattern, so I always recommend stopping the pill at least three months before you want to conceive.

As we learned in chapter 4, the birth control pill is commonly prescribed for legitimate medical issues but without an evaluation for potential causes of abnormal cycles (as in Hazel's case). I see women all the time who were placed on the pill for irregular cycles (is it PCOS?), severe pain (is it endometriosis?), or heavy bleeding (is it uterine fibroids?). When you stop the pill and your underlying issue still exists, you can be left more confused than before. This is why it's important to get to know your real cycle before you start trying to conceive.

### Depo-Provera ("The Birth Control Shot")

Depo-Provera is an injectable progesterone that provides contraception for up to three months. However, the dose of progesterone is so high that it can prevent ovulation for up to eighteen months. This means that one injection of Depo-Provera a year ago can be causing your ovulatory issues right now. If there is any chance you want to conceive in the next two years, switch to a shorter-acting form of contraception.

### Progesterone Intrauterine Device (IUD)

A progesterone-based IUD is a reliable long-term contraceptive option, since it has a low failure rate and doesn't rely on user compliance. With an IUD, progesterone is slowly released into your bloodstream through your uterus. The local impact of progesterone thins the lining to a point where many women have no or very light periods. About half of women with an IUD will still ovulate even if they do not bleed, as progesterone levels are not always enough to suppress ovulation.

Due to the endometrial changes seen with long-term progesterone exposure, time to pregnancy can be longer after a progesterone IUD, especially the longer the IUD has been in place.[6] I have seen women with a very thin lining for months after removal. It is important to understand this potential risk if you desire conception soon. In general, the longer you have a progesterone IUD, the greater the endometrial impact will be and the earlier you should consider removal.[7] Remove a progesterone IUD at least six months before you desire conception.

### Copper IUD

A copper IUD works by creating an inflammatory uterine environment, which is toxic to sperm, preventing implantation. Most women with a copper IUD will still have regular periods but may have an increase in bleeding due to the inflammation. After removing a copper IUD, inflammation decreases and resumption of fertility appears to be immediate, with no change to fertility.[8] This means that if your cycles are regular, you can remove a copper IUD when you are ready to conceive.

## Common Questions

**Does birth control cause infertility?**

Birth control does not increase the rate of infertility or harm your future fertility. Claims that hormonal contraceptives decrease your egg count are false, and as discussed in chapter 3, your egg count continues to drop regardless of whether you are on hormonal contraception (you lose eggs every month). Birth control may temporarily suppress AMH levels, but this does not reflect a true reduction in egg count. In a review of 14,884 women stopping birth control, there was no higher rate of infertility (defined as failure to conceive after twelve months of trying).[9]

## Schedule a Preconception Visit

Once you've stopped birth control and waited the recommended amount of time, the next step is to schedule a preconception visit with your doctor. A preconception visit is an opportunity for your doctor to review pregnancy next steps with you. Do not try to squeeze this into your annual exam; call your doctor's office and schedule a specific appointment for this purpose. Any preexisting medical problems will be reviewed, along with strategies to optimize health before pregnancy, especially if you have high blood pressure, thyroid disease, or diabetes, as we know these worsen throughout a pregnancy. All medications should be reviewed with your doctor to confirm they are safe for pregnancy. Many of my patients need to switch to pregnancy-safe alternatives.

A preconception visit will also include testing your immunization antibody levels and genetic carrier screening, in addition to a health screening and a review of medical problems.

### Check Immunizations

When you are pregnant, exposure to certain infections can cause devastating birth defects. Both rubella (MMR) and varicella (chicken pox) can pass the placenta and result in a congenital infection. Although you may have been vaccinated against rubella and varicella as a child, not everyone develops an appropriate immune response to last into adulthood. Checking antibody levels for both diseases is recommended, and if you are not immune (low antibody levels), you should receive the vaccine prior to conceiving. Since the vaccines for both are live-virus vaccines (the virus lives in your body for a short time), you should wait one month after getting a booster before conceiving. If you have never received these vaccinations, a two-dose series (each is one month apart) is recommended, which would need to start two months prior to conception.[10]

### Get Genetic Screening

Preconception genetic carrier screening is blood testing to see if you carry a disease that can potentially be passed on. Most of these diseases are autosomal recessive, meaning both parents must have the gene in order to pass it on. Both you and your partner need to be tested. If you get a positive result, you are a carrier. If a child inherits a copy from each parent, they will then have the disease.

When we know both partners carry the same gene, we can test the embryos before implanting them into your body in a process called preimplantation genetic testing (PGT). Since there are hundreds of possible diseases, and we only get five to ten embryo cells to test, it is impossible to test for each disease at the embryo level. However, one vial of your blood has thousands of cells, so we can test for many diseases at one time.

Genetic testing has expanded, and you can now test for more than seven hundred disorders at one time. The minimum recommended genetic testing for everyone includes cystic fibrosis, spinal muscular atrophy, and fragile X. If you have Jewish ancestry, there are additional recommended tests.

Genetic screening also includes looking at family history for diseases known to be caused by a single gene disorder, which can be tested. Cancer genes, such as BRCA, and autosomal dominant diseases, such as Huntington's disease, can be passed on with only one copy of the gene, as there are no carrier states. Diseases like these can be eliminated from your family line with genetic testing of embryos. This can be life-changing for someone who watched a family member die from a genetic disease. The decision to test yourself for an autosomal dominant disease that runs in your family is complex, and I recommend working with a genetic counselor to best understand your options. I know some people may not want to discover they carry a gene that would shorten their life or lead to progressive disability.

No carrier test or genetic screening result will force you to do IVF or mean that you can't get pregnant. I had patients who found out they both carried a gene for congenital deafness. They made the decision not to do IVF but to learn sign language and prepare themselves for potentially having a non-hearing child. I have also had patients in the exact same situation decide to proceed with IVF and PGT to test for the gene. Both of these decisions are appropriate and reasonable, but you should be the one deciding what is right for your family. Without carrier screening, you don't have all the information you need to make an educated choice.

The saddest cases I have had were with couples who had no idea they both carried a genetic disease until they conceived and had an impacted child. Some of these diseases are devastating and incompatible with life. Losing a child this way is heartbreaking and sets you back significantly on your journey to grow your family.

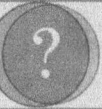 **Common Questions**

**Is an at-home genetic ancestry test the same as genetic screening?**

Most ancestry tests are not the same as genetic carrier screening. These tests often identify ancestry, traits, and linking family members. Although some of these tests may include genetic screening, it is typically only offered with more expensive options and a limited panel. Testing through your doctor is likely cheaper and will expedite partner testing. If you are both carriers, your results will be sent to a PGT company that will want official genetic carrier screening (not an ancestry test). Ancestry testing that includes carrier screening is reliable but limited, and you should consider expanded testing before you conceive.

## Start Taking Prenatal Vitamins

You should start taking a prenatal vitamin to build up cellular stores of important nutrients for pregnancy at least three months before you want to conceive. In a perfect world, you would get all your nutrients from your diet. But since pregnancy requires so many nutrients, it's worth taking a prenatal vitamin to ensure your body has everything it needs. Thankfully, it is an easy and low-risk intervention.[11]

One essential ingredient in a prenatal is at least 400 mcg of folic acid. Folic acid is a B vitamin (B9) required for cell division. Folic acid deficiency has been associated with neural tube defects (NTDs), including incomplete brain development (anencephaly) and spinal cord formation (spina bifida). Most neural tube defects can be prevented with folic acid supplementation. If you are on medication to prevent seizures or have had a pregnancy with a prior NTD, the recommendation for folic acid is ten times higher at 4 mg a day. Folate is available through food sources, but the consequence of a neural tube defect is so severe that I don't recommend relying solely on food as your source of folate.

There is no one perfect prenatal, but many include various nutrients important for pregnancy. Below is an outline of these key nutrients. If you do not have the recommended amount in your prenatal or you know you have deficiency, do not double your prenatal, as this will result in toxic levels of some nutrients. Instead, you can find single-nutrient supplements if they are needed or recommended.

**PRENATAL NUTRIENT RECOMMENDATIONS**

| Nutrient | Daily Dose | Purpose | Food Source |
|---|---|---|---|
| Folic acid (B9) | 400 mcg | Cell growth, prevents NTD | Leafy greens, fortified grains, peanuts, beans |
| Vitamin D | 600 IU | Bone growth and teeth development | Sunlight, fortified milk, fatty fish |
| Calcium | 1,000 mg | Bone growth and teeth development | Milk, cheese, yogurt, leafy greens |
| Omega-3 fatty acids (DHA/EPA) | 300 mg | Brain development | Flaxseed, chia seeds, walnuts, edamame, fish, seaweed |
| Choline | 450 mg | Brain development | Milk, eggs, peanuts, soy, organ meat |
| Vitamin A | 770 mcg | Healthy skin, eyes, and bones | Leafy greens, carrots, sweet potatoes |
| Vitamin B6 | 1.9 mg | Red blood cell formation | Meat, grains, bananas, potatoes, chickpeas |
| Vitamin B12 | 2.6 mcg | Nervous system development and red blood cell formation | Meat, eggs, dairy *Vegans need to supplement* |
| Iodine | 220 mcg | Brain development | Iodized salt, dairy, seafood, meat, eggs |
| Iron | 27 mg | Red blood cell formation | Beans, lentils, meat, leafy greens, fortified cereal |
| Vitamin C | 85 mg | Immune system development, iron absorption | Citrus, broccoli, strawberries, tomatoes |

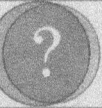 **Common Questions**

**Is methylated folate the same as folic acid?**

Many new prenatal vitamins containing methylated folate instead of folic acid have entered the market. Methylated folate is a downstream metabolite of folic acid. Although some people may have a genetic variant interfering with folate metabolism, it is very important to realize that *only* folic acid has been shown to prevent NTDs. Despite methylated folate supplementation resulting in sufficient blood folate levels, there is no study proving that methylated folate prevents NTDs or comparing methylated folate with folic acid. No study like this will ever exist, because when something clearly prevents a bad outcome, like a birth defect, there is never a reason to allow a group of pregnant people to be at risk. I recommend you take at least 400 mcg of folic acid, in the form of folic acid. If you love a prenatal that has methylated folate and are trying to conceive, please take an additional folic acid supplement to prevent NTDs.

## GET PREGNANT FASTER

You've come off birth control, had a preconception visit with your doctor, done genetic screening, and started taking a prenatal vitamin with folic acid to get your body ready for pregnancy. You're ready to start trying to conceive. In order to get pregnant faster, you need to time intercourse with your fertile window.

Thankfully, by this point we've covered several cycle tracking methods for determining your fertile window. Regardless of which you choose, trying to conceive will be less stressful if you know you are timing intercourse with ovulation.

After ovulation, the egg is released into the abdominal cavity and captured by the fallopian tube within fifteen to twenty minutes.[12] The egg only lives for twenty-four hours. But as we've learned, sperm can live up to five days in the cervix and uterus, though most sperm will swim through the reproductive tract and out the end of the fallopian tube within forty-eight hours.

The fallopian tube is where fertilization occurs. The embryo rapidly divides and develops while traveling through the fallopian tube, entering the uterine cavity around five days after ovulation. So more than just a passageway for the egg, sperm, and embryo, the fallopian tubes contract and help propel the embryo to the uterine cavity. Implantation typically occurs seven to nine days after ovulation, known as the implantation window.[13]

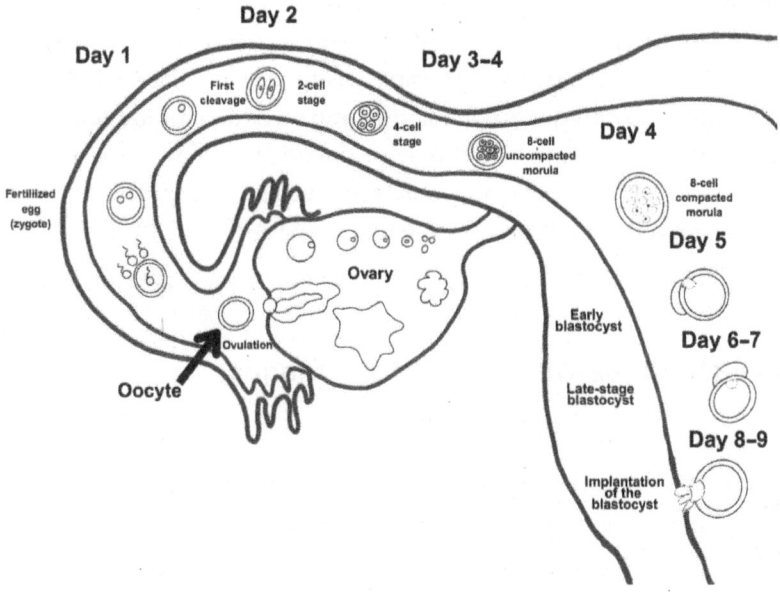

**Fertilization and Implantation Timeline**

The implantation window of the uterus is narrow and directly controlled by progesterone. Your uterus needs between five and seven days of progesterone to allow implantation. Remember Maple from chapter 2, who was placed on daily progesterone to treat her "estrogen dominance"? Daily progesterone closes the implantation window, and this is one of the ways that progesterone is an effective contraceptive option.

Let's go over how to take advantage of your fertile window, including when to time intercourse, the frequency with which you should or should not have intercourse, and coital practices that can impact conception.

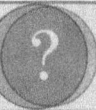 **Common Questions**

**Can you get pregnant with just one fallopian tube?**

One interesting fact is that the ends of the fallopian tubes, called the fimbriae, are not actually connected to the ovaries. This means that eggs are released into the abdominal cavity prior to being captured by the fallopian tube. Further, your fallopian tubes move around (unless they are damaged), which means the fimbria from a tube on one side can move closer to an egg that is ovulating on the other side. Since the eggs are released into the abdominal cavity, and the tubes move inside your body, you can get pregnant after you've had one tube removed—even when you ovulate from the ovary on the other side. Depending on the reason for tube removal, your fecundability may still be the exact same even after you have had one tube removed.[14]

## Time Intercourse with Your Fertile Window

Even though sperm can live for up to five days, having intercourse closer to ovulation day improves the odds of getting pregnant. The highest rates of fecundability are the two days before ovulation and the day of ovulation.[15] This is why knowing when you are ovulating will improve your odds of getting pregnant.

A common recommendation is to have intercourse every other day in your fertile window and then target the day of ovulation.[16] The premise is that sperm should be constantly presented to the egg in the fertile window, based on the idea that you might miss your ovulation day, and getting sperm into the reproductive tract earlier is better than nothing. But I find this method to be frustrating and imprecise, because we know that intercourse closer to ovulation is more effective. Why not use cycle tracking to be more accurate about when you're ovulating?

## FERTILITY AWARENESS METHODS DETERMINATION OF OVULATION DAY

| FAM | Ovulation Day |
| --- | --- |
| Calendar method | Average cycle length (days)—14 days |
| Basal body temperature (BBT) | 3 days prior to first temp elevation of at least 0.4°F (which remains elevated for at least three days) |
| Cervical mucus monitoring (CMM) | Last day of Type 4 cervical mucus (egg white, sticky, stretchy) |
| Ovulation predictor kit (OPK) | Day after the positive OPK (day after LH surge) |

That said, if you have regular cycles, you may not need a tracking plan to conceive. The second week of most women's cycles will be their most fertile week. Cycle day twelve has a 58 percent chance of being in the fertile window.[17] You could simply target intercourse for the second week of your cycle and not worry about tracking. An even easier option would be to simply have intercourse every two to three days, two to three times a week (I call this the 2–3 method). Since sperm live up to five days in the female reproductive tract, and the egg can live for twenty-four hours, having intercourse two to three days apart and two to three times a week will make sperm present on ovulation day. However, if you have infertility or are trying to conceive over the age of thirty-five, targeting intercourse with FAM is advantageous.

Remember, the best FAM for conception is the one you will consistently use. OPK use has been shown to improve pregnancy rates by 10 percent compared with results for those who do not use tracking.[18] Tracking CMM has consistently been shown to decrease time to pregnancy as compared with no tracking.[19] Multiple methods are better than any one option alone, and the highest fecundability was with calendar tracking and the use of *both* CMM and OPK.[20]

## Optimize Frequency of Intercourse

Many people think that daily intercourse isn't conducive to pregnancy, or that they should abstain and "save up" sperm to have a higher deposit on the day of ovulation. However, around 1,500 sperm are made each second, meaning 200 million sperm are made every day. In one single act of intercourse, 200 to 300 million sperm will be deposited in a single ejaculate, but only a few hundred actually reach the egg.[21] Daily ejaculations do not decrease available sperm and may even improve the number of motile sperm.[22] In fact, many sperm will die if not ejaculated, resulting in a large amount of debris.

Imagine a highway full of cars. The normal moving sperm are cars on the highway, but the dead sperm are cars stalled randomly in the lanes. With all these obstacles, it's harder for the normal sperm to get where they are going. Keeping the road clear by having frequent intercourse if you are trying to conceive will make the path easier for the sperm to get to the egg.

Daily intercourse has the highest probability of pregnancy, with very similar pregnancy rates seen with intercourse every other day.[23] This means that although you do not have to have daily sex, there is absolutely no need to decrease sex if you want to get pregnant. If you are an everyday sex couple, keep at it. The need to determine your ovulation day is less important if you are having daily intercourse.

Most people do not have sex daily, so timing with your fertile window can decrease stress levels and help you get pregnant faster.[24] My recommendations for timing intercourse are as follows:

1. Track your cycles and mark your expected fertile window.
2. Try to have intercourse *at least once* during the first three days of your fertile window.
3. Then, choose either OPK or CMM (or both) to determine your ovulation day.
    a. OPK: Begin testing once per day between 10 a.m. and 2 p.m. each day starting the first day of your expected fertile window.

    *Target intercourse on the day of the positive OPK and the next day.*

b. CMM: Begin observing CMM starting the first day of your fertile window.

*Target intercourse any day with Type 4 cervical mucus.*

## Common Questions

**Can having intercourse before or after ovulation determine the sex of my child?**

The Shettles method claims that you can control the sex of your baby based on the weight and speed of sperm.[25] Male sperm are lighter because the Y chromosome is smaller and not as heavy as the X chromosome. If you want a boy, the idea is to abstain before ovulation and have intercourse on ovulation day so male sperm have the highest chance of getting to the egg (presuming lighter sperm are faster sperm). If you want a girl, have sex a few days before ovulation and then abstain during ovulation, as male sperm will less likely be present three days later. Although this theory is intriguing, it has not held true in any study.[26] It can be something fun to do if you desire a girl or a boy, but the day you have intercourse does not impact the sex of your baby.[27] If you have infertility, I would not recommend having less intercourse on purpose, as is recommended with these techniques.

## Improve Coital Practices for Conception

Nothing will make you analyze every single thing about sex more than trying to get pregnant. There are so many myths out there about how to have sex for conception that it can put a lot of pressure on how you actually do the deed. I am asked daily about best sexual positions, lubrication, and what to do after intercourse to increase the chances of conception. The reality is, the most important thing you can do to help yourself get pregnant is to have intercourse at the right time in the fertile window. Other coital practices have very little impact on conception rates.

That said, there are a few things worth considering.

## Choose a Position Based on What You Prefer

Sexual position preferences are personal and do not impact conception. Although you may hear that deeper penetration is better, no evidence supports one position over another. Whichever position satisfies both partners and can result in ejaculation is the best one to use. Female orgasm may help facilitate faster sperm movement toward the egg but does not increase conception rates.[28]

There is also no need to adjust intercourse position based on uterus orientation. Your uterus can have different orientations inside your body, named for the direction the top of the uterus is tilted. Your uterus can be anteverted (aimed upward) or retroverted (aimed backward). These are normal variants, like having red or blond hair. Although uterine orientation can sometimes be induced by external forces, causing scar tissue, an anteverted or retroverted uterus does not impact your fertility.[29]

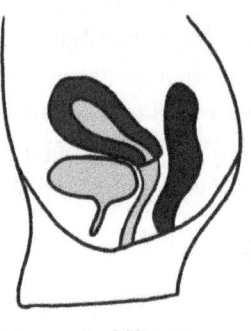 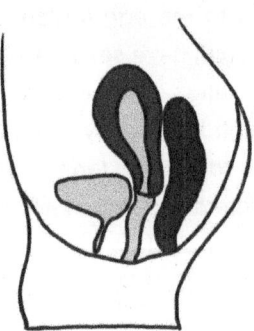

**Anteverted Uterus**  **Retroverted Uterus**

Uterine Orientation

## Use Lubrication If Needed

Intercourse should never be painful. Using a vaginal lubricant can make having sex easier and more pleasurable—and therefore more frequent. No lubricant, even if marketed to "improve fertility," will improve your odds of pregnancy.

All lubricants affect sperm in some way. The ejaculate has an alkaline pH to protect the sperm from the acidic pH of the vagina. Lubricants mimicking the pH of the cervical mucus at the time of ovulation (pH 7.2 to 8.5) appear to have the least impact on sperm survival in the lab.[30] Many lubricants are outside this pH range or have artificial ingredients that can be toxic to sperm, resulting in reduced motility and an increase in sperm DNA damage.[31] Most lubricants are water based, and a good rule of thumb is that those that are glycerin based are toxic, while those that are hydroxyethylcellulose based appear more fertility friendly. Oil-based lubricants can alter the vaginal pH and microbiome, and most common oils (olive, coconut) have limited evidence for or against their use. Saliva is harmful to sperm motility as it has an acidic pH and the salivary enzyme amylase, which is spermicidal.[32]

All lubricants present an additional barrier for sperm to swim through—no lubricant *improves* sperm survival or motility. If you are trying to get pregnant, my recommendation is to avoid lubricant if you do not need it. But if you have vaginal dryness or discomfort with intercourse, you should use lubricant to help improve your experience and frequency. Below is a summary of the best and worst options for lubricant use on sperm survival. I would recommend choosing a lubricant in the "Best" column if you are trying to conceive.

**VAGINAL LUBRICANTS AND FERTILITY**

| Type | Best | Worst |
|---|---|---|
| Water | hydroxyethylcellulose-based (Pre-Seed, Conceive Plus) | glycerin-based (K-Y Jelly and Astroglide) |
| Oil | mineral oil, canola oil | sesame oil, baby oil |
| Other | | saliva |

## After Intercourse

After intercourse, you do not need to try to trap the sperm in your vagina. There is no need to lie flat after intercourse or elevate your pelvis. You do not need to put your legs up in the air for any amount of time. The sperm will move through the cervical mucus in seconds.

Urinating after intercourse can decrease the risk of urinary tract infection and does not decrease your chances of getting pregnant.[33] Sperm is deposited in the vagina and urine comes out the urethra, so you do not need to worry about peeing out the sperm. Yes, you may see ejaculate when you wipe, but remember, the ejaculate protects the sperm and is not the sperm itself. If you go to the bathroom, the sperm is well on its way through the cervical mucus.

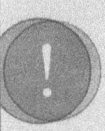

## *Important Study Findings:* Intercourse and Implantation

"Peri-Implantation Intercourse Does Not Lower Fecundability"[34]

- **Study basics:** Uterine contractions from intercourse have been hypothesized to impact implantation. The study observed 2,606 possible conception cycles from women without infertility to evaluate the impact of peri-implantation sex (post-ovulation days five to nine) on pregnancy rates.
- **Results:** No connection was seen between the frequency of peri-implantation intercourse and fecundability.
- **Conclusion:** There is no need to recommend abstinence after ovulation or during the implantation window.

## AFTER CONCEPTION

So you've done everything needed to conceive and now you're starting to get pregnancy symptoms. You're tired, bloated, nauseated, and have sensitive breasts. What's next?

### Confirm with a Pregnancy Test

Once an embryo begins to implant, it secretes hCG, which can be detected on a pregnancy test. Implantation typically occurs seven to nine days after ovulation, so this is usually the earliest you can see a positive pregnancy test. Different pregnancy tests have different sensitivity levels for how high hCG must be to turn the test positive. Each pregnancy test box will tell you the level of hCG needed (lower = more sensitive and can detect earlier). I always tell patients that many inexpensive pregnancy tests work just fine—any line at all is a positive test, even if it is very faint! Once you get a positive pregnancy test, call your OB-GYN to schedule your first appointment, which will usually fall between nine and thirteen weeks of pregnancy.

As the pregnancy develops, hCG will increase, a sign that the pregnancy is progressing normally. If you are taking pregnancy tests, you should notice the line getting darker. If you went through fertility treatment, see your doctor for a blood hCG level. Your hCG levels should approximately double every two days, which is a very reassuring sign that the pregnancy is viable. However, hCG levels only follow this pattern very early on. The minimal rise of hCG that is associated with a normal pregnancy is a 49 percent increase over forty-eight hours, identifying 99 percent of all early viable pregnancies.[35]

One important fact about pregnancy tests and fertility treatments: If you used a trigger shot with fertility treatments, it was an hCG injection. Make sure that you don't take a pregnancy test while the trigger shot is still in your system (typically ten to fourteen days after injection) or you will get a positive test. Some women "test out their trigger," where they check a pregnancy test until it turns negative (confirming the trigger is gone) and then begin to test for a possible pregnancy.

## Determine Your Due Date

Before ultrasounds and ovulation detection, the only way to know your gestational age was to count backward to your last period and assume that ovulation took place on day fourteen. If you go to any online pregnancy calculator today, that is exactly what their formula will calculate, unless you provide a more accurate day of ovulation.

A full pregnancy is forty weeks in length—not nine months! One way to calculate your due date is to take the first day of your last period and add forty weeks. Another way to do this is to take the first day of your last period, then subtract three months and add seven days. For example, if the first day of your last period was August 1, your due date will be May 8. Now, if you have short or long cycle lengths or irregular cycles, this calculation definitely may not be accurate.

If you think about it, counting back to your period is a little crazy, because you certainly were not pregnant when your period started. The moment you have an egg fertilized by sperm, you are "two weeks" pregnant by standard calculators. When you miss your period and take a pregnancy test, you are "four weeks" pregnant. We call this the estimated gestational age (EGA). For consistency, EGA is still referenced this way even though we know it is not truly accurate for fetal age. You can see that if you are "six weeks pregnant," you probably only found out about your pregnancy two weeks ago at most.

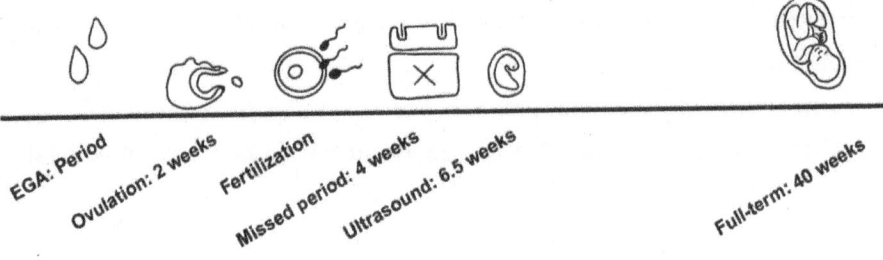

**Gestational Age Timeline**

For fertility treatments or cycle tracking, we have a more precise measurement of your due date that uses your ovulation day or embryo transfer day to determine your EGA. You will typically have your first ultrasound around six weeks, which should show a gestational sac with a small fetal pole and heartbeat. If you did not need fertility treatments or your last menstrual period (LMP) is unknown or less certain, your due date may be moved if ultrasound disagrees with your EGA. Ultrasound is an imperfect art, and we allow a one-week difference in the first trimester, a two-week difference in the second trimester, and a three-week difference in the third trimester.

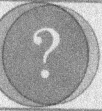 **Common Questions**

### Am I having a miscarriage?

If you are pregnant and bleeding, please call your doctor. Sometimes bleeding in pregnancy is due to a blood clot between the placenta and the uterus, known as a subchorionic hematoma (SCH), which can be seen on ultrasound. I recommend pelvic rest (no intercourse or vigorous exercise) and talking to your doctor about stopping any blood thinners you may be taking. An SCH is typically followed with subsequent ultrasounds to make sure the pregnancy is developing appropriately. On the other hand, sometimes bleeding can be due to a pregnancy loss. A biochemical pregnancy is one where you had a positive pregnancy test, started bleeding, and now your pregnancy test is negative. This is a pregnancy loss but does not need further evaluation. However, other potential etiologies could include ectopic pregnancy or a missed miscarriage (the pregnancy has stopped growing but is still in the uterus), and any positive pregnancy test with bleeding warrants a call to your doctor.

---

When Violet came to see me, she had been trying to get pregnant for over nine months, with two early losses. We went ahead with fertility testing and found out that she was born with a birth defect of her uterus, known as a uterine septum. A uterine septum is associated with a much higher rate of miscarriage, and Violet had no idea she had this birth defect until we evaluated her anatomy.[36] In her case, the uterine septum didn't cause any symptoms until she became pregnant.

After surgery to remove the septum, Violet conceived quickly and stayed pregnant. She couldn't believe that she didn't even know that birth defects of the uterus were possible, let alone that she had one that caused infertility and pregnancy loss. She was so thankful that she went to a fertility doctor instead of waiting six more months and suffering who knows how many more losses.

Many of us will struggle to get pregnant. I was one of those people. Infertility can happen to anyone, and it is not your fault if you find yourself in that position. When you try to conceive, you can't control the outcome, but you can control your actions during the process. My goal is for you to know that you are optimizing your chances of getting pregnant each month, and if you do not conceive, at least you will be able to move on to fertility testing and/or treatment more confidently. We'll talk about this next.

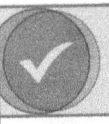 *Facts to Remember*

- You should take a prenatal vitamin with 400 mcg folic acid before you conceive.
- A preconception visit with your doctor can help confirm you are in the best health for pregnancy.
- Tracking your cycle and timing intercourse will help you get pregnant faster.
- Do not have less sex if you are trying to conceive.
- The earliest you can take a pregnancy test is seven to nine days after ovulation.
- When you miss your period, you are four weeks pregnant.

# 7

# Navigating Infertility

Sometimes, even when you're tracking your cycle and timing intercourse, you may not be able to conceive. Six months go by, maybe a year, maybe more, and nothing. You feel like you've tried everything—and you've definitely tried a lot. I know how frustrating this can be. So many patients come to my office feeling this way. I've felt this way. Infertility can be a debilitating experience. It's also a very common one.

As we've learned, infertility is defined as the inability to get pregnant after twelve months of regular, unprotected intercourse. It is something nobody is prepared to experience. But the hardest experience for me is seeing patients in my office later than I should. It's extremely important to know how long is too long and to learn to identify the signs that you should get a fertility evaluation sooner rather than later.

When Ruby came to see me, she was thirty-two, healthy, and her cycles were regular, occurring every twenty-eight to twenty-nine days. She could easily detect ovulation with CMM and a temperature shift, and she and her husband had no problem having intercourse. But when she'd seen her doctor, she was told they needed to be trying to conceive for a year before having fertility testing. So, they'd kept trying. After another six months, Ruby still wasn't pregnant.

After a full year of tracking and trying, Ruby went back to her doctor and fertility testing was ordered. Her partner had a semen analysis as part of their testing, and when the results returned, they were shocked to find out he had no sperm. Ruby couldn't believe they had been trying for so long, putting so much effort into tracking and timing, and the entire time there was zero chance of pregnancy.

Unbeknownst to him, Ruby's husband had a birth defect that resulted in him not having a vas deferens, important in sperm transport from the testes in ejaculation. It is like being born with a vasectomy—permanent birth control that he never knew he had! They would have to do IVF with a surgical procedure for her husband if they wanted to conceive.

Here is the truth: You can call a fertility clinic and get an appointment with a fertility doctor anytime. You do not have to wait for anyone to tell you that you need to schedule an appointment. I don't need your doctor to send a referral. We will get your medical records if you have had any testing completed. Don't let time make a decision for you.

My goal as a fertility doctor is to make the infertility journey less scary. I went into this field because I love it—understanding the hormone puzzle and forming deep connections with my patients make being a fertility doctor truly special. But this job is not all rainbows and sunshine. It is hard, full of emotions and tears, and there are days I am reminded of just how unfair life can be.

My own experience with infertility has forever changed how I approach patients. I didn't want to admit we had infertility, and I delayed getting testing or seeing a doctor myself. I wanted the problem to fix itself so I could move on to that next chapter of life. Seeing a doctor felt like an acknowledgment of my failure. What if nothing worked? My own denial held me back. If you are there, know that I have been there too.

The unknown of infertility is often the scariest part. We can't always control the outcome, no matter what we do. This means it is important to focus on what you can control:

1. The way you understand your body
2. That you know what you are doing and why
3. That you are confident in the plan

We can't rewind the clock. I wish we could. What we can do is know we made the best decision we could with the data we had. No matter how this journey ends, we can leave with the knowledge that we would not have done anything differently.

## FERTILITY TESTING AND EVALUATION

You should not be forced to wait any amount of time or prove you have infertility in order to have fertility testing. My dream is that fertility becomes proactive, with early testing and preventative measures emphasized. You should not have to fail first before seeking care. If your periods are irregular, extremely painful, or you have difficulty with intercourse, you should seek evaluation now. If you feel like something is wrong, trust your gut.

Over 70 percent of couples who will conceive do so in the first six months of trying.[1] Although it is fine to wait until you hit that one-year mark of trying to get a fertility evaluation, it is also perfectly reasonable to do so before then. Due to the impact of age on fertility, women who are thirty-five or older should get an evaluation after six months of trying.[2]

Your initial fertility consultation is nothing to be nervous about. Your doctor will start by reviewing your medical history. Be prepared to walk through your goals, history, and prior testing or treatment. The majority of the first consultation will be educational, and a fertility doctor will discuss the standard evaluation and appropriate next steps. Preconception testing (reviewed in chapter 6) will typically be ordered at this time if it wasn't completed prior to your fertility consult.

Standard fertility testing includes:

1. Evaluation of ovulation
2. Ovarian reserve testing
3. Anatomic evaluation
4. Semen analysis

## Evaluation of Ovulation

The best way to confirm ovulation is a great menstrual history. Regular, predictable cycles with a normal luteal phase indicate no further testing is needed. If you have cycle tracking data with any inconsistencies, please be sure to let your doctor know. We covered the various causes of ovulatory dysfunction in chapter 4, but below are potential tests that may be ordered for irregular or absent cycles.

**EVALUATION OF OVULATION**

| Test | Potential Cause |
| --- | --- |
| FSH, LH, estradiol | Hypothalamic amenorrhea (HA) <br> Diminished ovarian reserve (DOR) <br> Ovarian failure |
| TSH | Hypothyroid <br> Hyperthyroid |
| Prolactin | Hyperprolactinemia |
| Testosterone | PCOS |
| Mid-luteal progesterone | Confirmation of ovulation |
| Ultrasound | Confirmation of ovulation <br> PCOS <br> DOR |

## Ovarian Reserve Testing

In chapter 3, we learned that ovarian reserve testing is an approximation of how many eggs you have remaining. Individual levels should be reviewed based on age. All patients getting a fertility evaluation should have their ovarian reserve tested, as it can significantly impact treatment plans.

**EVALUATION OF OVARIAN RESERVE**

| Ovarian Reserve Test | Levels Suggestive of DOR |
|---|---|
| Anti-müllerian hormone (AMH) | <1.5 ng/mL |
| Antral follicle count (AFC) | <10 follicles |
| Day 3 FSH and estradiol | FSH > 10 IU/L or E2 > 60 pg/mL |

## Anatomic Evaluation

A typical anatomy evaluation begins with a transvaginal ultrasound (TVUS) to evaluate the ovaries and the uterus. Additional tests will be required to evaluate the inside of the uterine cavity and the fallopian tubes, often a hysterosalpingogram (HSG), known as an X-ray dye test, or an ultrasound-based evaluation, known as sono-hysterosalpingography (sono-HSG). Below are other possible imaging options.

**IMAGING OPTIONS FOR ANATOMIC EVALUATION**

| Imaging Option | Description | Potential Diagnosis |
|---|---|---|
| Transvaginal ultrasound (TVUS) | The best way to evaluate the ovaries and the uterus | AFC, ovarian cysts, fibroids, endometriosis, adenomyosis, uterine birth defects |
| Hysterosalpingogram (HSG) | Dye injected into the uterus with X-ray to see the uterine cavity and fallopian tubes | Polyps, fibroids, uterine birth defects, scar tissue, fallopian tube blockage, hydrosalpinx |
| Sono-hysterosalpingography (sono-HSG) | Water-infused TVUS to see the inside of the uterine cavity with bubbles, foam, or flow through fallopian tubes | Uterine birth defects, polyps, fibroids, scar tissue, adenomyosis, fallopian tube blockage, hydrosalpinx, ovarian cysts |
| Saline infusion sonogram (SIS) | Water-infused TVUS to see the inside of the uterine cavity | Uterine birth defects, polyps, fibroids, scar tissue, adenomyosis, ovarian cysts, AFC |

| Imaging Option | Description | Potential Diagnosis |
| --- | --- | --- |
| Pelvic MRI | MRI to look at uterus and ovaries | Uterine birth defects, fibroids, endometriosis, adenomyosis, hydrosalpinx, ovarian cysts, AFC |
| Hysteroscopy | Surgical procedure where a camera is inserted into the uterus | Polyps, fibroids, uterine birth defects, scar tissue |
| Laparoscopy | Surgical procedure where a camera is inserted into the abdomen to look at the uterus and ovaries | Endometriosis, ovarian cysts, blocked fallopian tubes, uterine fibroids, uterine birth defects |

## Semen Analysis

A semen analysis is an evaluation of sperm parameters, including volume, pH, concentration, motility, and morphology (shape). For a semen analysis, we want two to three days of abstinence prior to sample collection. Longer abstinence intervals are not recommended unless specifically requested by your clinic, as this can increase the amount of debris and dead sperm. If the semen analysis is normal, no further testing is usually needed. Abnormal results may necessitate repeat semen analysis, hormone testing, genetic evaluation, or urology referral, pending the specific abnormality.

It's important to note that the low end of normal and the ideal sperm parameters for conception are different. If all the sperm parameters are barely above the minimal threshold for normal, the semen analysis may be called "normal" but fertility will be reduced.[3]

**SEMEN ANALYSIS PARAMETERS**

| Parameter | Low-End Normal | Ideal for Conception |
|---|---|---|
| Volume (mL) | ≥1.5 | ≥1.5 |
| pH | 7.2–7.8 | 7.2–7.8 |
| Concentration (million/mL) | ≥15 | ≥40 |
| Motility (forward progression) | ≥40% | ≥60% |
| Morphology (Kruger/strict) | ≥4% | ≥14% |
| Total motile sperm count (million) | ≥20 | ≥50 |

One way to evaluate the reproductive potential of a semen analysis is to calculate the total number of moving sperm in the sample, called the total motile sperm (TMS). The TMS is calculated by the following formula: volume (mL) × concentration (million/mL) × motility (%). A TMS count above fifty million moving sperm is ideal for conception.[4]

Sperm concentration is a sign of proper communication between the brain and testes and represents hormonal function. Motility and morphology are factors that may be influenced by the structure of the testes themselves or the environment. If your partner has an inability to achieve or maintain an erection or failure to ejaculate, that information needs to be disclosed so a bigger evaluation can be completed.

## TOP CAUSES OF INFERTILITY

The most common causes of infertility are ovulatory, tubal, and male factor, with 85 percent of patients having one of these three diagnoses.[5] Many patients actually have more than one cause of infertility. Around one third of infertility is caused by female factors, one third is caused by male factors, and one third is caused by a combination of male and female factors.[6] Other causes of infertility are related to age, endometriosis or uterine conditions, recurrent pregnancy loss, or are unexplained.

## Ovulatory Factor

Remember, having regular, predictable periods is a sign that you are ovulating.[7] If you track your cycles and realize that your periods have changed, or if you have concerns about short luteal phase or irregular ovulation, please tell your doctor. Lifestyle optimization and ovulation induction are standard treatments.

## Tubal Factor

The fallopian tubes capture the egg and are the site of fertilization and early embryo development. All mechanisms of tubal damage are due to inflammation and unfortunately are often permanent.

Tubes can be blocked at their opening (proximal) or in the midportion or the end (distal). Proximal tubal obstruction can sometimes be caused by tubal spasm, and unilateral proximal blockage can be evaluated by surgery to determine if it is real. Mid- and distal blockage is almost always due to inflammatory changes and is an indication for IVF.[8]

A blocked and dilated tube is known as a hydrosalpinx. Pregnancy rates are 50 percent lower and miscarriage rates are two times higher in patients who have a hydrosalpinx at the time of embryo transfer.[9] A hydrosalpinx needs to be surgically removed even if you are doing IVF.

## Male Factor

Sperm development takes about seventy days in the testes and up to twenty-one days to move through the reproductive tract. Since sperm are constantly produced, an environmental change has the potential to have a big impact. Sperm are highly sensitive to their environment, and inflammation is especially detrimental. Sperm counts have decreased more than 50 percent in fifty years due to an increase in toxins, poor lifestyle factors, and an increase in overall poorer health.[10]

The production of sperm is a hormonally controlled process, similar to ovulation. In men, GnRH stimulates FSH and LH from the pituitary, which are important in testicular production of sperm and testosterone. Low testosterone levels may present with fatigue, weight gain, and low libido. However, testosterone is not the appropriate treatment if you are trying to conceive. Sperm and testosterone are made at the same time, so when a man takes testosterone, it prevents FSH and LH release, and therefore sperm production. Essentially, testosterone is male birth control. Even after stopping testosterone use, 20 percent of men will never resume sperm production.[11]

Men can also have anatomical reasons impacting conception, such a history of undescended testes, testicular trauma, birth defects, and dilated blood vessels—known as varicoceles. A complete medical history is key as some of these factors may have treatment options while others do not.

Just like egg quality, sperm quality is also very important for fertility. On a semen analysis, motility and morphology both give insight into sperm function. In addition, a sperm DNA fragmentation test can give greater insight into the DNA quality inside each sperm. This test is not part of a routine evaluation, but may be considered in certain cases of recurrent pregnancy loss, recurrent implantation failure, or unexpected poor outcomes with treatment (such as failure of embryo development).[12] A high level of fragmented DNA inside the sperm is an indication of poor sperm quality and function.[13]

Treatment for male factor should be individualized but can include medications to improve sperm concentration, surgical removal of a varicocele, intrauterine insemination (IUI), consideration of IVF with intracytoplasmic injection (ICSI) for fertilization, and potential testicular sperm extraction. Since the sperm lifespan is approximately three months, lifestyle changes to decrease inflammation should always be considered, as they can have a major impact on sperm quality. These are discussed in depth in part III.

## INFLUENCE OF LIFESTYLE FACTORS ON SPERM QUALITY

| Beneficial | Harmful |
|---|---|
| Vitamins | Environmental toxins |
| Antioxidants | Inflammation |
| Sleep | Smoking |
| Exercise | Marijuana |
| Normal weight | Alcohol |
| Increased blood flow | Stress |
| Fiber | Obesity |
| Fruits and vegetables | Chronic illness |
| Whole grains | Processed food |
| Healthy fats | External heat |

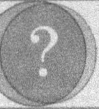

## Common Questions

### Does paternal age impact fertility?

Testosterone production and sperm production both decrease with age. Male age contributes to infertility as infertility rates are two to three times higher for men over forty as compared with men under age forty.[14] Paternal age over fifty is associated with increased genetic abnormalities. Increased damage of the DNA inside the sperm head can lead to new autosomal dominant mutations, such as dwarfism or Marfan syndrome.[15] Overall, these mutations are rare, as autosomal dominant diseases are rare. Due to genetic changes, miscarriage rates are also increased with paternal age over 40.[16]

## Age-Related Infertility

As we learned in chapter 3, increased age is associated with a decrease in pregnancy rates and increase in miscarriage. Age-related fertility becomes more significant after age thirty-seven. It is important to know that your personalized testing and treatment recommendations may differ based on your age.

## Endometriosis

Endometriosis is an inflammatory disease characterized by implants of endometrial-like tissue outside the uterus, discussed in detail in chapter 4. Endometriosis can cause infertility from chronic inflammation or scar tissue formation. The probability of pregnancy in patients with endometriosis is significantly lower than it is for age-matched peers, with an estimated fecundability of 2 percent to 10 percent per month. Although women with stage I/II disease may conceive with less aggressive treatment, those with stage III/IV disease often need IVF.[17]

## Uterine Factor

Uterine factors that contribute to infertility include uterine polyps, uterine fibroids, uterine scar tissue, adenomyosis, endometritis, and uterine birth defects. The majority of these conditions present with abnormal cycles and are reviewed in chapter 4. Uterine birth defects are typically asymptomatic and often present with pregnancy loss over infertility. Treatment can include surgery or IVF.

# RECURRENT PREGNANCY LOSS

Recurrent pregnancy loss (RPL) is defined as two or more pregnancy losses.[18] As someone who had RPL, I know how hard it can be to keep losing pregnancies. Pregnancy loss occurs in 15 to 25 percent of all pregnancies, with an increasing risk as you age.[19] A full workup is indicated for

RPL, even though testing often comes back normal. Treatment should always focus on decreasing inflammation where you can, as many causes of RPL increase inflammatory markers. Further treatment is indicated based on specific diagnosis, so the best thing you can do is advocate for testing to try to get to the root cause of RPL. Potential causes include:

- Genetic factors
- Endocrine disease
- Uterine birth defects
- Clotting disorder
- Autoimmune disease
- Toxin exposure

### Genetic Factors

Random genetic abnormalities, called aneuploidy, are the top cause of miscarriage. Aneuploidy can be detected at the embryo level with IVF, but there is no test to see if an egg is genetically normal (just as there is no test for egg quality).

A balanced translocation is a specific genetic abnormality that can cause miscarriage. This occurs when two of your chromosomes have switched spots. When an egg's chromosomes split in half, a patient with a balanced translocation may end up with an egg without all the chromosomes it needs. Since a balanced translocation can impact both eggs and sperm, both partners should be tested by getting a blood test called a karyotype. People who have a translocation have a very high percentage of miscarriage for their age and often need IVF with genetic testing to identify the translocation.

### Endocrine Disease

Endocrine diseases associated with pregnancy loss include diabetes, thyroid disease, elevated prolactin, and luteal phase defect (LPD). Preexisting thyroid disease and diabetes should both be controlled prior to conception in order to decrease pregnancy complications. Lab work typically ordered to check for endocrine causes of RPL includes TSH, PRL, and HbA1c (or another test for insulin resistance). Treating the underlying endocrine disorder often improves pregnancy outcomes. If LPD is identified, treating this with ovulation induction, with or without progesterone supplementation, can help improve ovulatory pattern.

## Uterine Birth Defects

Your uterus is formed from two different buds of tissue called the Müllerian ducts, which become the top third of the vagina, cervix, uterus, and fallopian tubes. Prior to your birth, these Müllerian buds elongate, fuse together, and the midline connecting tissue will reabsorb, leaving the central cavity of the uterus, cervix, and vagina. Failure of any portion of this process will result in a uterine birth defect, collectively known as Müllerian anomalies.

The most common Müllerian anomaly is a uterine septum, which is a failure of the midline connecting tissue to reabsorb; this is the condition Violet had in chapter 6. A patient with a uterine septum has up to a 77 percent chance of miscarriage. Luckily, your miscarriage rate decreases after surgical resection.[20] Surgery is not routinely recommended for any Müllerian anomalies except a uterine septum.

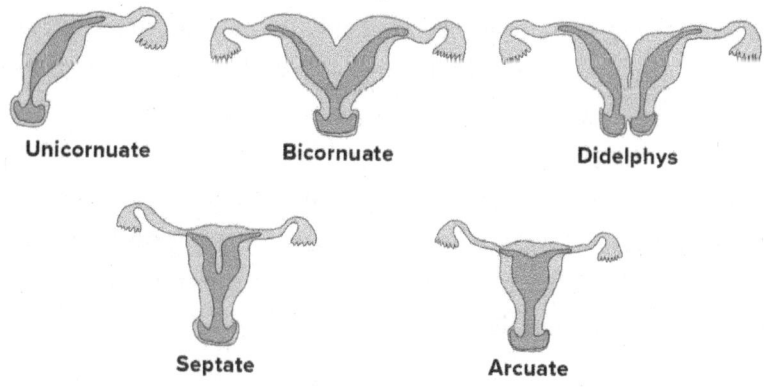

Müllerian Anomalies

Five percent of all women are born with a birth defect of the uterus, and 13 percent of women with recurrent pregnancy loss will be found to have a uterine abnormality.[21] Most women who have abnormal uterine development have no idea anything is wrong. Patients with Müllerian anomalies have an increased risk of endometriosis and pain, but most patients are asymptomatic. Anatomical evaluation can help identify Müllerian anomalies.

## Clotting Disorder

The blood vessels of the placenta are very small. If you have a blood clotting disorder, small blood clots can block the placental blood vessels and result in miscarriage. The standard evaluation is testing for a clotting disorder called antiphospholipid syndrome (APS) with blood work. I describe APS as an autoimmune clotting disorder that activates only when you are pregnant, meaning you are unlikely to have a blood clot outside of pregnancy. If you have a history of blood clots, such as deep vein thrombosis or a pulmonary embolism, and you now have pregnancy loss, you need a more extensive evaluation for other clotting disorders as well. Clotting disorders are treated with blood thinners, like aspirin and/or Lovenox.

## Autoimmune Disease

There are other autoimmune diseases in addition to APS that can contribute to pregnancy loss. Current recommendations are not to test for autoimmune disease in women with RPL unless they have other symptoms or a family history. However, many autoimmune diseases have been shown to have a significant risk of miscarriage and long-term health implications.[22] If you have RPL, I recommend you look at these potential causes and research the symptoms to see if anything may be going on that you didn't know. Also, talk to your family members about autoimmune diseases and include them in your family history.

## POTENTIAL AUTOIMMUNE CAUSES OF RPL

| | |
|---|---|
| Celiac disease | Systemic sclerosis |
| Autoimmune thyroid disease | Psoriasis |
| Lupus | Endometriosis |
| Rheumatoid arthritis | Adenomyosis |
| Sjögren's syndrome | |

Autoimmunity is characterized by a persistent inflamed state, so many symptoms of chronic inflammation will be present prior to diagnosis. Autoimmune disease takes years to diagnose from symptom onset. Infertility or RPL may be your warning sign that something is going on behind the scenes like it was for me. Even if you don't receive a diagnosis, lowering your inflammation can improve your health and fertility. Part III reviews how to decrease chronic inflammation, and part IV has my anti-inflammatory protocol.

## Toxin Exposure

Many toxins are associated with a higher rate of miscarriage. Some exposures carry risk even if the male partner is the only one exposed to toxins such as marijuana and smoking.[23] We'll go over this in depth in part III.

## TOXIC EXPOSURES AND RPL

| | |
|---|---|
| Smoking | Alcohol (3 glasses/week) |
| Marijuana | Caffeine (over 200 mg) |
| Cocaine | Heavy metals |

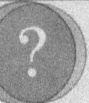

### Common Questions

**Did low progesterone cause my miscarriage?**

When an embryo implants and makes hCG, it "rescues" the corpus luteum, allowing it to continue making progesterone. Unfortunately, not every pregnancy is genetically normal. Since abnormal pregnancies do not divide and grow normally, they make lower levels of hCG that cannot stimulate enough progesterone. This low progesterone is the embryo's way of communicating to the body that it is not normal, likely resulting in a miscarriage. Most of the time, low progesterone is a sign that the pregnancy is abnormal. However, some women may have a luteal phase defect resulting in low progesterone production, reflecting a form of ovulatory dysfunction. Progesterone supplementation may benefit some with RPL and likely has the greatest impact in patients with multiple prior losses or current vaginal bleeding.[24] If progesterone is to be used for RPL, I recommend starting supplementation after ovulation is confirmed (in the luteal phase) as opposed to a positive pregnancy test.

## UNEXPLAINED INFERTILITY

Unexplained infertility is defined as infertility despite regular cycles, open fallopian tubes, and normal sperm counts. I believe unexplained infertility is undiagnosed infertility. This doesn't mean we will never know what is causing your infertility, but it doesn't fit into one of the big three categories of ovulation, tubal, or male.

Top causes of unexplained infertility are linked to inflammation, including endometriosis, adenomyosis, autoimmune disease, poor egg/sperm quality, and fertilization failure. Unexplained infertility may be a symptom of chronic inflammation or the preclinical stage of autoimmunity. If infertility is your symptom, you may not be able to fully diagnose the disease until you are "sicker." I don't believe that we should accept unexplained infertility without at least looking for inflammatory symptoms or associated factors. Treatment includes lifestyle optimization, ovulation induction with IUI, or IVF.

 **Common Questions**

**We don't know what is causing my infertility. Do I need fertility treatments?**

Unexplained infertility is a hard diagnosis to receive. With no specific reason for your infertility, pregnancy is unlikely but possible. The chance of conception is only 2 to 4 percent per month, significantly lower than natural fertility rates.[25] Since inflammation is a common link between conditions causing unexplained infertility, I view this as an opportunity to actively decrease inflammation. I always say that 2 to 4 percent is low but not zero. Some patients will get pregnant without treatment, but the longer you have been trying, the lower the odds are for natural conception. Ultimately, this is not an efficient way to grow your family.

## PREPARING FOR INFERTILITY TREATMENTS

There is no one-size-fits-all fertility treatment plan. Your goals play a big role in your treatment recommendations. Depending on your diagnosis, there may be only one treatment option available. Other times, your doctor may present you with choices.

Fertility treatments are a balance of four things: (1) your time, (2) your money, (3) your physical health, and (4) your emotional health. At different points in your life one aspect may be more valuable than another, and no one treatment fulfills all needs.

With infertility, your odds of getting pregnant are lower than your age-related rates. In vitro fertilization (IVF) is the only treatment that will exceed age-based success rates. Others will never match or exceed it. This does not mean you have to do IVF—every situation is unique. At the end of the day, you should be given the data you need about your fertility to make this decision for yourself.

I strongly believe that nobody should be denied more effective treatment or be forced to fail less aggressive treatment first. Unfortunately, insurance companies and corporate medical practices often institute protocols and policies requiring a set number of cycles of less-effective treatment before moving on to IVF. My job as a fertility doctor is to help you use your resources wisely and understand your options.

The treatment options we'll be discussing are:

- Ovulation induction (OI)
- Intrauterine insemination (IUI)
- In vitro fertilization (IVF)
- Third-party reproduction
- Surgery
- Lifestyle changes

## Ovulation Induction

Ovulation induction (OI) is the use of medication to stimulate ovulation. This can be done with oral medications or injectable hormones. OI is recommended if you have ovulation issues, such as PCOS, hypothalamic amenorrhea, or LPD, and for unexplained infertility.

Oral medications (clomiphene, letrozole) work by lowering estrogen levels. Your brain will sense a lower estrogen and send out a stronger signal of FSH to grow an egg. Medications have a 7 to 10 percent chance of producing multiples, such as twins, and a small chance of triplets.[26] Clomiphene binds to estrogen receptors and may occasionally result in a thin lining, making letrozole a better choice for some patients.

Gonadotropins are injectable hormones, typically a synthetic FSH or a combination of FSH and LH, that directly stimulate the ovary. Interestingly, we don't have the ability to synthetically make LH, but since women in menopause have high levels of FSH/LH, their urine can be purified and used as a source of LH and FSH. Gonadotropins have up to a 36 percent risk of multiples and a much higher cycle cancellation due to overresponse.[27]

## MEDICATIONS OF OVULATION INDUCTION

| Type | Medication (Brand) | Action |
| --- | --- | --- |
| Oral | clomiphene citrate (Clomid) | binds estrogen receptors |
|  | letrozole (Femara) | breaks down estrogen in bloodstream |
| Injectable | FSH (Follistim, Gonal-f) | gonadotropin |
|  | FSH/LH (Menopur) | gonadotropin |

Always ask your doctor how they will determine your response to treatment—whether via ultrasound, OPK, or a luteal progesterone level—and the next steps if you do not respond. A personalized approach should always be prioritized. Not everyone will respond to a medication the way that they hope. I always say that OI cycles begin as a trial. With my patients, I use the data available to me to pick the best medication, but I don't know how their ovaries will actually respond. Canceled cycles or dose increases are an expected part of the process. If you do respond and ovulate, remember that not every cycle will result in pregnancy, as you will never exceed your age-related chances of pregnancy with these medications. Discuss how many cycles you will plan before reviewing with your doctor or crafting a new plan.

First-line medication is based on diagnosis. Let's go through each of these.

## FIRST-LINE OI MEDICATION BY DIAGNOSIS

| Condition | First-Line Medication |
| --- | --- |
| PCOS | Letrozole |
| HA | FSH/LH |
| Short luteal phase | Clomid |
| Unexplained infertility | Clomid + IUI |

### Polycystic Ovary Syndrome (PCOS)

Letrozole is the drug of choice for patients with PCOS.[28] If there is no response to letrozole, other options include a trial of Clomid or gonadotropins. The goal of OI with PCOS is to get one to two eggs to grow. If this goal cannot be achieved, IVF is the next best option. OI for PCOS should always be combined with lifestyle modification to decrease inflammation and insulin resistance.

### Hypothalamic Amenorrhea (HA)

If your brain is already not responding to a low estrogen level, an oral medication with a mechanism of lowering estrogen will be ineffective. Gonadotropins are used for ovulation induction with HA, specifically FSH/LH since the brain is not making either hormone. The risk of overresponse, multiples, and cycle cancellation is high with gonadotropins, as it is often difficult to get just one or two eggs to respond. Many of my patients with HA will find OI frustrating, and moving on to IVF is often the safest option.

### Luteal Phase Defect (LPD)

A short luteal phase is a sign of LPD and often reflects ovulatory dysfunction. If no cause can be found after an evaluation, treatment with ovulation induction can help the brain send out a stronger signal of FSH, improving the quality of the follicle and ovulation. Clomid is typically my drug of choice for LPD.

### Unexplained Infertility

Treatment with OI for unexplained infertility is based on the goal of ovulating two or more eggs to increase the opportunity for sperm and egg to meet. OI alone does not improve pregnancy rates with unexplained infertility (2 percent to 4 percent per cycle), but there is a small benefit of OI combined with intrauterine insemination for women under age thirty-eight (5 percent to 8 percent per cycle).[29] Studies confirm that gonadotropins add minimal additional benefit (over Clomid) in unexplained infertility, and the recommended medication for OI is typically Clomid.[30]

In women age thirty-eight and older with unexplained infertility, a large study evaluated success rates with OI and IUI versus IVF. In this study, known as FORT-T (Forty and Over Treatment Trial), women were randomized to receive either Clomid with IUI, gonadotropins with IUI, or IVF. After two cycles of IUI, pregnancy rates were 21.6 percent with Clomid and 17.3 percent with gonadotropins, as compared to 49 percent after one round of IVF.[31] Over 84 percent of all pregnancies in the study came from IVF, leading to the recommendation that women aged thirty-eight and older should consider limiting the number of OI and IUI cycles or bypassing them completely and moving faster to IVF.

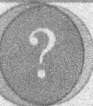 *Common Questions*

**Can metformin be used for ovulation induction?**

Metformin is a medication used to improve insulin resistance. Since insulin resistance is an important component in the metabolic changes seen with PCOS, around 30 percent of women with PCOS will ovulate in response to metformin treatment alone.[32] Metformin treatment improves live birth rates in women with PCOS over placebo.[33] Although metformin alone may not be sufficient in all patients with PCOS, it can be considered as a potential first-line treatment option or an adjunct treatment with additional ovulation induction medications.

## Intrauterine Insemination (IUI)

IUI, sometimes called "artificial insemination," is used to treat mild male factor, unexplained infertility, or for donor sperm conception. Sperm is processed to concentrate and remove debris, then placed into a small catheter and injected into the uterus. This is a quick procedure done in the office, similar to a Pap smear. In IUI, we are trying to get the sperm closer to the egg. I always use an analogy of a football field. An IUI is letting your best players start farther downfield, but it doesn't guarantee they will score or win the game.

### Male Factor

Live birth rates with IUI will never exceed maternal age–related fertility rates. Highest IUI success rates are seen when the number of total moving sperm in the insemination is at least ten million.[34] Since approximately 50 percent of the sperm is lost in the IUI processing, we ideally want a TMS of at least twenty million on semen analysis to be a good candidate for IUI.

Abnormal sperm morphology is not a contraindication for IUI, but highest live birth rates are seen with normal sperm morphology.[35,36] As abnormal morphology is often associated with high inflammatory states, lifestyle interventions should always be reviewed.

### Unexplained Infertility

IUI can be used in combination with ovulation induction as a potential treatment for unexplained infertility. Up to three cycles of OI with IUI can be considered in women under age thirty-eight. If pregnancy is not achieved after three cycles, I recommend a follow-up with your doctor to discuss the best next steps, as progressing on to IVF may be more cost-effective, pending your situation.[37] As discussed earlier, women thirty-eight and older should consider skipping IUI and proceeding right to IVF.[38]

### Donor Sperm

IUI is an excellent treatment option for donor sperm conception, and success rate matches age-expected fertility rates. I always recommend a complete fertility evaluation prior to purchasing donor sperm. Depending on age, if pregnancy has not occurred after four to six IUI attempts, IVF is often recommended.

 *Common Questions*

**Do I need to lie flat after my IUI?**

Sperm will rapidly swim through the fallopian tubes and will not travel back down through the cervix or out the vagina. One study found no

> difference in pregnancy rates when comparing lying flat for fifteen minutes after an IUI versus immediate movement.[39] I like to have my patients rest for a couple of calm minutes just for stress reduction prior to leaving, but you can feel free to get up and go.

## In Vitro Fertilization (IVF)

In vitro fertilization has revolutionized fertility treatments and is often the best option for many conditions, especially when all fertility factors and family planning goals are considered. In IVF, we want to get all the eggs outside the vault to grow instead of just one. This means that each person will be limited by their own ovarian reserve. Since we can only get the eggs outside the vault to grow, we are not tapping into the vault or decreasing your total egg count—meaning IVF does not harm your future fertility or your ovarian reserve.

**POTENTIAL INDICATIONS FOR IVF**

| | |
|---|---|
| Age | Recurrent pregnancy loss |
| Tubal factor | Genetic disease |
| Male factor | Egg donation |
| Hypothalamic amenorrhea | Reciprocal IVF |
| PCOS | Sperm donation |
| Unexplained infertility | Gestational carrier |
| Endometriosis | Fertility preservation |
| Adenomyosis | Sex selection |

During IVF, gonadotropin injections are used for approximately eight to twelve days to stimulate egg growth. You will see a doctor for monitoring appointments every two to three days with ultrasounds and blood work. Because IVF requires overriding the normal communication between the brain and ovaries, a medication must also be used to suppress ovulation. The combination of suppression and stimulation medication is called the

"IVF protocol," and protocols are named based on the type of suppression used. If a second cycle is needed, the first cycle should be reviewed to see if any changes are needed.

Once the eggs reach maturity, determined by ultrasound size and estrogen level, you will use a "trigger" medication to help the eggs finalize the process of maturity. Since we don't have an isolated LH medication, the trigger is either hCG or Lupron—both work by mimicking LH or sending out LH.

The leading two protocols are a GnRH agonist (Lupron protocol) or a GnRH antagonist (antagonist protocol). Stimulation is typically with FSH but can include FSH/LH, Clomid, letrozole, and even Lupron. Within each of these options are many different variations depending on clinical circumstance, but your IVF protocol should be personalized and made based on ovarian reserve, age, medical history, and prior cycle response.

1. **Lupron protocols:** With Lupron, the pituitary gland releases all stored FSH/LH and prevents further production, called "downregulating" the pituitary. These are known as "long" protocols as Lupron must be started before stimulation, in the luteal phase or overlapping with birth control. Lupron is a great option for patients with lower than average ovarian reserve, endometriosis, or autoimmune disease. Patients using Lupron must use hCG for a trigger and are at risk for ovarian hyperstimulation syndrome (OHSS). There are many variations in timing, dose, and length of Lupron use.

2. **Antagonist protocols:** GnRH antagonists block release of gonadotropins, but they are expensive and very short-acting. These are excellent protocols if you have high ovarian reserve (like PCOS), as Lupron can be used for a trigger over hCG, decreasing the risk of OHSS. Many antagonist protocols are first primed with birth control pills, estrogen, progesterone, or even testosterone. Mini-stim protocols are antagonist protocols that use lower gonadotropin doses for stimulation; this may be advantageous for some women, but it can dramatically understimulate the ovaries and result in a poor outcome for most women.

After a trigger, we extract the eggs in a procedure called the egg retrieval. This is performed under anesthesia using a needle attached to a vaginal ultrasound. The needle is inserted into each follicle, the follicular fluid is drained, and the eggs are then identified in the lab. After retrieval, the eggs are combined with sperm for fertilization, either with conventional fertilization or intracytoplasmic sperm injection (ICSI).

**FERTILIZATION OPTIONS FOR IVF**

| Fertilization Type | Description |
| --- | --- |
| Conventional | Sperm and egg are placed in a dish to incubate; sperm must fertilize eggs on their own |
| Intracytoplasmic sperm injection (ICSI) | Single sperm is injected into an egg under a microscope; best for male factor, genetic testing, failed fertilization |

The fertilized eggs are now embryos and will grow in the lab for the next five to six days until they reach the implantation stage, known as a blastocyst. At the blastocyst stage, embryos can be transferred into the body, frozen, or biopsied for genetic testing.

One of the most difficult aspects of IVF is the attrition. Not every egg will be mature, fertilize, become an embryo, or be genetically normal (euploid). The table on the following page shows average attrition, but remember what average means: Some people will have higher rates, while others will have lower rates. As expected, the percentage of genetically

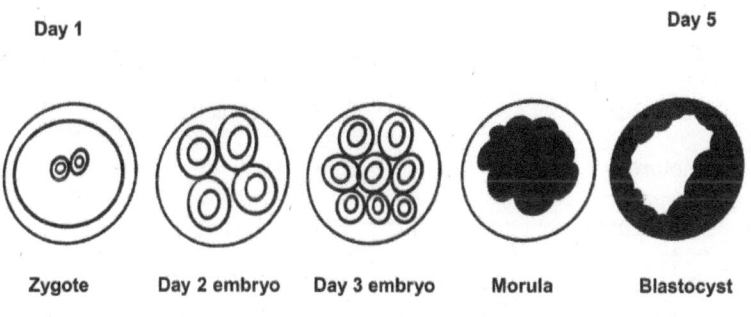

Stages of Embryo Development

normal embryos declines with age, with a more significant drop at age thirty-seven and beyond.[40]

Preimplantation genetic testing (PGT) is the sampling of five to ten cells from the outer layer of the embryo (known as the trophectoderm) and then sending these cells off for sampling to determine the rate of euploid (genetically normal) embryos. PGT-A is utilizing PGT to check for aneuploidy— or an abnormal chromosome number. Embryos can result neither euploid or aneuploid but mosaic (cells exhibit both normal and abnormal results). Mosaic embryos are further defined as either low-level mosaics (most the cells are normal) and high-level mosaic (most the cells are abnormal). A euploid embryo has the highest odds of live birth, around 65 percent per transfer, while mosaic embryos have the potential for live birth, but at lower rates.[41] PGT can also be used to test for single gene disorders, known as PGT-M (for monogenetic disease) or for balanced translocations, known as PGT-SR (for structural rearrangement).

Importantly, older studies are frequently quoted providing relatively high rates of euploidy from technology prior to detecting mosaic embryos. This doesn't reflect true patient experience. However, once we account for aneuploid and mosaic embryos, the euploid rate per age bracket (seen in the table below) is reflective of what we see in clinical practice.[42,43] PGT-A is not needed for all patients, but is encouraged as women get older and have fewer embryos to test. Further, I think PGT-A is very helpful in family planning. If you knew you had no genetically normal embryos, would you do another cycle? If you have the resources, the answer is likely yes. If you are freezing embryos now with the intent to use in the future, knowing the number of genetically normal embryos is essential information to aid in your decision-making.

**AVERAGE ATTRITION IN IVF CYCLES BY STAGE**

| Milestone | % of Stage Before |
| --- | --- |
| Mature | 80% |
| Fertilization | 75% |
| Blastocyst development | 50% |

| Milestone | % of Stage Before |
|---|---|
| Euploid % by age (years) ≤35 | 65% |
| 35–37 | 56% |
| 38–40 | 45% |
| 41–42 | 30% |
| >42 | 21% |

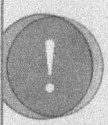

## *Important Study Findings:* How Many of Your Embryos Are Normal?

"Aneuploidy Rates and Likelihood of Obtaining a Usable Embryo for Transfer Among In Vitro Fertilization Cycles Using Preimplantation Genetic Testing for Monogenic Disorders and Aneuploidy Compared with In Vitro Fertilization Cycles Using Preimplantation Genetic Testing for Aneuploidy Alone"[44]

- **Study basics:** This study evaluated over 75,522 IVF cycles with biopsied embryos to determine euploid rates in patients doing both PGT-A compared to PGT-M.

- **Results:** The percentage of genetically normal embryos decreases with age, just as egg quality decreases. At age thirty-five and younger, 65 percent of embryos are genetically normal, 56 percent are normal between thirty-five and thirty-seven, 45 percent are normal between thirty-eight and forty, 30 percent are normal between forty-one and forty-two, and 21 percent are normal at forty-three and beyond.

- **Conclusion:** At age thirty-five, around half your eggs are already genetically abnormal, and the percentage of abnormal embryos increases each subsequent year.

Your odds of IVF success depend on age, ovarian reserve, and egg and sperm quality. In any one cycle we may not have success, but that does not mean success is not possible. One of the advantages of IVF is the ability to more efficiently utilize the eggs available in a given month to find any genetically normal embryos. This has a huge advantage as women age.

To put this in perspective, let's compare an average forty-year-old and thirty-year-old, assuming both have an average follicle count and attrition in an IVF cycle.

**EXAMPLE AVERAGE IVF CYCLE OUTCOMES BY AGE**

| Development Stage | 30-Year-Old | 40-Year-Old |
|---|---|---|
| Follicle count | 20 | 10 |
| Mature eggs | 16 | 8 |
| Fertilized | 12 | 6 |
| Blastocysts | 6 | 3 |
| Euploid | 3 | 1 |

For one IVF cycle, the thirty-year-old would end up with three normal embryos while the forty-year-old would end up with one normal embryo. You can easily see how a forty-year-old may end up with no normal embryos if they have a lower AFC or fall below average on any aspect of a cycle. That doesn't mean the forty-year-old will never have a normal embryo, but she may need more cycles to have success.

### Embryo Transfer

Once you're ready to become pregnant, an embryo transfer is needed. This is when an embryo is placed into the uterus. This is a simple, in-office procedure like a Pap smear. You can expect to come to the office with a full bladder, review the embryo with the lab, and then your doctor will use an abdominal ultrasound while watching a small catheter advance into the uterus to place the embryo. The process takes less than five minutes and is my favorite procedure to do.

When IVF was first discovered, all embryo transfers were "fresh" transfers, meaning the embryo was not frozen but put into the uterus immediately after developing in the lab. As embryo freezing has improved, the vast majority of embryo transfers are now frozen.

Frozen embryo transfers (FETs) result in improved live birth rates, especially in women over age thirty-seven, due to the ability to synchronize the stage of the embryo development with uterine receptivity and normalize the uterine hormonal environment. FETs are needed for all women with preimplantation genetic testing (PGT) to determine which embryos are genetically normal. Embryo freezing techniques are now extremely successful, with 97 percent of blastocysts surviving the freeze-thaw process.[45]

FET protocols grow the uterine lining in preparation for implantation and are either a modified natural cycle or a medicated cycle. For a modified natural cycle, OI medications are used to induce egg growth; the egg makes estrogen, which grows the lining, and then the transfer timing is based on when ovulation occurred. A "true" natural cycle simply tracks ovulation. Vaginal progesterone supplementation is started after confirmed ovulation. In a medicated cycle, estrogen is given to grow the lining, and progesterone is started once the lining looks appropriate. Estrogen can be oral, vaginal, in patches, or injectable (none are superior to others). Lupron can be used with a medicated cycle and is advantageous for endometriosis, adenomyosis, and implantation failure. Progesterone is not being made in medicated cycles and needs to be administered intramuscularly to provide enough replacement.[46]

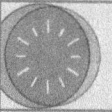 *Top Tip*

**What to do after embryo transfer**

I tell my patients that embryos implant in the wild while you are out living your regular life. That said, here are my tips:

1. Bed rest is not needed and can decrease success rates.[47] A full bladder (needed for transfer) can cause uterine contractions after a sustained length of time. Early ambulation can improve blood flow. You can get up immediately to go to the bathroom after transfer.

2. Laughing after transfer can improve success, demonstrated in a study bringing clowns into the office post-transfer.[48] Carve out time to use laughter to lower stress and improve your odds.

3. Continue to take your medications. They are just as important after transfer.

4. Eat a diet high in fruits, vegetables, and nourishing foods. Plan a great meal for dinner. Cook more in the two-week wait. Stay hydrated.

5. Continue to move your body, but listen to it and rest when needed. I'm a big fan of nightly walks after dinner.

6. Avoid things that would be harmful in pregnancy. No smoking, drinking alcohol, or cannabis—you are pregnant until proven otherwise.

Transfer success rates largely depend on age and genetics, as seen in the following table based on national US statistics.[49] Without genetic testing, age is a significant factor for success, with the highest live birth rate of approximately 40 percent per embryo transfer in women under age thirty-five. After this, a significant decline is seen in each age group. However, euploid embryos have similar live birth rates across age groups, reflecting the utility of genetic testing as a treatment for age-related infertility. These are average US success rates, and individual clinics or other countries may have different results. You should always ask (or be told) your clinic's rate of success per euploid embryo.

**LIVE BIRTH RATE PER EMBRYO TRANSFER (ET) BY AGE**

| Age (Years) | Fresh ET (No PGT) | Frozen ET (No PGT) | Frozen ET (PGT) |
|---|---|---|---|
| <35 | 39.2% | 39.8% | 52.4% |
| 35–37 | 28.4% | 32.2% | 51.5% |
| 38–40 | 11.3% | 23% | 50% |
| 41–42 | 4.7% | 16.9% | 48.7% |
| >42 | 1.5% | 12.7% | 44.4% |

Reported national statistics are typically lower than those we see in clinical practice and studies (due to challenges with how we must report). Most people will have success with IVF if they have enough euploid embryos, as recurrent implantation failure—defined as no pregnancy after three euploid transfers—occurs less than 5 percent of the time.[50] Cumulative live birth rate with a single euploid embryo is 65 percent after the first transfer, 83 percent after two transfers, 93 percent after three transfers, 96 percent after four transfers, and 98 percent after five embryo transfers.[51] I usually tell patients to anticipate needing at least two to three euploid embryos per child they wish to have. Most women will need multiple IVF cycles if they desire more than one child.

Although recurrent implantation failure exists, the data presented here suggests that most patients do not need extreme measures to conceive. I approach implantation failure as an undiagnosed inflammatory issue—endometriosis, adenomyosis, autoimmune, or anatomic factors—and I personalize a protocol based on a full evaluation and patient scenario. In patients with recurrent implantation failure and endometriosis, improved live birth rates can be seen with prolonged suppression with a GnRH agonist (Lupron), GnRH agonist and an aromatase inhibitor (Lupron and letrozole), or an oral GnRH antagonist (Orilissa) in order to decrease inflammatory markers with endometriosis.[52,53] For patients with recurrent implantation failure, I think it is essential to also decrease inflammation with lifestyle optimization, as reviewed in part III. For questions to ask during IVF, and especially if you are not having success, see "Navigating Your Fertility Appointments" in the appendix.

 **Common Questions**

**Why do people recommend McDonald's fries after an embryo transfer?**

This is an old recommendation that has hung around even though the way we do IVF has changed completely. In the early days of IVF, all cycles included a fresh embryo transfer; sometimes we would even transfer two to four embryos at a time. A fresh transfer put patients at risk for OHSS, which is when your estrogen levels get so high that your blood vessels begin to leak out the water component of blood. This can result in ascites (fluid in your abdomen), pleural effusions (fluid in your lungs), thickening of the blood, increased risk for blood clots, kidney failure, infection, and serious illness. OHSS is worse after a successful embryo transfer because the pregnancy stimulates the ovaries to continue to make estrogen, increasing the risk and duration of symptoms.

In modern practice, OHSS is quite rare as we often freeze all embryos for a later FET and we can select improved stimulation protocols that decrease this risk. However, when fresh transfers were commonplace, patients were encouraged to eat salty foods at the time of embryo transfer to try to decrease symptoms of OHSS. Water is attracted to salt, so when you consume more salt, the water component of blood is more likely to stay inside your blood vessels. McDonald's fries quickly became a favorite of the infertility community on transfer day because of the high salt content. Most people having an FET today have very little risk of OHSS. Thus, the fries are really a nod to a prior time in IVF history.

## Third-Party Reproduction

Sometimes you go through countless IVF cycles. Maybe you can't make any euploid embryos or you've had multiple embryo transfers without success. You may have a scarred uterus or a medical condition leaving you unable to carry a pregnancy. Maybe you are in a relationship with someone who doesn't have any sperm or you went into premature ovarian failure. Perhaps you are single and want to pursue parenthood, or you are madly in love with someone of the same sex. These are all reasons you might look toward third-party reproduction to have a family.

Third-party reproduction involves the help of another person to conceive, including donor eggs, sperm, embryos, or a gestational carrier. There may be different testing requirements before proceeding, and a psychological evaluation is strongly recommended prior to selection of donor gametes. All known donor relationships require a legal agreement. Although third-party conception is a complex topic, you can find a high-level overview of different options below.

## THIRD-PARTY REPRODUCTION TREATMENTS

| Treatment Option | Description |
| --- | --- |
| Donor sperm | Donated sperm is frozen to be used for IUI or IVF. |
| Donor eggs | IVF using eggs from a donor can be combined with sperm to make embryos. Donor eggs can be fresh (donor actively goes through IVF cycle) or frozen (egg bank). |
| Donor embryos | Donated embryos can be transferred with a FET. Embryo donation programs vary, and embryo quality should be reviewed. (Should not be called embryo adoption.) |
| Reciprocal IVF | In a same-sex partnership, one partner is the egg source for IVF and the other partner has the transfer and carries the pregnancy. |
| Gestational carrier | A gestational carrier (GC) is not a genetic source of the pregnancy carried. (Should not be called surrogacy.) Intended parents go through IVF, and the GC has an FET. |

Prior to proceeding with third-party reproduction, I recommend a complete evaluation of all parties involved, especially for same-sex couples. I've seen women who have been told just to buy donor sperm and "go for it"; these women can end up having many IUIs only to later find out they had blocked fallopian tubes. They are left without success after spending thousands of dollars, going through many sperm vials, and losing time trying a treatment option that would never work.

Your clinic should be up front with you about how they work with sperm and egg banks, what options exist, and what may be best for you. Ethical decisions will be made about identified (known) or non-identified (anonymous) donation, and these decisions will significantly impact your child down the road. There is no one "right" way to have a family, and even if third-party reproduction was not your first choice for conception, please know that it is a beautiful option.

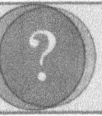

### Common Questions

**Will I still bond with a child that is not genetically mine?**

I can speak from over a decade of experience—genetics are the least important factor when it comes to having a family. I hear this concern frequently, and I understand the fear. Choosing to pursue third-party reproduction is not a failure, it is an opportunity. Holding that baby at the end of a long struggle will make all the prior attempts that didn't work feel like an important part of your journey—because it led you to right now. Third-party reproduction will not be right for everyone, but I've never had a patient feel like this was not the child they were meant to have.

## Surgery

Both hysteroscopy and laparoscopy are surgical procedures that can be used for diagnosis and treatment of infertility, depending on the situation. Surgery is rarely the only treatment needed and is often used in conjunction with other options.

In a hysteroscopy, a camera is placed through the cervix into the uterus. It is typically a quick procedure with a fast recovery. More extensive hysteroscopic procedures may require a short period of recovery time prior to conception attempts. Indications for hysteroscopy include uterine polyps, fibroids, scar tissue, and septum.

Laparoscopy is a more extensive surgery where a camera is placed through the belly button, the abdomen is filled with carbon dioxide gas, and instruments are inserted to operate. Laparoscopy is often an outpatient surgical procedure but has increased risks and a longer recovery. Indications for laparoscopy include hydrosalpinx, endometriosis, ovarian cysts, fibroids, and pelvic pain.

No surgery is without risk. A review of potential risks and benefits should always include a discussion of the full fertility picture, as surgical intervention is not always the solution. There are indications for surgery beyond fertility (pain, bleeding, quality of life), but I often see patients at a place where fertility is our top goal. The three scenarios where I always consider surgery are normalizing the uterine cavity (polyp, fibroid, scar, septum), removing a hydrosalpinx, or implantation failure. You should have a complete fertility evaluation prior to proceeding with surgery.

## Lifestyle Changes

You can't control everything with infertility, but you can improve your success by decreasing inflammation. With chronic inflammation, our immune system is continuously activated, working on fighting inflammation instead of carrying out other important body functions. Inflammation creates a toxic environment, which impacts all aspects of reproductive health, including ovulation, ovarian reserve, egg quality, anatomy, and fertility.[54] Inflammation also decreases your chance of success with fertility treatments.[55,56] Even with IVF, high levels of inflammatory markers are associated with lower live birth rates.[57] Insulin resistance, which we know is highly inflammatory, decreases IVF success rates even in women who do not have PCOS.[58] Chronic inflammation is especially harmful in embryo transfer cycles.[59,60]

Decreasing inflammation is an opportunity to improve your chance of conception even with fertility treatments. In part III, we will dive into all the lifestyle factors impacting fertility, from stress, sleep, and exercise to toxins, diet, and supplements. In part IV, I will provide my step-by-step plan to implement changes.

 **Common Questions**

**Is it time to stop fertility treatments?**

I tell my patients they have four main resources to spend when it comes to their fertility: time, money, emotional energy, and physical energy. Nobody has an unlimited amount of all of these resources. And once you run out of one resource, your journey will likely come to an end. Although money is often a rate-limiting step in fertility treatments, the emotional toll of infertility is what causes the majority of people to stop pursuing treatment. If your doctor is telling you there is nothing more that can be done, and you don't feel comfortable with this decision, please consider a second opinion. The decision on when to stop fertility treatments is difficult for everyone. Letting go of a dream will always be hard, and facing a future that looks different than you planned can be overwhelming. You should know that you are not alone, and I encourage you to seek resources to help. I highly recommend Lana Manikowski's book *So Now What?*

---

Ruby was frustrated that she didn't listen to her gut or push harder to get answers for her infertility. Luckily, Ruby's husband still made sperm, and we were able to do IVF and a sperm extraction. It turned out that he carried the gene for cystic fibrosis (associated with absent vas deferens), and after genetic carrier screening, we discovered Ruby carried it as well. Ruby went through three rounds of IVF to make enough embryos for their desired family size after genetic testing for cystic fibrosis. She was thankful they found out and were able to have a healthy child, but she wishes she had known earlier. Would they have had an easier time with IVF? We can't know for sure, but she certainly could have saved time and heartbreak.

Infertility can be overwhelming, but knowing what to expect will help you make the best decisions for your treatment. One way to combat the uncertainty and fear that can come with infertility is to be prepared and proactive—and that is what this book is all about. Ultimately, what's most important is that you understand your fertility, control the lifestyle variables impacting inflammation, and are confident in your plan moving forward.

### Facts to Remember

- Infertility is no pregnancy after twelve months of trying to conceive.
- If you are over age thirty-five, you should start a fertility evaluation after no more than six months of trying.
- Both partners need to be evaluated.
- Typical fertility testing includes blood work, imaging, and semen analysis.
- Fertility treatments should be personalized.
- Decreasing inflammation can improve success with all fertility treatments.

# PART III

# NATURALLY BALANCE YOUR HORMONES AND IMPROVE YOUR FERTILITY

# 8

# Create a Strong Foundation

## *Stress, Sleep, and Exercise*

As we've been learning throughout this book, inflammation—more than age-related factors—is the biggest contributor to rising infertility. Chronic inflammation interferes with many essential parts of reproduction, including hypothalamic function, ovarian hormone production, ovulation, and implantation.[1] If your body is fighting inflammation, it's harder for the brain to interpret and respond properly to hormone signals, which are essential for both normal hormone production and conception. To set yourself up for a successful pregnancy, you must stop the incoming inflammation and create a healing environment to reverse any damage already caused.

Remember, our inflammatory burden is directly correlated to the exposures we have on a daily basis, from what we eat and drink to the toxins in our food, products, and more. The first step to combating inflammation is creating a strong foundation for your day. Although much emphasis is placed on decreasing inflammation with diet and supplements (and we will discuss this in chapter 9), the single biggest thing you can do for your hormonal health is not found in a pill but in how you structure your day and life—meaning your stress levels, sleep, and exercise.

June was a high-energy thirty-eight-year-old who decided she was ready to be a mom. She didn't have a partner but was excited to pursue single motherhood with donor sperm. She'd had a progesterone IUD for the past five years, and after a few months with the IUD, she'd stopped having a period. However, after her IUD was removed, her cycle didn't return. She presumed it was normal but went to see her OB-GYN just in case. Her doctor thought it may have been from not ovulating and suggested Clomid. June purchased donor sperm, was excited for this next chapter, and started Clomid. She was told to check OPKs and call the office with a positive test.

When June didn't get a positive test, she got worried. The clinic said it was fine and to keep checking. After forty-five days, they brought her in to check her progesterone level, which was low (indicating she had not ovulated). Her doctor increased her dose of Clomid, but her progesterone was low again. At this point, June felt off. She had low energy, weight gain, and brain fog. She knew her hormones were out of whack, but her doctor made it seem like no big deal. Frustrated, June scheduled an appointment to come and see me.

June was hardworking, high stress, and had recently run a marathon. It would have been easy to dismiss her symptoms as simply due to the IUD, but her evaluation told another story. June had a thin endometrial lining on ultrasound, which was not surprising given her five years on the IUD, but she also had low FSH and E2. June had hypothalamic amenorrhea—which had nothing to do with the IUD.

Three years prior, June had started restricting her calories. Around her thirty-fifth birthday, she started fasting, counting calories, and working out to get in better shape. She lost twenty pounds and felt great, but she became obsessed with food and exercise. June knew that overexercising was unhealthy, and she had worked to improve her caloric intake and change her exercise routine over the past year. Unfortunately, despite improving her habits, June was still suffering from undiagnosed hypothalamic amenorrhea.

Once the body has decided it has had too much stress and the hypothalamus shuts off, it can take years for it to turn back on. June was thirty-eight. She wanted to have a child, and she didn't have time to wait for her hypothalamus to get it together.

If left unchecked, inflammation will get to a tipping point where your body will stop trusting you. Your brain will misinterpret hormone signals. Your ovaries will become more stubborn. Unless you break the pattern, this will continue, with worsening inflammation resulting in disease, unbalanced hormones, and an overall unhealthy state. The good news is that you are the one who gets to build your foundation, and you can start fresh tomorrow.

Your lifestyle choices do not need to be perfect. There will always be off days. Some days you will stay up late, get stressed, and not exercise. But if you have a strong routine as your foundation, you will be able to recover from the inevitable challenges that arise. Making poor choices day after day and not taking care of yourself results in your body not being able to handle any additional burden.

Your behavior impacts your body's ability to heal and function normally, and it is time that you really start thinking about how you use your most valuable commodity—your time. When thinking about how you structure your days, I want you to ask yourself:

1. Can I better manage my stress?
2. Am I getting the best sleep that I can?
3. Is my exercise routine hormone friendly?

## MANAGE YOUR STRESS

Our bodies are beautifully wired to respond quickly to acute stressors. Just think about the fight-or-flight response. When you get in a car accident or hear a sudden boom, your stress response activates, turning on the hypothalamic-pituitary-adrenal (HPA) axis. Similar to the hypothalamic-pituitary-ovarian axis, the pituitary sends out adrenocorticotropic hormone (ACTH) to stimulate the adrenal glands to make cortisol and adrenaline. When these hormones are activated, everything shifts into short-term survival mode. Your heart, lungs, and muscles get an influx of energy. Your digestion slows. The brain stops sending out FSH and LH because you don't need to ovulate right now. You need to run from the bear.

Our immune response is tightly connected to our level of stress. Remember, your hypothalamus adjusts hormone release based on the signals it receives from the world around you. The brain cannot see what is really happening, and stress directly interferes with this communication pathway. In addition to interfering with communication, increased cortisol activates the immune system as an adaptation mechanism, resulting in chronic inflammation and insulin resistance.[2] This means chronic stress directly contributes to chronic inflammation.[3]

We are not meant to exist with constant stress. Of course, throughout history and even now, humans have lived through extremely and unceasingly stressful times, including famines and war. To survive, the body shifts all its energy toward essential functions, favoring your heart, lungs, and brain, while ignoring less critical systems, such as hormone production. Cortisol stimulates an increase in circulating glucose levels by directing the liver to break down stored glucose (called gluconeogenesis) and by promoting cellular insulin—this ensures there is adequate energy for cellular function needed to handle an acute stressor such as running from a bear.[4] If we did in fact run from a bear, we would use up this glucose and our hormones would return to normal, but with chronic stress we perpetuate a high-insulin environment without ever giving our body a way to recover.

We are living in difficult times, with a recent global pandemic, a heated political climate, and devasting wars. Furthermore, with high-stress jobs, financial debt, and hustle culture, many people have normalized living with constant stress. This continued stress activation results in elevated cortisol and increased inflammation. And all of this is bad for fertility.

Chronic stress can cause chronic inflammation, hypothalamic disruption, insulin resistance, and hormone imbalance.[5] Stress changes hormone production, increasing the risk of irregular cycles and a longer time to pregnancy.[6] In fact, high cortisol lowers progesterone production—and we now know how crucial progesterone is for conception.[7] In IVF cycles, chronic stress has a negative impact on all cycle parameters, including a decrease in live birth rates.[8] Chronic stress creates such an inflammatory response that it can even lower your ovarian reserve.[9,10]

Self-reported stress levels are shown to be a better measurement of your stress than lab testing.[11] I don't need a lab test to tell me something that you already know. Unless we are concerned about a disease process making too much cortisol (such as an adrenal gland tumor making cortisol), I recommend intervening based on your own interpretation rather than checking lab levels. Actively working to decrease chronic stress is an important part of improving your hormonal health.

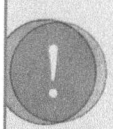 ***Important Study Findings:***
***Stress and Fertility***

"Preconception Stress Increases the Risk of Infertility: Results from a Couple-Based Prospective Cohort Study—the LIFE Study"[12]

- **Study basics:** 501 couples trying to conceive naturally had their hormones checked and tracked their cycles. The stress hormones alpha-amylase and cortisol were measured prior to conception attempts.

- **Results:** Women with the highest level of alpha-amylase had a 29 percent reduction in monthly fecundability and double the risk of infertility.

- **Conclusion:** In women without infertility, higher baseline levels of chronic stress are associated with decreased pregnancy rates. This shows us that infertility isn't causing their stress, but stress is contributing to their infertility.

Nobody wants to be stressed, and I hope that reading this doesn't make you stressed about being stressed. But the best thing you can do for your future health is to start making behavior changes now. You don't have to start big. Just start where you are. What works for me may not work for you. Release yourself from the idea that you "must" do something and instead evaluate how your body feels. You are not meant to live in a constant state of stress, and when you do, your hormones pay the price.

We like to joke about toxic coping mechanisms, but alcohol and food will not improve your stress. You may get a temporary dopamine boost, but you are doing more harm than good. Sleep and exercise are two important components of stress reduction and hormone regulation that I will go over later in this chapter, but for now, here are some of my favorite recommendations for stress reduction.

### STRESS-REDUCTION OPTIONS

| | |
|---|---|
| Personal time | Yoga |
| Mindfulness | Acupuncture |
| Meditation | Time with others |
| Boundaries | Exercise |
| Journaling | Sleep |

## Personal Time

My top recommendation to reduce stress begins with setting aside thirty minutes just for you. Most of us spend the majority of our days catering to everyone else's needs, whether at work or at home. Take some time to prioritize yourself. Make sure you're alone so you're not bothered and can truly achieve stress reduction. You can allot 2 percent of your day to your health, but it won't happen unless you decide to do it. Find something that makes you feel *better*. Think about what calms you, what grounds you, what lowers your cortisol.

If nothing comes to mind immediately, start here: Clench your hands and your jaw, shrug your shoulders up, hold for five seconds, then relax it all. Do you feel that *aaah* calming sensation once you let go of the tension? That is the feeling you are looking for—how can you find time for that during your day?

The cheapest and easiest way to do this is to go outside alone. Stand in your backyard in the morning. Feel the grass between your toes. Take a walk in the evening. My personal favorite is having a cup of tea on the back porch in the morning while I practice a mindfulness exercise.

## Mindfulness

Mindfulness is a coping technique to reduce stress by becoming aware of the present moment while calmly acknowledging and accepting your feelings, thoughts, and bodily sensations without judgment. You are opening yourself up to you, being vulnerable and honest with yourself. Even if what you feel is discomfort or fear.

I recommend mindfulness to all my patients, as it can lower cortisol levels and decrease anxiety. In an IVF study, women who attended a mindfulness program had more self-compassion—and even ended up getting pregnant faster.[13]

Mindfulness can be practiced anywhere and anytime. You may be in a room of people and nobody would even know. Here are my steps for practicing mindfulness:

1. Pause.
2. Bring your awareness to this moment.
3. Acknowledge your feelings and name them.
4. Clearly say why you feel this way, without judgment and with honesty.
5. Accept that your feelings are valid.

## MEDITATION

Similar to mindfulness, meditation is the purposeful clearing of your mind. It is a proven coping technique to reduce stress, lower heart rate, slow breathing, and improve mental clarity—in addition to lowering inflammatory markers.[14]

I love meditating in my bed at night. It took me a while to allow my brain to calm down, and I would have to redirect my brain multiple times at first. Know that this is normal. As you train your brain to step away from the stress, it will lower your cortisol. To meditate, try to:

1. Find your position (straight back with legs crossed or lying down).
2. Focus on your breath. I like a simple four-second process: breathe in for four seconds, hold for four seconds, exhale for four seconds.
3. Begin to focus on each body part from your toes up. How do they feel? What are they touching? Acknowledge any discomfort.
4. When you get to the top of your head, allow yourself space to acknowledge your emotions and stress. Do not go through your to-do list but instead say to yourself, "I am feeling . . ."

## Boundaries

The boundaries you set determine how you spend your time. Every "yes" that you say is a "no" to something else. It might be a "no" to something important to you—meaning you are living your life out of line with your priorities. Your internal self knows this. Trying to balance what you need to do and what you want to do will cause anxiety and even more stress.

Please take things off your plate. Say no to things that you don't want to do or do not have time for, even if it's for someone else. Let go of any guilt. Use this as an opportunity to uplift someone else! I often say no to great opportunities, and I will suggest another colleague who may love that chance. Learn to gracefully say no. Glamorizing doing it all will have reproductive consequences.

## Journaling

I also love journaling as a form of stress reduction, especially brain dumping. For years, I have kept a document on my desktop called "Life Planning," which is where I always dump my ideas, thoughts, feelings, and plans. It helps me put my emotions into words. Reading back through this document is also a great form of stress reduction in that I can see how far I have come and put into perspective my current worries. Many of my creative ideas start in the Life Planning document.

## Yoga

Yoga is the practice of posture, breath, exercise, and meditation that changes the neuroendocrine axis by lowering cortisol and decreasing stress.[15] Practicing yoga actively decreases inflammation, and it can decrease stress and anxiety in women undergoing fertility treatments.[16,17] In women with PCOS, yoga decreases androgen levels and improves ovulation.[18]

Yoga can be a very intimidating practice to start. I remember walking into my first yoga class feeling so out of place. I had no idea what to do. I am sure I looked like a fool, but in reality, nobody cared but me. Yoga is for you. It is a personal practice, and I think everyone can benefit. There are now so many options for you to learn yoga basics online and decrease the barrier to start.

## Acupuncture

Acupuncture involves needle insertion into specific points to decrease inflammation, improve circulation, and promote relaxation. Acupuncture decreases stress and anxiety for many people, especially in stressful situations like IVF.[19] It can improve uterine blood flow in women with implantation failure.[20] Women with low ovarian reserve may also see an increase in number of eggs retrieved in their IVF cycle.[21] If you are having unexpected or poor outcomes in your fertility journey, I encourage you to consider acupuncture as an option.

There is, however, an IVF study that has shown no benefit of acupuncture over "sham" acupuncture (non-insertion of needles, pressure only) during stimulation.[22] This doesn't mean that acupuncture won't help, but it likely is an individual response. That said, sham acupuncture may have its own benefits as well—making it hard to detect a significant difference in outcome. In both cases, stress is likely reduced because you're not on your phone or answering emails but in a calm space and alone with your thoughts. You have nothing to do but be present.

Acupuncture is certainly something you can consider trying, but if you don't have a reduction in cortisol afterward (no *aaah* feeling), then do not feel like it is something you *need* to do.

## Time with Others

An unspoken stressor with infertility is the isolation and the feeling of no longer belonging in your friend group. My patients will often say they feel left behind or like a bother to their friends. I felt the exact same way during my infertility journey. Thankfully, my absolute best advice is also backed by studies: Sharing your journey with a friend and getting support can decrease the stress associated with infertility.[23]

It is more stressful to walk this road alone. Your friends can't show up and support you if you don't let them in and give them a chance. Stop worrying about how you might be perceived or your burden to them and instead believe that they want the opportunity to be there for you during this difficult season.

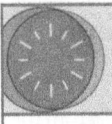 **Top Tip**

**How to reduce stress**

1. Set aside thirty minutes a day to decrease stress.
2. Go outside daily.
3. Incorporate morning mindfulness and evening meditation.
4. Consider creating your own journal and brain dump.
5. Explore other stress-reduction techniques, including yoga, acupuncture, journaling, and therapy. Not every technique will be for you.
6. Don't forget the importance of community. Share your stress with someone you trust.

## SLEEPING BETTER AND MORE CONSISTENTLY

The single most important thing you can do for your health, hormones, and fertility is improve your sleep quality. If this book inspires you to change one thing, let it be this. Sleep is an essential function that allows your body time to repair and decrease inflammation. It can be much harder to get pregnant if you are not sleeping well.

Unfortunately, over 30 percent of adults get less than six hours of sleep per night.[24] Women need seven to nine hours to function properly. Sleep deprivation can be caused by multiple physical factors, including insomnia and sleep apnea. But the top cause of sleep deprivation is our behavior: use of electronics and TV before bed, alcohol, and poor sleep habits (going to bed late and getting up early). How many times have you stayed up late to finish a project, scroll the internet, or watch Netflix? We live in a world where our sympathetic nervous system is always turned on and ramping us up.

Regardless of the cause, poor sleep is detrimental to your health in numerous ways. Sleep disturbances significantly affect your hypothalamus, resulting in metabolic changes, abnormal hormone response, and, of course, inflammation.[25] Sleep is a crucial time for your body to return to homeostasis. Your body uses glucose for cellular functions; insulin levels decrease in response to this improving insulin sensitivity. Even short-term sleep deprivation is associated with an increase in insulin resistance.[26] In an attempt to conserve energy, not knowing when you will get proper sleep again, your hypothalamus signals to the adrenal glands that you are "stressed," and more cortisol is released. Your brain responds to this stress and the hypothalamic signal to the ovaries (FSH and LH) is suppressed, impairing ovulation and hormone production, resulting in low progesterone and luteal phase defects.[27] In fact, women with poor sleep have double the risk of infertility.[28] In a study of IVF cycles, for every hour of sleep a woman lost, she had 1.5 fewer eggs retrieved.[29]

Sleep and stress are deeply intertwined, as cortisol and melatonin—the hormone released in response to darkness, signaling to your body it's time to sleep—work in tandem.[30] When you wake, cortisol levels are at their natural highest and decline throughout the day. At night, when cortisol is low, melatonin is released. Think of it as a scale. When one is high, the other is low. An imbalance can lead to a dysfunctional stress-sleep cycle: If you are stressed and have more cortisol, you will have less melatonin and it will be harder to sleep, which will increase your stress and cortisol.[31]

Decreased production of melatonin is not beneficial to our health and fertility. Melatonin is an important regulator of your circadian rhythm, your internal clock that regulates your sleep-wake cycle. Melatonin release varies throughout the menstrual cycle, with an increase around ovulation to decrease oxidative stress to the egg.[32] In fact, supplementation with melatonin during IVF has been shown to improve egg quality.[33] Disruptions to your circadian rhythm are associated with abnormal hormone production, decreased fertility, and poor pregnancy outcomes.[34] Higher day-to-day sleep variability is associated with longer time to pregnancy.[35]

Sleep is essential not only to women's fertility—men are affected too. Testosterone and sperm production increase during sleep, so having a short sleep interval also results in lower testosterone.[36] Poor sleep quality decreases sperm production and fertility in men.[37] Couples have lower pregnancy rates even when only the male partner is sleep deficient.[38]

You cannot be your healthiest self if you are not sleeping. In addition to increased inflammation, stress, and insulin resistance, lack of consistent sleep also leads to an inability to heal and decreased immune function.[39] When you have less time to sleep, you also do not have time to make the hormones your body needs. Your gonadotropins are increased at night, human growth hormone is secreted at night, and insulin and cortisol decrease overnight. Getting proper sleep is essential for proper hormonal function and balance.

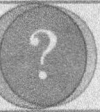

## Common Questions

**Does shift work increase my risk for infertility?**

Shift work interferes with your circadian rhythm and HPO axis, resulting in hormone imbalance and irregular cycles.[40] Night-shift work itself has been associated with abnormal ovulation and stress.[41] In IVF cycles, shift workers had fewer eggs retrieved.[42] Although shift work may contribute to infertility, there is a clear association with poor pregnancy outcomes. Evening and night-shift workers have two to four times the rate of early pregnancy loss.[43]

I'm well aware that not everyone can control their schedule, and I have definitely had schedules that involved night-shift work. However, if you have infertility, pregnancy loss, or are going through IVF, it is important to know that sleep is a variable you can change. Can you swap schedules? If not, what changes can you make? You absolutely must prioritize sleep when you get off: blackout curtains, a sleep mask, white noise, and saying no to daytime responsibilities so you can get seven to nine hours of sleep. It may be hard, but you can do it.

There will be seasons of life where getting proper sleep is near impossible. For me, it was during residency and fellowship when my schedule was not my own. Life changes and poor sleep behaviors are temporary, but you need to make sure you don't let your bad habits carry on. Just because you can survive on little sleep does not mean you should.

Your sleep pattern is also impactful. People who go to bed early and wake up early (following the natural sun pattern) have the lowest risk of infertility.[44] Setting a good sleep pattern and maintaining your circadian rhythm are important. I recommend starting with:

1. Ruling out medical problems
2. Setting a sleep routine
3. Creating a restful environment

### Ruling Out Medical Problems

Many medical problems—thyroid disease, sleep apnea, heartburn, and more—may present with sleep disruptions. Snoring is not normal and is a sign that something may be wrong. Sleep apnea (snoring and gasping at night) is a huge sleep disruptor and can interfere with the brain getting oxygen.

### Setting a Sleep Routine

Your body likes a schedule, and the best thing you can do is be consistent (and closer to the sun in your area, if possible). Wake up at a set time every day (even on weekends), open the curtains, see the sunshine, and step outside. Give yourself enough time to get ready so you don't have to rush out the door. Work backward and give yourself at least eight hours of sleep time. Get in bed thirty minutes before the estimated time each night.

### Creating a Restful Environment

Set the stage for success with a cool, dark room and regular sleep routine. You should limit exposure to electronics in the evening or when it's dark.

I'm bad at this myself, and I've been trying really hard to plug my phone in across my room. You want your body to get the external message (from light) that it is time for bed. Your body's ability to see darkness is a huge stimulus for a normal circadian rhythm.

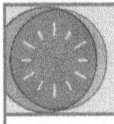 *Top Tip*

**How to improve your sleep routine**

1. Set a schedule; your body likes routine.
2. Establish a goal of seven to nine hours of sleep at night.
3. Limit exposure to electronics in the evening or when dark outside.
4. Make your room dark; use curtains or a sleep mask.
5. Keep your bedroom cool and use white noise.
6. Start a nighttime meditation routine.
7. Stop eating two hours before bed. Avoid caffeine, alcohol, and nicotine in the evening.
8. Consider taking 3 mg of melatonin thirty minutes before bed each night.

## REDUCING INFLAMMATION WITH EXERCISE

Physical activity is important for more than just your overall health. Building skeletal muscle benefits every aspect of your fertility by lowering inflammation, improving insulin sensitivity, and decreasing fat.[45] When you build muscle, your metabolism and sleep improve. Exercise also improves how your body handles stress by changing your hormone response and neurotransmitter release. Dopamine and serotonin, neurotransmitters released after you exercise, can elicit a euphoric state known as a runner's high. I may procrastinate working out and dread it, but afterward I am always in a better mood and feel better.

You don't have to do much to reap the benefits of exercise. Just twenty to thirty minutes a day can lead to calmness that lasts for hours—talk about a great way to manage stress! The WHO recommends that adults engage in at least 150 minutes of moderate-intensity activity and two days of strength training a week, but most adults get significantly less.[46] Non-exercise time is often sedentary—sitting at a computer, a couch, or a desk—which has detrimental effects on your health. Women are often told they need to avoid exercise if they are trying to conceive, but we know that physical activity improves fecundability.[47]

That said, not all exercise is created equal, and too much or the wrong type may be harmful to your fertility. Before you start, take an honest assessment of your body's needs and craft a plan that will optimize your hormonal health and decrease inflammation. The type of activity you choose matters, whether it's vigorous, moderate, low-impact, or strength training. Each has a different effect on your fertility.

**PHYSICAL ACTIVITY TYPES**

| Activity Type | Activity Description | Examples |
| --- | --- | --- |
| Vigorous | Significant sweating, shortness of breath, can only speak 1–2 words | Swimming, running |
| Moderate | Some sweating and shortness of breath, can talk but only short sentences | Brisk walking, cycling |
| Low-impact | Easy to carry on a conversation, do not break a sweat | Walking, housework |
| Strength training | Improves strength and posture, can talk, light sweat | Lifting weights, resistance bands, Pilates, yoga |

If you are trying to set yourself up for pregnancy, I recommend you focus on building muscle and make strength training the core of your exercise plan. Strength training has a clear advantage for your hormone health—by increasing skeletal muscle you can decrease insulin resistance and inflammation.[48] With exercise, glucose is able to move into the muscle cells via a pathway that does not require insulin because muscle contraction increases the action of glucose transporters (known as GLUT4).[49] This means that when you build and use skeletal muscle, you can lower your blood glucose and improve insulin sensitivity throughout your body—decreasing inflammation.

One type of exercise you should be careful about is vigorous activity. Vigorous exercise for more than two hours per week appears to decrease pregnancy rates, with a more severe impact seen with increasing hours of activity.[50] For example, 58 percent of runners have a luteal phase defect or menstrual irregularity, all of which impedes fertility.[51] Overexercising can lead to chronic inflammation and underfueling. One study showed that vigorous exercise did not impact pregnancy rates, as long as calorie intake also increased.[52] As vigorous activity for sixty minutes a day or more will increase stress and cortisol, again leading to chronic inflammation, my recommendation is to limit the total amount and frequency of vigorous activity to only thirty minutes at a time, one to two times per week.[53] This means that vigorous activity can actually worsen your body's metabolic state.

High-intensity interval training (HIIT) is a popular type of vigorous activity that can increase cortisol and result in a fight-or-flight response. It is meant to be stressful and to force your body to adapt to meet the challenge. However, HIIT has been shown to improve insulin resistance and metabolic health, especially in women who have PCOS or are trying to lose weight while trying to conceive, and can be incorporated into a workout plan—in addition to strength training.[54] For other women, I recommend that you limit HIIT to one time per week if you are trying to conceive.

If you are undergoing fertility treatments, always talk to your doctor about exercise. There is no reason for you to be sedentary or to completely stop all activity during treatment cycles. During IVF, for example, any movement is better than time spent sedentary. Women with increased screen time and decreased activity have been shown to have fewer eggs retrieved and fewer embryos per cycle.[55]

However, you will need to modify your behavior in order to prevent ovarian torsion—the twisting of your ovary around its blood supply—which is a surgical emergency. This means no running, jumping, plyometrics, or inversions.

I always tell my IVF patients to imagine their ovaries are water balloons. I want them to stay in their pelvis. Anything that would move the water balloon is a no. If you are preparing for an embryo transfer, you will need to understand your protocol to guide restrictions. Overall, moderate activity and strength building, such as weight training, walking, cycling, and yoga, are encouraged.

## Cycle Syncing Your Exercise

If you're not ready to start trying to conceive but do want to optimize your hormones and health, syncing your exercise needs with your menstrual cycle phase can be an excellent place to start. The central focus for exercise should be to build skeletal muscle and use it with strength training at least three times per week. For me, cycle syncing is when you learn to listen to your body and modify the activity you do on other days of the week. At the end of the day, any exercise is better than no exercise—and it is OK if cycle syncing is not for you.

**CYCLE SYNCING YOUR EXERCISE**

| Cycle Phase | Exercise |
| --- | --- |
| Menstrual phase | Low-inflammatory movement. Walks, slow yoga, resistance training. Listen to your body. |
| Follicular phase | Better glucose usage and aerobic performance. Excellent time for heavier weights, HIIT training, and long runs. Try for a personal best; you can build more muscle. |
| Luteal phase | Higher baseline heart rate with less variability. Focus on moderate activity and sustained movement such as Pilates, yoga, stretching, low-intensity training. |

### During the Menstrual Phase

The low estrogen and progesterone levels of the menstrual phase have been shown to be loosely associated with a decrease in exercise performance.[56] During this time, you should move your body, but focus on low-impact activities that keep your heart rate lower. Don't try to go for a personal best, and don't push your body to exhaustion.

### During the Follicular Phase

When estrogen levels rise, it is the time to go on the long run, do the HIIT workout, and lift the heavier weights. Estrogen improves your cardiovascular function, resulting in both an increase in your heart rate variability and dilation of your blood vessels for improved oxygen delivery. Estrogen also promotes glucose uptake into the muscles, while progesterone antagonizes glucose uptake, meaning that times of unopposed high estrogen are your optimal metabolic state, where muscle can more readily use glucose.[57] The lower basal temperature in the follicular phase also improves metabolic rate. Weight training in the follicular and ovulation phases build more muscle than in the luteal phase.[58]

### During the Luteal Phase

The rise in progesterone during this phase decreases aerobic capacity, heart rate variability, and athletic performance, so allow your body to nourish a potential pregnancy.[59] Take it easy and don't divert your energy. In fact, 40 percent of elite athletes report a decrease in performance ability in the luteal phase.[60] Limit HIIT or trying to achieve new personal bests during the luteal phase. Instead, focus on moderate activities.

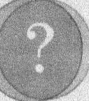

## Common Questions

### Does my weight impact my fertility?

If you are overweight, you have extra inflammation and hormone dysfunction. Losing weight by prioritizing healthy choices and decreasing inflammation can make a large difference in reproduction. A normal body mass index (BMI) is best for hormonal function, and at both ends of the spectrum, your fertility is impacted by hormonal changes and inflammation. An average BMI is 19 to 25, and being underweight or overweight increases your time to pregnancy and risk of infertility and pregnancy loss.[61] Women with a BMI under 19 take four times as long to conceive, while women with a BMI over 35 take twice as long to conceive. I don't love BMI for many reasons, but science shows weight is tied to hormonal health.

## Make an Exercise Plan

Exercise is a way to show your body how thankful you are for it. The goal is to build muscle, improve core strength and posture, increase cardiovascular endurance, and reduce stress—all of which reduces inflammation and is beneficial to our hormones. Creating a weekly exercise plan can help. You don't need to spend time thinking, "What exercise should I do today?" Instead, establish a routine that works for you.

My recommended weekly exercise plan includes a combination of strength training and moderate activity. I like to plan for an activity every day, without an off day. This allows me more freedom for when (not if) I do miss a day. You may need to rearrange days due to your schedule. Of course, always consult with your doctor if needed.

**THE FERTILITY FORMULA EXERCISE PLAN**

| Day of the Week | Suggested Activity |
| --- | --- |
| Monday | Strength training (arms/chest focus) |
| Tuesday | Moderate activity (hiking, brisk walking, low-impact cycling) |
| Wednesday | Strength training (legs/glutes focus) |
| Thursday | Pilates or Yoga (vinyasa, focus on strength) |
| Friday | Strength training (full-body focus) |
| Saturday | Moderate or vigorous activity (hiking, jogging, cycling, interval training) |
| Sunday | Yoga (hatha, focus on flexibility) |

Exercise is not all or nothing. If you stop exercising for a week because you are sick, I am proud of you for taking care of your body. No guilt, no gaslighting, and no starting over. You will pick back up once you are well. We are not exercising for a one-time goal. This isn't to be skinny or run a marathon or get pregnant. We are exercising to decrease insulin sensitivity, improve inflammation, and to benefit our hormonal health.

If you are not exercising at all now, start at twenty minutes a day. Work to increase the strength-training days to thirty minutes. Afterward, start to increase some days to at least thirty minutes. A good goal is to exercise thirty minutes each day. You don't need to go crazy or have hour-long workouts. If you only have fifteen to twenty minutes one day, then only do fifteen to twenty minutes. Just don't be sedentary.

Remember to adjust for your circumstances. If you have weight to lose, incorporating HIIT and more vigorous activity may be beneficial. If you are undergoing fertility treatments, modify your activities accordingly. Different seasons of life will have different needs, and I want you to be OK with that. You only have one body. Control how you treat it.

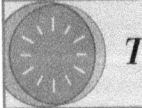 *Top Tip*

**How to incorporate exercise into your day**

1. Aim for thirty minutes a day, but any movement is better than no movement.
2. Make strength training your top priority to build skeletal muscle.
3. Incorporate yoga or stretching.
4. If you miss a day, keep going.
5. Increase time on your feet. Track your steps and try to get ten thousand a day. Get a standing desk. Take the stairs.

Your daily decisions impact your hormones and your health. When June had her IUD in place, she developed hypothalamic amenorrhea from overexercising and undereating. This made getting pregnant difficult. June and I first tried gonadotropin injections for ovulation induction, but she had five mature eggs and her cycle was canceled due to risk of quintuplets—yikes! June decided to proceed with IVF so we could give gonadotropins, take out her eggs and fertilize them, and then only replace one embryo. She now has a child from IVF and has frozen embryos for a possible second.

June has also worked hard on improving her calories and decreasing her stress and exercise burden. After the birth of her daughter, her cycle returned! She still can't believe that the impact of her caloric restriction and overexercising lasted for years and affected her ability to conceive.

I wish I could tell you why so many doctors—my own included—say that lifestyle doesn't matter. The evidence is clear that lifestyle factors—especially sleep, stress, and exercise—and fertility are connected. You have the power to make a difference in your own health. You deserve to be the one making decisions that will determine your future. You can choose right now to start with a strong foundation for your day.

### Facts to Remember

- Create a strong foundation for your day with stress management, adequate sleep, and prioritizing exercise.
- Decrease stress and set aside time for yourself. Figure out what works for you.
- Stop "escaping" your stress with alcohol, smoking, marijuana, and processed foods. These do not help your stress and are toxic.

- Sleep is the most important thing you can do for your health. Create a proper environment for sleep.

- Move your body—not to lose weight or look a certain way but to build strength and improve your health.

# 9

# Eat to Boost Fertility

Four years ago, Daisy easily conceived in her first month of trying and had a great pregnancy, resulting in her beautiful daughter. After breastfeeding for a year, she and her partner decided to start trying for their second. But after two years, she still wasn't pregnant.

Daisy was ready to get some answers. Her OB-GYN ordered blood work, an ultrasound, an HSG, and a semen analysis. Surprisingly, Daisy was informed that everything was normal. She was diagnosed with unexplained infertility and told to see a fertility doctor. Daisy couldn't believe it. She had gotten pregnant so easily before. Could she really have infertility now? She was convinced they would get pregnant once they started fertility treatments, but ovulation induction and IUI didn't work either. Daisy decided to move on to IVF.

Despite being thirty-four with normal ovarian reserve, Daisy had no normal embryos after IVF with genetic testing. She was devastated, shocked, and embarrassed. She was healthy—in fact, she owned a fitness studio and she helped women improve their fitness every day. When she asked her doctor about next steps, all she was told was that she must have "bad eggs." There was nothing she could do.

When she came in for a second opinion, Daisy told me she had no medical problems. But when I ran through the symptoms of chronic inflammation, she revealed she had fatigue, difficulty sleeping, brain fog, abdominal weight gain, bloating, GI distress, painful periods, and pain with intercourse. In fact, these symptoms had been worsening since her daughter's birth!

After more questions, Daisy admitted that she had fallen into some bad habits. In order to lose weight postpartum, she had severely restricted calories.

She was eating processed food on the go and ordering takeout, and her diet was lacking diverse nutrients. Daisy was also not getting enough sleep and often had a glass of wine in the evening to relax after a stressful day.

Even though she appeared healthy on the outside, she was caught in a cycle of inflammation that was resulting in harm. Daisy's unexplained infertility and her failed IVF cycle were red flags that her body was past the point of being able to mask the chronic inflammation and cellular damage.

In addition to being a poor source of nutrients, poor diets are one of the most common causes of chronic inflammation.[1] Eating to decrease inflammation and improve gut health is essential to optimizing your fertility. However, food choice is just that—a personal choice. There is no all-or-nothing approach in this chapter. Some advice you will take, and some may not be right for you. And that is OK. There is no perfect diet or single food that will result in pregnancy. Rather, the sum of our choices matters most. Every decision you make is a step toward improved health and fertility.

To help you better understand the connection between food, your gut, and your fertility, I'll be answering the following questions in this chapter:

1. What is gut health?

2. How can food decrease inflammation?

3. What is the best diet for your fertility?

## THE IMPORTANCE OF GUT HEALTH

The foods you eat contain essential nutrients that provide the basic building blocks for all your body's functions. But in order to use nutrients, they must be broken up and absorbed through the intestines. Inflammation interferes with this process.

My favorite way to think about it is to imagine brewing coffee. The coffee beans are the food you eat, but they need to be ground and brewed correctly before you can sit down with your cup of coffee.

We once had a coffee maker that would grind the beans and brew the coffee immediately (we don't have this one anymore because of plastic—more on this in chapter 10). This coffee maker was easy to use, but somehow, I always messed it up. You were supposed to put in the beans, water, and a filter. The beans would grind, water would heat and pour over the beans, and then the filtered coffee would go into the pot.

My fatal flaw with the coffee maker was that I would put in the filter wrong. Inevitably, there would be little ground bits of coffee and water all over the kitchen counter. The coffee in the pot was concentrated and full of grounds, gritty and completely undrinkable (don't ask how I know that). Without a functioning filter, you can't properly make coffee.

Your intestines are the coffee filter of your gut. At twenty feet long, they work to provide a barrier between the internal function of your body and the outside world. They play a vital role in getting your body all the nutrients it needs, as well as keeping out things that shouldn't be there. If the filter is damaged, things go haywire.

Inflammation directly damages your intestinal "filter." Chronic inflammation results in gaps between our intestinal cells, allowing more than just the nutrients we need to pass into our bloodstream. This is known as "leaky gut."[2]

The symptoms and conditions associated with a leaky gut are all related to inflammation, and include cramping, constipation, brain fog, fatigue, and weight loss or weight gain. Stress can also increase intestinal permeability, leading to leaky gut.[3] Because a leaky gut results in increased systemic inflammation and insulin resistance, it increases the risk of infertility. Even more significant, a leaky gut changes the gut microbiome—which is essential for proper hormone function.

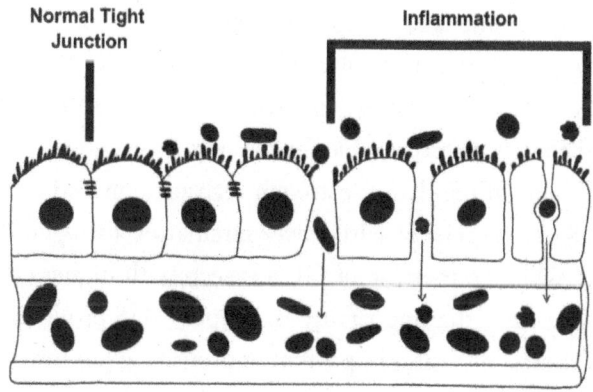

**Normal vs. Leaky Gut**

## SYMPTOMS OF A LEAKY GUT

| | |
|---|---|
| Gas | Overstimulation |
| Bloating | Weight loss or gain |
| Cramping | Headaches |
| Diarrhea | Acne |
| Constipation | Eczema |
| Heartburn | Rosacea |
| Sugar cravings | Asthma |
| Fatigue | Food allergies |
| Brain fog | Joint pain |
| Mood instability | PCOS |
| Depression | PMS |
| Anxiety | Increased infections |

## The Gut Microbiome

Your gut has a natural microbiome made up of bacteria and microbes important to immune regulation and hormone metabolism. Inflammatory foods, as well as toxins and stress, increase intestinal permeability and alter the gut microbiota, leading to an increase in systemic inflammation, altering estrogen metabolism, and worsening fertility.[4]

The gut microbiome is an endocrine system and is an essential component of estrogen metabolism, known as the estrobolome. Excess estrogen is metabolized in the liver to be excreted through bile, urine, and stool. The microbiota of the gut is responsible for making β-glucuronidase (GUS), an enzyme important in regulating estrogen reabsorption and excretion. Low levels of GUS are associated with lower circulating estrogen levels (lower reabsorption), while an increase of GUS is seen with higher circulating estrogen—highlighting the importance of proper GUS production from the estrobolome.[5] Estrogen is also important in protecting gut integrity, and low estrogen states (menopause) result in increased intestinal permeability.[6]

The gut microbiome is extremely important in immune function and inflammation. The gut bacteria secrete by-products, largely butyrate and propionate, which improve insulin sensitivity, suppress inflammation, and decrease gut permeability.[7] Many inflammatory diseases impacting hormonal health and fertility, such as PCOS and endometriosis, are associated with gut dysbiosis.[8] Patients with recurrent pregnancy loss are more likely to have an altered gut microbiome.[9] Your gut is more than a gatekeeper for nutrients—it is a dynamic system important in hormonal health and immune regulation.

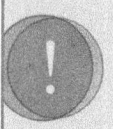

### Important Study Finding: Gut Microbiota and Infertility

"Distinct Gut and Vaginal Microbiota Profile in Women with Recurrent Implantation Failure and Unexplained Infertility"[10]

- **Study basics:** Gut and vaginal microbiome profiles in fertile women were compared to those with unexplained infertility and recurrent implantation failure (RIF).

- **Results:** Infertile women had more abnormal gut microbiota than controls, with different microbiome profiles for unexplained vs. RIF. Vaginal microbiota were normal in infertile women compared with controls.

- **Conclusion:** Gut dysbiosis does not appear to impact the vaginal microbiome. Abnormal gut microbiota is seen with infertility while abnormal vaginal microbiota is more likely to be seen in controls. Normalizing the gut microbiome is important to optimize fertility.

The microbiota of our gut depends on fiber. Many of us are familiar with fiber being good for us without understanding how. Fiber is not digested but passed through our intestines, feeding our gut microbiota and bulking up our stool. Foods without fiber can't feed our gut microbiota, leading to an imbalance in gut flora, known as gut dysbiosis. Abnormal gut microbiota is associated with increased inflammation, insulin resistance, and altered hormone metabolism.[11] Many, but not all, of the factors associated with abnormal gut microbiota are choices we can control, from processed food intake to alcohol, stress, and lack of sleep.

**FACTORS CONTRIBUTING TO AN ALTERED GUT MICROBIOTA**

| | |
|---|---|
| Processed foods | Environmental toxins |
| Sugar and artificial sweetener | Medications |
| Low fiber | Infections |
| Stress | Genetics |
| Lack of sleep | Age |
| Alcohol | Childhood factors |

## FIGHTING INFLAMMATION WITH FOOD

Since inflammation damages the intestinal lining, your health and fertility depend on maintaining a healthy gut. Most of us need to start by healing the damage chronic inflammation has caused to our gut health by stopping the influx of inflammatory substances, especially ultra-processed foods.

Although some food is processed (altered from its natural state) to last longer or for easier use, ultra-processed foods are completely foreign to our bodies. They have had intense manufacturing, with additives, preservatives, dyes, and ingredients that are not natural. Ultra-processed foods are inexpensive, ready to eat, and addictive. They include soft drinks, fast food, processed bread, breakfast cereals, pastries, and processed meats. Most are very low in nutritional value, high in caloric density, and have chemicals and additives. Consumption of ultra-processed foods also results in lower intake of fruits, vegetables, and fiber, which are beneficial to our gut microbiome.[12]

In addition to being poor in nutrient composition, ultra-processed food worsens inflammation and intestinal permeability, opening up passageways for undigested food and toxins to pass through the intestinal barrier.[13,14] This results in immune system activation, increasing inflammation even more to try to get rid of these foreign invaders.[15]

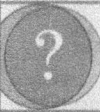 **Common Questions**

**Is fasting beneficial for fertility?**

Fasting may be a strategy to help decrease insulin resistance, but not all fasting is created equal. Intermittent fasting typically describes longer periods of fasting (of more than twelve hours, typically sixteen hours or more) while time-restricted eating refers to limiting your eating window to a set time during the day (twelve hours of restriction or less). When you restrict food, glucose is utilized by your cells, helping to fight insulin resistance and inflammation. However, concern exists about the negative impact of fasting on women's health, specifically by increasing stress and decreasing caloric intake and therefore suppressing the hypothalamus.[16] Women with PCOS who followed a time-restricted eating pattern decreased insulin resistance and androgen production while improving menstrual regularity.[17] I recommend time-restricted eating with a twelve-hour eating window (and twelve hours of fasting), in conjunction with your circadian rhythm. In addition, try to make sure your last eating interval is at least three hours before bed. This allows you to properly augment natural melatonin release and lower evening cortisol, improving sleep and decreasing chronic inflammation.[18]

All nutritional studies have limitations because it is hard to control all variables of someone's diet. This is why I always say there is no perfect diet for everyone. Your microbiota and mine are different. Your needs and my needs are different. However, there is compelling evidence that:

1. Our dietary choices contribute significantly to gut dysbiosis via inflammation.
2. The composition of our diet directly impacts our fertility.
3. Ultra-processed foods are not part of an inflammatory-fighting diet.

You have the ability to change how you approach nutrition and prioritize your own health, starting with your gut. Let's go through the major categories of food and the impact of each on your body.

## Fruits and Vegetables: Your Best Friends

The bulk of your diet should come from a variety of fruits and vegetables, which are whole foods. This means they are eaten in their natural state (raw or cooked) without processing. Whole foods are rich in healthy antioxidants and nutrients, which decrease inflammation.[19] There are no "bad" fruits or vegetables. You should aim to eat as many colors and varieties of fruits and veggies as possible, as different colors provide different phytonutrients and antioxidants, which work together to decrease inflammation.

Fruits and vegetables are a main dietary source for fiber and are essential to a healthy gut microbiota. Although fruit has fructose, a natural sugar, the reaction in the body is much different than with artificial or added sugar. The fructose from fruit is balanced with fiber, which slows intestinal absorption of sugar. Three servings of fruit a day (or more) is associated with a decreased time to pregnancy.[20]

A fiber intake of at least 25 grams a day is associated with improved fertility, but most women eat much less than this.[21,22] Eating more fiber can improve infertility. Increased fruit and vegetable intake is directly associated with increased fiber intake and improved fertility, including decreased miscarriage rates, improved sperm parameters, and improved embryo quality in IVF.[23,24,25,26]

**FIBER CONTENT PER SERVING OF COMMON FRUITS AND VEGETABLES**

| Fruit | Fiber (g) | Vegetables | Fiber (g) |
|---|---|---|---|
| Raspberries | 8.0 | Green peas | 8.8 |
| Blackberries | 7.6 | Brussels sprouts | 6.4 |
| Pear | 5.5 | Sweet potato | 6.3 |
| Apple | 4.8 | Broccoli | 5.2 |
| Orange | 3.7 | Avocado | 5.0 |
| Blueberries | 3.6 | Cauliflower | 4.9 |
| Banana | 3.2 | Carrots | 4.8 |
| Strawberries | 3.0 | Spinach | 4.3 |

A plant-rich diet is the best way to reduce your inflammation and heal gut permeability. This does not mean plant only, but plants should be the mainstay of your diet. I recommend the following:

- Two servings of fruits/vegetables at every meal
- A goal of 25 g of fiber a day
- Eat the rainbow
- Buy organic when you can
- Wash all produce completely

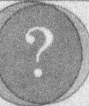

### Common Questions

**Will eating pineapple core help me get pregnant?**

Pineapple core is high in the enzyme bromelain, which reduces inflammation and is a mild blood thinner. Essentially, bromelain is nature's version of aspirin. Since decreasing inflammation and thinning blood may aid in implantation, eating pineapple core around implantation is a well-known fertility tradition. Although no study has shown that pineapple core improves fertility, pineapple has many other benefits—as a source of fiber, vitamin C (an antioxidant), and B vitamins (essential for reproduction), so go ahead and eat pineapple core if you want to (or avoid it if you don't) during your implantation window.

## Proteins: Your Building Blocks

Amino acids from proteins are important building blocks of the body. The recommended daily allowance for dietary protein is 0.8 g/kg of body weight per day.[27] This is a minimum amount needed for daily activity, and many women do need higher levels, especially if they are trying to build muscle, are pregnant, or are breastfeeding. Most women need at least fifty to seventy grams of protein a day, and you should target at least twenty grams of protein per meal. Although very-high-protein diets are popular, they can increase inflammation, especially when animal-based protein sources are largely consumed.[28] This means you need to be selective about your protein sources and increase the amount of plant protein you consume daily.

Many people mistakenly believe that animal meat is the only way to get protein and is therefore good for you. But animal meat has no fiber—it does not benefit your gut microbiota and is highly inflammatory. Animal meats are also high in advanced glycation end products (AGEs), which are toxic. AGE accumulation causes cellular damage and results in poor egg and embryo development and lower pregnancy rates.[29] Animal protein even increases insulin-like growth factor 1 (IGF-1), resulting in insulin resistance.[30]

All animal-based protein, including poultry, decreases ovulation rates.[31] Red meat and processed meat (such as hot dogs, sausage, ham, and bacon) have been clearly linked to an increase in inflammation and cancer.[32] Red meat especially is associated with infertility, endometriosis, and poor embryo development in IVF.[33,34] Men who consumed red meat had a decrease in sperm parameters and lower fertilization rates and pregnancy rates with IVF.[35]

If you consume meat, consider purchasing higher-quality "free-range" beef or "pasture-raised" poultry. Although it is more expensive, it is better for your health. Typical farming and processing practices significantly decrease the quality of meat by feeding animals a high-grain diet, treating them with hormones and antibiotics, and keeping them in very poor habitats.

Unlike meat, fish are high in omega-3 fatty acids and can decrease inflammation. Consuming fish over other animal-based protein sources is associated with an improvement in health, sperm parameters, and reproductive outcomes.[36,37] However, high levels of fish intake increase the risk for mercury toxicity and neurologic damage, so I recommend limiting fish to three times per week or less.

Eggs are another good option. They are high in vitamin B12, vitamin E, vitamin A, vitamin D, and choline, although they do not have a large impact—positive or negative—on inflammation for most people.[38] Eggs may have a potential anti-inflammatory benefit for people who consume plant-based diets.[39]

Plant-based protein is a source of protein that decreases inflammation and improves fertility with little to no downside. Increasing servings of plant-based proteins like lentils, beans, and soy, which are high in fiber, decreases inflammatory markers.[40] Many plant-based foods have higher protein levels than most of us realize and should be incorporated more frequently into our diet. You can meet your protein needs without animal-based products.

**PLANT-BASED PROTEIN SOURCES PER SERVING**

| Plant-Based Food | Protein (g) |
|---|---|
| Tempeh | 17 |
| Seitan | 17 |
| Tofu | 10 |
| Lentils | 9 |
| Hemp hearts | 9 |
| Black beans | 9 |
| Peanuts | 9 |
| Edamame | 9 |
| Chickpeas | 8 |
| Potato | 8 |
| Almonds | 8 |
| Green peas | 8 |
| Sunflower seeds | 7 |
| Lima beans | 7 |
| Chia seeds | 5 |
| Spinach | 5 |
| Quinoa | 5 |
| Asparagus | 4.5 |
| Avocado | 4 |
| Broccoli | 4 |

Even replacing one animal-based protein serving with a plant-based protein is shown to improve inflammatory markers and fertility.[41] IVF outcomes, for example, were improved with higher intake of plant-based protein.[42] In addition, plant-based protein intake is directly associated with progesterone production in the luteal phase, supporting the protective benefit of plant-based protein on hormonal function and ovulation.[43]

When planning out your protein, I recommend the following:

- Incorporate plant-based protein into every meal.
- Aim for at least 50 to 70 g of protein a day.
- Consume up to three servings of fish per week.
- Limit animal meat to one serving a day.
- Do not eat processed meat.
- Limit consumption of red meat to once per week.
- Animal meat should be sustainable—no factory farming.
- Eggs are neutral, potentially beneficial in plant-based diets.

## Common Questions

### What about soy?

Soy has isoflavones, which have estrogen-like properties, known as phytoestrogens. Some people have concerns that soy-based products may impair endocrine function, but soy has not been associated with an increase in estrogen excess or hormonal imbalance. Actually, soy intake in women with PCOS resulted in an improvement in gut microbiota and insulin resistance.[44] Increased soy intake is associated with improved IVF outcomes.[45] Soy is also protective against damage from BPA exposure.[46] In men, soy intake does not decrease sperm counts or testosterone levels, even with high intake.[47,48] Soy is a great dietary option for protein.

## Fat: Your Hormone Fuel

Fat is an important nutrient for your body, as cholesterol—found in fat—is essential for hormone production. However, not all fats are created equal. Some dietary fats can stimulate inflammation while others have anti-inflammatory properties.

Different types of fat include:

- Unsaturated fats: from plant-based sources and fish
- Saturated fats: from animal products
- Trans fats: artificial fat to keep products shelf-stable

Unsaturated fats help fight inflammation and are the healthiest fat choice.[49] They include both monounsaturated fatty acids (MUFAs) and polyunsaturated fatty acids (PUFAs) and are important in improving your good cholesterol and lowering your bad cholesterol.

MUFAs, also known as omega-9 fatty acids, are found in nuts, olives, olive oil, and avocados. Women with higher preconception MUFAs have higher pregnancy rates and a shorter time to pregnancy.[50,51]

PUFAs are omega-3 and omega-6 fatty acids and are known as essential fatty acids, because you need to get them through diet. Increased PUFA intake is associated with improved ovulation and progesterone production.[52] Omega-3 fatty acids are high in fish, flax, algae, walnuts, and chia seeds, and they are anti-inflammatory. A diet high in omega-3 fatty acids can improve pregnancy rates and egg quality, and may even help improve reproductive longevity.[53] Omega-6 fatty acids can be found in healthy food sources, like eggs and nuts, but they are also used in inflammatory ultra-processed foods like seed oils.

Saturated fats, on the other hand, are found in animal products and increase harmful cholesterol levels. Saturated fats upregulate genes, increasing inflammation, worsening insulin resistance, and altering the gut microbiota.[54] A diet high in saturated fat increases the odds of infertility.[55]

Trans fats are industry-made fats, typically identified with the words "partially hydrogenated oils," and should be avoided. They are found in ultra-processed foods and have no positive health benefits. Trans fats are clearly linked to increased inflammation, cellular damage, and infertility.[56,57]

**DIETARY FAT SOURCES**

| Type of Fat | Food Sources | Reproductive Implication | Recommendation |
|---|---|---|---|
| Unsaturated fats | avocados, olives, olive oil, nuts, fish | higher live birth rates and embryo development (especially omega-3) | encourage MUFAs and omega-3 fatty acids |
| Saturated fats | red meat, chicken, dairy, butter, and eggs | associated with worse IVF outcomes | limit |
| Trans fats | fried food, processed food, margarine, microwave popcorn | harmful to all health parameters and fertility | avoid |

Healthy fats from whole foods are an important part of your diet. I recommend the following:

- Incorporate unsaturated fats from whole foods, especially omega-3 fatty acids.
- Limit saturated fats.
- Avoid trans fats.

 **Common Questions**

**What oil should I cook with?**

Many cooking oils have a combination of fats. The best oils to cook with include those with a high ratio of omega-3 to omega-6, such as olive and avocado. Extra virgin olive oil, EVOO, is less processed, more expensive, and has a higher nutrient profile. At high temperatures, oils can break down and release free radicals, causing inflammation. In general, EVOO is better for dressings and lower-temperature cooking as it breaks down at a lower temperature. When cooking at high temperatures (roasting, sautéing), avocado oil is a better choice. If you need oil for baking, I recommend either using melted butter or canola oil, which has MUFAs, PUFAs, and the lowest amount of saturated fat, providing a better taste profile for baked goods. I recommend avoiding oils with high levels of processed omega-6 fatty acids—known as seed oils—including corn, peanut, safflower, and sunflower oil.

## Carbohydrates: Your Energy Source

Carbohydrates are an important energy source. Many carbohydrates contain fiber, which is important in combating insulin resistance. However, it is the quality of carbohydrates that makes a huge impact on your health and fertility.

Complex carbohydrates, such as whole grains and legumes, take longer to digest and provide a stable energy source, which improve insulin sensitivity. The glycemic index (GI) is a ranking of carbohydrates based on how fast they raise your blood sugar (a higher number is reflective of a greater increase in blood sugar). Complex carbohydrates with a low GI are associated with higher total fiber intake and reduced time to pregnancy.[58]

Refined carbohydrates, known as high GI foods, cause a spike in your blood sugar. These carbohydrates include breakfast cereals, white rice, and white bread, and they increase insulin resistance, inflammation, and infertility.[59] Ultra-processed carbohydrates are associated with an increase in miscarriage.[60] Whenever possible, you should look to swap out high GI foods with lower GI options.

**GLYCEMIC INDEX (GI) CARBOHYDRATE SWAPS**

| High GI Food | Lower GI Substitute |
| --- | --- |
| White rice | Brown rice |
| Baked potato | Sweet potato |
| White bread | Whole-grain bread |
| Corn | Peas |
| Cornflakes | Bran cereal |
| Instant oatmeal | Steel-cut oats |
| Flour tortilla | Corn tortilla |

Low-carbohydrate diets can help those with diabetes or insulin resistance prepare their bodies for pregnancy. Diabetics often "carb count" to adjust their insulin dose to the appropriate expected glucose rise. However, low- and no-carb diets have become popular as a way to lose weight. Although these diets can aid in short-term weight loss for those who are overweight or have insulin resistance, they should only be used when medically indicated. Low- and no-carb diets can cause nutritional deficiency and are not recommended during pregnancy.[61]

Carbohydrates are a necessary part of your diet, but carbohydrate composition matters. I recommend the following:

- Limit processed and refined carbohydrates.
- Include whole grain, complex carbohydrates that are high in fiber.
- Choose low-GI carbs over high-GI carbs.

 **Common Questions**

**What about gluten?**

There is no need for the majority of people to be gluten-free for life, but there are exceptions. Undiagnosed celiac disease, for instance, is a risk factor for infertility and miscarriage.[62] Celiac disease is treated with a gluten-free diet to decrease inflammation and improve reproductive outcomes. Some people have a sensitivity to gluten without celiac disease, and this can result in an inflammatory response to gluten. When your gut is already inflamed, it is more sensitive to possible triggers like gluten. For my own infertility, restricting gluten decreased my symptoms of inflammation well before I was ever diagnosed with celiac disease. The majority of people do not need to be gluten free, but restricting gluten for a short period of time and then adding it back in can allow you to see how your body responds.

## Dairy: Your Frenemy

Dairy products are foods made from animal lactation, such as milk, butter, yogurt, and cheese. Dairy provides protein and fat while also being an important dietary source of calcium and vitamin D.

Dairy itself may or may not cause inflammation, depending on composition and tolerance.[63] It may lower risk of endometriosis, especially full-fat dairy consumed in adolescence.[64] However, increased dairy consumption has been linked to impaired ovulation, low ovarian reserve, and low estrogen levels.[65,66] Low-fat or fat-free dairy products may be more harmful than previously thought, as they increase inflammatory markers more than whole-fat dairy.[67] Studies are mixed on the relationship between dairy and sperm production, but higher total dairy intake is associated with decreased sperm parameters.[68]

The impact of dairy consumption differs from person to person. Since the majority of adults have difficulty digesting dairy, I recommend eliminating it, reviewing your symptoms, and then deciding if it makes sense to reincorporate it into your diet. I recommend the following:

- Eliminate dairy for at least thirty days.
- When adding it back, consume in moderation and monitor symptoms.
- Consume dairy once per day, at most.
- If you do consume dairy, choose full-fat products.

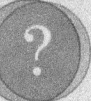 **Common Questions**

**What about plant milk?**

Plant milk has become a common alternative to cow's milk. There are many available plant milks on the market, with soy milk having the most nutritional value due to its antioxidant properties and protein content (8 g per serving, the same as cow's milk). Other popular milks have a lower protein content: oat (3 g), hemp (3 g), almond (2 g), coconut (1 g). Plant milks are excellent sources of calcium and vitamin D, and some types (soy, oat) can have added anti-inflammatory properties. Beware of added sugar and sweetener in plant milk and always read the label.

## Sugar: Your Nemesis

There is no way around it: Sugar is toxic to your fertility.[69] Eating sugar results in high glucose levels, insulin resistance, fat storage, and chronic inflammation—all of which are detrimental to fertility. All sugary food has limited nutritional value while worsening intestinal permeability and gut dysbiosis.[70] Just one sugary drink per day can decrease your fecundability.[71] In other words, one Diet Coke or pumpkin spice latte can make it harder to get pregnant. In IVF studies, sugar is associated with a lower number of eggs retrieved, decreased fertilization, and fewer embryos.[72] Sperm concentration also decreases with increased sugar intake.[73]

I don't believe that you should never have sugar, but it should absolutely be limited, especially if you are preparing for pregnancy. I recommend the following:

- Do not drink sugary beverages, especially those containing high-fructose corn syrup and soda.
- Limit foods that have added sugar.
- Prioritize real sugars—honey, maple syrup, and dates—when needed.

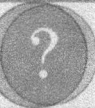 **Common Questions**

**What about alternative sweeteners?**

Nonnutritive sweeteners cause gut inflammation and gut dysbiosis, resulting in decreased fertility.[74] Artificial sugars, like aspartame (Nutra-Sweet, Equal), saccharin (Sweet'N Low), and sucralose (Splenda), have no positive benefit to your body and only increase inflammation. Even sweeteners promoted to be "healthier" or naturally occurring can be problematic. Stevia is a calorie-free natural sugar that alters gut microbiota and likely reduces fertility.[75] Zero-calorie alternative sugars are hundreds of times sweeter than real sugars and can change the sensitivity of your taste buds and increase sugar cravings! I see no benefit to alternative sugars.

## THE ROLE OF SUPPLEMENTS

You should aim to get as many nutrients through your diet as possible, but there are certain situations where additional supplementation may be necessary. I always review supplements with my patients and personalize recommendations. You should always discuss supplements with your doctor.

### Folic Acid

As we learned in chapter 4, folic acid, also known as vitamin B9, is essential for DNA synthesis and cell division. Grains are typically fortified with folic acid, but with an avoidance of processed grains, many people need other dietary sources and supplementation. If you are trying to conceive, folic acid is essential to prevent neural tube defects. Supplement with at least 400 mcg of folic acid a day.

Food sources of folic acid include:

- leafy vegetables, mainly spinach
- brussels sprouts
- asparagus
- oranges
- avocado
- milk
- yogurt
- nuts
- beans

## Coenzyme Q10 (CoQ10)

Coenzyme Q10, or ubiquinol, is an antioxidant important in growth and repair. CoQ10 supports the mitochondria, the energy factory of the cells, and may slow down reproductive aging.

CoQ10 has been shown to improve the number of eggs retrieved and embryo quality in IVF cycles.[76] Pregnancy rates are higher in IVF cycles with CoQ10 supplementation.[77] CoQ10 supplementation also improves sperm parameters.[78] Although CoQ10 is found in low levels in some foods (meat, nuts, fish), it is not enough to raise blood levels, and supplementation is often beneficial.

## Vitamin D

Vitamin D is a fat-soluble vitamin well-known for its role in calcium metabolism and bone growth. Vitamin D decreases inflammation and improves glucose metabolism. It has been associated with improved natural fertility, IVF outcomes, and a reduction in pregnancy loss.[79]

Goal Vitamin D levels are >30 ng/mL a day. I always like to check my patients' vitamin D and target treatment. As more than 50 percent of adults are vitamin D deficient, many women need additional supplementation.

Food sources of vitamin D:

- fatty fish
- fortified milks
- mushrooms
- eggs
- cheese
- animal meat

## Omega-3 Fatty Acids

Omega-3 fatty acids decrease inflammation with their antioxidant properties. Omega-3 fatty acids include alpha-linolenic acid (ALA), eicosapentaenoic acid (EPA), and docosahexaenoic acid (DHA). Women taking omega-3 supplements had 1.5 times the odds of conceiving naturally.[80] Many people need to supplement since food sources are limited.

Food sources of omega-3 fatty acids:

- fish
- algae
- walnuts
- chia seeds
- flax

## Dehydroepiandrosterone (DHEA)

Dehydroepiandrosterone (DHEA) is a precursor hormone to estrogen and testosterone made by the adrenal glands. In patients with low ovarian reserve, DHEA may provide a hormone substrate to potentially improve the number of eggs available and IVF outcomes.[81] DHEA increases androgen side effects, such as oily hair and acne, and should not be taken by everyone. There are no food sources for DHEA.

## Melatonin

Melatonin is well-known as a sleep aid, but it is also an important antioxidant. Melatonin improves progesterone production and egg quality.[82] However, melatonin is not a "more is more" supplement. Doses that are over 3 mg can impact brain signaling and be harmful. Many supplements have well over the recommended amount of melatonin.

Food sources of melatonin:

- tart cherries
- pistachios, almonds, cashews
- white rice
- corn
- bananas
- pineapple
- oats
- eggs
- fish
- milk

## Vitamin C

Vitamin C is an antioxidant that improves immune function and is important in egg selection and ovulation. Higher vitamin C intake decreases inflammation in women with endometriosis, improves egg quality in IVF, and decreases time to pregnancy.[83,84] Vitamin C supplementation can improve progesterone production, ovulation, and sperm parameters.[85,86]

Food sources of vitamin C:

- red and green peppers
- oranges
- grapefruit
- broccoli
- strawberries
- brussels sprouts
- cantaloupe
- cauliflower
- potatoes
- tomatoes

## Vitamin E

Vitamin E is a powerful antioxidant that decreases inflammation. Vitamin E may improve fertility by improving embryo quality, increasing endometrial thickness, and decreasing the pain from endometriosis.[87,88,89] Vitamin E supplementation can improve sperm parameters and pregnancy rates.[90]

Food sources of vitamin E:

- walnuts
- hazelnuts

- almonds
- sunflower seeds
- pistachios
- spinach
- broccoli

### Vitamin B12

Vitamin B12 is an antioxidant found in animal products and fortified foods. Unless fortified, no plant food contains significant amounts of active vitamin B12. If you do not eat animal products, you should supplement with 3 mcg a day of vitamin B12.

Low levels of vitamin B12 may cause clotting and anemia; it may also increase the risk of having a miscarriage, while higher levels are associated with improved live birth rate and IVF outcomes.[91] Men with lower B12 levels also have lower testosterone levels.[92]

Food sources of vitamin B12:

- meat
- fish
- eggs
- dairy
- nutritional yeast
- fortified grains
- plant-based milks

### Myo-Inositol (MI)

Myo-inositol (MI) is important in cell communication and participates in insulin and gonadotropin signaling. MI is an antioxidant that improves insulin sensitivity and menstrual cycle regularity in PCOS.[93] In IVF, MI improved outcomes in poor responders.[94] MI supplementation also improves sperm parameters.[95]

Foods sources of myo-inositol:

- cantaloupe
- oranges
- grapefruit
- nuts
- quinoa
- brown rice
- oatmeal
- beans
- chickpeas

## N-Acetylcysteine (NAC)

N-acetylcysteine (NAC), a derivative of natural amino acid L-cysteine, is a potent antioxidant that can reduce DNA damage. NAC can improve ovulation in PCOS and pregnancy rates in unexplained infertility, in addition to decreasing miscarriage rate.[96,97] In IVF studies, NAC improved embryo quality in women over age thirty-five.[98] In endometriosis, NAC decreased pain and size of endometriomas.[99] Sperm parameters in infertile men improved after NAC supplementation.[100] NAC is not found in food.

## Magnesium

Magnesium is an important cofactor in many enzyme reactions, including the functions of the aromatase enzyme, which converts androgens to estrogens. In addition, magnesium is important for DNA repair, decreasing inflammation and improving fertility outcomes.[101] Magnesium is important in optimizing insulin sensitivity and has shown benefits in improving insulin resistance in patients with PCOS.[102]

Food sources of magnesium:

- green leafy vegetables
- nuts
- seeds
- whole grains

## Zinc

Zinc is an antioxidant important in egg maturation and ovulation. Zinc deficiency can contribute to poor egg and embryo quality.[103] Lower zinc levels have been seen in patients with endometriosis, representing a potential therapeutic option to improve inflammation in these women.[104]

Food sources of zinc:

- meat
- dairy
- nuts
- whole grains

## Selenium

Selenium is important in DNA synthesis and thyroid function with antioxidant properties. Selenium deficiency can result in miscarriage and low birth weight.[105] Selenium impacts both male and female fertility, crucial in sperm development and follicular growth.[106] Although low levels have been seen in women with unexplained infertility, high selenium may be toxic to egg development, and supplementation should be considered only if deficient.[107]

Food sources of selenium:

- Brazil nuts
- meat

- seafood
- tofu
- eggs
- dairy
- fortified grains

## Calcium

Calcium is well-known to be important for bone health, but it is also crucial in hormone metabolism. Calcium is required for neurotransmitter production, which regulates GnRH release from the hypothalamus and is crucial in the LH surge release essential for ovulation.[108] Calcium is also important in follicular development, egg maturation, embryo development, and implantation.[109]

Food sources of calcium:

- leafy greens
- fortified dairy
- fortified grains

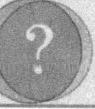 **Common Questions**

**What about vitex?**

The herb vitex, also known as chasteberry, is the fruit from a chaste tree. Vitex decreases prolactin and has potent estrogen-like properties that impair the brain's interpretation of normal ovarian signals. It was even used by monks to decrease sexual desire! Although this might help improve symptoms in some low-estrogen states like anovulation or menopause, the benefit for fertility or PCOS has not been definitive.

> Animal studies have actually shown harm to fertility, but vitex may alter endometrial receptivity, and I do not recommend it in anyone trying to conceive.[110]

## THE FERTILITY FORMULA PLAN FOR HEALING YOUR GUT

As we've been learning, the foods you eat affect your inflammation, gut health, and fertility. If you have symptoms of chronic inflammation or infertility and suspect your diet is behind it but don't know where to start, consider following the Fertility Formula plan for healing your gut.

My approach to healing your gut includes:

1. Elimination—reduce dietary sources of inflammation
2. Nutrition—eat nutrient-rich foods for cellular repair
3. Supplementation—develop a focused supplement plan

### Elimination Phase

The first step is to heal your gut. Reduce all potential sources of inflammation and allow your gut to rest. Start with four weeks of extremely clean and anti-inflammatory eating: no sugar, processed foods, refined carbohydrates, red or processed meat, dairy, or gluten. Also, no alcohol, smoking, or marijuana, and caffeine up to two cups in the morning only. Beware of added sugar in your coffee. We often consume these foods so frequently, especially dairy and gluten, we may not even realize the low level of chronic inflammation they are causing.

Although it may feel restrictive to completely eliminate food, remember that you are trying to break the cycle of chronic inflammation and allow your gut microbiota to repopulate and intestinal permeability to repair. This is a reset for your gut and is not meant to be restrictive forever. I want you to stop drinking for at least twelve weeks as a part of your elimination.

After this, you can decide what works for you. If you do decide to drink alcohol, I recommend drinking only for special occasions and not more than two drinks a week.

**FOODS TO AVOID IN PHASE 1: GUT REST (4 WEEKS)**

| | |
|---|---|
| Sugar | Fried food |
| Alcohol | Processed meat |
| Processed foods | Red meat |
| Trans fats | Dairy |
| Refined carbohydrates | Gluten |

After four weeks of gut rest, you can add back dairy for two weeks. If you do not have any inflammatory symptoms, you may continue to consume dairy. After two additional weeks to adjust, you can add gluten for a two-week trial. If you have any symptoms, rest your gut for two additional weeks. By the end of three months, you will know if you can tolerate dairy and/or gluten, and if they can stay in your diet or should be removed completely.

| Weeks | Elimination and Exposure Guidelines |
|---|---|
| 1–4 | Clean, anti-inflammatory—no exceptions |
| 4–6 | Add back dairy once per day max<br>Add back red meat once per week max, if desired |
| 6–8 | Tolerate dairy? Yes → OK to continue | No → remove dairy |
| 8–10 | Add back gluten once per day max |
| 10–12 | Tolerate gluten? OK to continue | No → remove gluten |
| 12+ | Add back celebration foods on occasion, only as long as there is no inflammatory response based on above testing |

The elimination phase is a short-term restriction. Remember this is gut rest. You are in charge of what goes in your body. Nothing is "off-limits" forever, but your body needs time to heal.

## Nutrition Phase

Greater adherence to healthy diet patterns, including emphasis on whole grains, fruits, vegetables, and olive oil, results in improved health and fertility. Every single day, I tell my patients that they already know what they should eat. We all know what is healthy, but it takes commitment to make change. Remember that every single positive choice is helpful! This is not all-or-nothing.

**THE FERTILITY FORMULA BASIC PRINCIPLES**

| Encourage | Avoid |
|---|---|
| Fruits | Sugar |
| Vegetables | Alcohol |
| Complex grains | Processed foods |
| Fiber | Refined carbohydrates |
| Healthy fats | Fried food |
| Plant-based protein | Processed meat |
| Vitamin D | Red meat* |
| Vitamin B12 | Dairy* |
| Omega-3 fatty acids | Gluten* |

*May be resumed after elimination

The Fertility Formula centers around plant-based eating with complex grains, fiber, healthy fats, vitamin D, and vitamin B12. Plant-based doesn't mean no animal products, but it does mean most of your food should come from plants. Of all the food categories, only plants have no "restricted" items because they are all good for you.

## THE FERTILITY FORMULA FOOD GROUP RECOMMENDATIONS

| Food Group | Recommendations |
|---|---|
| Fruits and Veggies | - 2 servings of fruits/vegetables at every meal<br>- 25 g of fiber a day<br>- Eat the rainbow<br>- Buy organic when you can; wash all produce completely |
| Protein | - Incorporate plant-based protein into every meal; soy is fine (tofu, soybeans); encourage lentils, beans, and other fiber-rich protein sources<br>- Aim for 50 to 70 g of protein a day<br>- Meatless Monday (no animal meat on Monday); max one serving of animal meat a day on other days<br>- Up to 3 servings of fish per week<br>- Limit red meat to once per week at most (none is better)<br>- Animal meat should be sustainable<br>- Eggs are neutral, potentially beneficial in plant-based diets |
| Fat | - Incorporate dietary sources of omega-3 fatty acids<br>- Encourage unsaturated fats from whole foods (avocado, olives, olive oil, nuts, seeds, fish) over trans fats |
| Carbohydrates | - Eliminate gluten for 8 weeks, then add back as per program<br>- Include complex, low–glycemic index carbohydrates that are high in fiber over high-glycemic refined carbohydrates and processed foods |
| Dairy | - Eliminate dairy for at least 4 weeks, then add back as per program and limit to once per day<br>- If you do consume dairy, choose full-fat products |
| Sugar | - Limit added or artificial sugars<br>- No high-fructose corn syrup<br>- Prioritize real sugars—honey, maple syrup, and dates—when needed |

## Supplementation Phase

First, we want to reset our gut. Then we create a good foundation of dietary choices. Finally, we supplement what is needed. Although it would be ideal if all your nutrients could come from your food, it isn't always realistic.

It is always important to talk to your doctor prior to taking supplements. In part IV, you can find details about supplement recommendations for certain scenarios. I recommend you use this as a guide to review with your doctor.

I recommend all women (regardless of life stage) consider supplementing with:

- Folic acid 400 mcg daily
- Vitamin D 1,000 IU daily
- Omega-3 fatty acids 300 mg daily
- Magnesium 250 mg daily

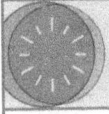 *Top Tip*

**How to know if a supplement is good**

Since supplements do not go through FDA approval, it is important to do your own research prior to choosing a supplement brand. Even if your doctor recommends supplements, not all brands are created equal.

1. Check to see if it is third-party certified. This means the ingredients have been verified, no harmful substances are added, and products are standardized in each batch. Look for labeling to include NSF, USP, BSCG, or ConsumerLab certified.
2. Look at the ingredient list to limit additives.
3. Confirm the dose needed.
4. Check the allergen labeling.

Daisy was told she couldn't do anything to improve her odds of success with fertility treatments, despite her symptoms of inflammation. But after changing her IVF protocol and switching to an anti-inflammatory diet, Daisy had huge success with her second IVF cycle. She was able to get multiple genetically normal embryos and is now pregnant after her first embryo transfer. Daisy was able to take charge of her fertility and improve her cycle success by changing her daily habits. She still needed IVF, but she was able to be more than a passenger on her journey.

There is no one perfect diet for everyone, but it is clear that the foods you eat set the stage for chronic inflammation, increased intestinal permeability, and an alteration of gut microbiota. These changes increase insulin resistance and ultimately result in hormonal imbalance and infertility. Being selective about the foods you consume is an essential component of taking charge of your fertility.

### Facts to Remember

- Your gut health is important for your fertility.
- Poor food choices can cause leaky gut, leading to chronic inflammation, insulin resistance, and gut dysbiosis.
- Your diet is the single most significant modifiable factor for your health.
- The best diet decreases inflammation by focusing on fruit and veggies; plant-based protein; complex, low-glycemic carbohydrates; and healthy fat sources.
- Gut healing requires both elimination for gut rest and proper nutrition.
- Supplement where you need to, but focus on getting most of your nutrients from food.

# 10

# Reduce Exposure to Endocrine-Disrupting Chemicals and Toxins

We are exposed to environmental chemicals, natural and manmade, every single day. With over eighty thousand registered chemicals in the US alone, it is unrealistic to ever imagine a world where you could avoid exposure. Toxins are present everywhere: in our food, water, air, and household items that we use every day. We also willingly ingest toxins in the form of alcohol, cigarettes, and other drugs.

Environmental chemicals directly affect our hormones and how our body functions. If you are trying to conceive, the toxins you are exposed to can not only limit your ability to get pregnant but also influence your child's life and overall disease risk. We now have clear evidence that children exposed to certain toxins in utero have a higher risk of obesity, mental illness, endocrine disorders, and even cancer.[1]

Morgan came to see me after two years of infertility. She was thirty years old, with regular periods and normal testing at her OB-GYN. She had a healthy lifestyle and tracked her cycles without any sign of an issue. Morgan was diagnosed with unexplained infertility and wanted to proceed directly to IVF.

Morgan's IVF cycle looked great. She had twenty eggs retrieved and sixteen fertilized. I then had to call and deliver the terrible news that despite expecting to send off around eight embryos for genetic testing, we had no embryos develop to the blastocyst stage.

Whenever I have a cycle outcome that is unexpected, I have a "WTF" appointment with my patients. Prior to the WTF appointment, I look at each data point, talk to the lab, and try to gather as much information as I can. The only thing that stood out was that Morgan's sixteen embryos all stopped developing around day three at the 6–8 cell stage. This is when the sperm genome kicks in, and a halt in development at day three is concerning for a male factor. This was very surprising because her partner's semen analysis was normal.

At the WTF visit, I asked about any toxic exposures that could be harming sperm quality. It turned out that Morgan's husband failed to mention he uses cannabis each night to wind down and go to sleep. This was not disclosed at our initial visit because he didn't think it was relevant, but it was causing damage to his sperm quality and contributing to their IVF failure.

Although much of the burden of infertility often rests on women, sperm are extremely sensitive to their environment. Unlike your eggs, which are inside your body your entire life, your partner will have an entirely new cohort of sperm in three months. If you are trying to decrease inflammation and get pregnant, you cannot ignore the environment and the world around you—and neither can your partner. It would be impossible to eliminate all toxic exposures, at least not without huge industrial reform. This means it is your responsibility to look at your daily life and understand how the environment you are exposed to is impacting your own health.

Changing behavior can be hard, but you can start by asking yourself the following questions:

1. What are endocrine-disrupting chemicals?
2. What other toxins impact hormones and fertility?
3. How can I remove toxins from my daily life?

## ENDOCRINE-DISRUPTING CHEMICALS

Endocrine-disrupting chemicals (EDCs) are found in the air, soil, water, plastics, food packaging, personal care items, and food and interfere with our endocrine system and normal hormonal function. Many can mimic or block sex hormones or their receptors, impacting hormone levels and fertility. EDCs are also directly responsible for an inflammatory environment, which contributes to a change in intestinal permeability and gut dysbiosis.[2]

There are a few different ways that EDCs can interfere with gut health. EDCs interfere with the gut enzyme GUS, important in estrogen metabolism. If estrogen is not cleared from the body, high levels of estrogen will interfere with brain function. Many EDCs enter our body via our gut, creating a "double hit"—one from the EDC directly and one from a change in your gut microbiota and function.

EDCs also impact brain function and health by interfering with the hypothalamus. After exposure to EDCs, hypothalamic inflammation can alter the release of GnRH, changing your ability to respond to hormonal stimuli. Hypothalamic inflammation may also be a contributing factor to numerous endocrine disorders that impact fertility, including PCOS and thyroid disease.[3]

More concerning, many EDCs are classified as "neurotoxic" and are associated with neurodegeneration, brain inflammation, and damage to the brain-blood barrier (the brain's protective layer).[4] This damage results in loss of brain cells and an increased risk of dementia, neurodegenerative diseases, and psychiatric illness. Every toxic exposure puts your health at risk.

Each endocrine disrupter acts on a different hormonal area of the body. Since many EDCs mimic estrogen, they can directly alter your cycles. EDC exposure can alter all stages of your reproductive life and influence development of many diseases. As many EDCs accumulate in fat cells, even a small exposure can have a lasting impact.

**EDC EXPOSURE ON WOMEN'S HEALTH**

| Condition | Result of EDC |
|---|---|
| Thyroid | EDCs compete with iodine and prevent uptake into the thyroid gland, making the thyroid unable to make enough thyroid hormone. |
| Puberty | Earlier age of puberty is associated with higher exposure to EDCs. |
| Abnormal cycles | EDCs that mimic estrogen can thicken the endometrial lining, causing heavier cycles, breakthrough bleeding, and irregular cycles. |

| Condition | Result of EDC |
|---|---|
| Endometriosis | Increased EDC levels are associated with worsening endometriosis. |
| PCOS | Exposure to EDCs mimicking estrogen increases the likelihood of developing PCOS. |
| Uterine fibroids | EDCs mimicking estrogen stimulate growth of uterine fibroids. |
| Menopause | EDC exposure is associated with earlier menopause. |
| Obesity | EDCs increase insulin sensitivity, resulting in increased stress. |

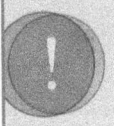

## *Important Study Findings:* Environment and Fertility

**"The Environment and Reproductive Health (EARTH) Study: A Prospective Preconception Cohort"**[5]

- **Study basics:** 477 couples trying to conceive were tested and evaluated, then followed for conception attempts through fertility treatments.

- **Results:** Higher levels of EDCs were associated with fewer eggs retrieved, decreased implantation, lower pregnancy rates, and increased risk of pregnancy loss after IVF (seen with both male and female exposure). Maternal soy and folic acid were protective for BPA exposure.

- **Conclusion:** Preconception exposure to EDCs negatively impacts IVF cycle outcomes and live birth rates, seen with both male and female exposure. Healthy diet patterns may be protective.

If you are experiencing infertility or trying to conceive, it's worth reducing your exposure to EDCs as much as you can. I tell patients every day that we can't undo past exposures, but we can make changes starting now.

The most concerning EDCs you should try to eliminate are:

- bisphenol A (BPA)
- phthalates
- perfluorinated compounds (PFCs)

## Bisphenol A (BPA)

Bisphenol A (BPA) is a hard, transparent plastic and a known endocrine disruptor interfering with hormones like estrogen, testosterone, and thyroid hormones. BPA has been removed from some, but not all, plastics. BPA exposure decreases egg quality and ovarian reserve, results in poor embryo development, lowers implantation and pregnancy rates, and interferes with egg maturation.[6]

The primary source of BPA for most people is their diet. It is especially prevalent when heating up BPA-containing products, like Tupperware, in the microwave, but also water bottles and canned goods.

**SOURCES OF BPA**

| | |
|---|---|
| Canned goods (lining) | Dental sealants |
| Thermal paper (receipts) | Food and beverage containers |
| Water bottles | Eyeglass lenses |

Tips to reduce BPA exposure:

- Don't microwave plastics.
- Look at labels for canned goods. They should declare there is no BPA or that the lining is made without BPA. Get rid of older canned goods (before 2019).
- Use glass, porcelain, or stainless steel for beverages.
- Decline thermal receipts or airline tickets (if you work in that industry, wear gloves).
- Avoid use of plastics #3 and #7.

## Phthalates

Phthalates are industrial compounds used as liquid plasticizers, which can increase flexibility. They are used in plastics, vinyl, cleaning products, nail polishes, and fragrances. Phthalates can cause high oxidative stress and have been associated with poor embryo development, lower pregnancy rates, higher miscarriage rates, endometriosis, and lower sperm counts.[7] Higher phthalate exposure is associated with hypothalamic inflammation and altered GnRH response, resulting in earlier puberty and irregular menses.[8]

Phthalate exposure often comes from food, water, and use of personal products, such as detergents and perfumes.

**SOURCES OF PHTHALATES**

| | |
|---|---|
| Food packaging | Fragrances |
| Take-out food containers | Toys |
| Cosmetics | Medical device tubing |
| Detergents | Plastic in coffee makers |

Tips to avoid phthalates:

- Choose fragrance-free products ("unscented" can be misleading as the product may contain chemicals to mask other fragrances).
- Stop using plastic bottles and storage containers.
- Reduce consumption of take-out food.
- Remove takeout from to-go containers and transfer into glass.
- Consider French press or pour-over coffee over a traditional coffee maker.

## Perfluorinated Compounds (PFCs)

PFCs are synthetic chemicals widely used to prevent binding in consumer goods, including food packaging, cookware, and textiles. PFCs build up in our body as "forever chemicals," and increased exposure is associated with a longer time to pregnancy and altered hormone secretion.[9] PFC exposure changes puberty onset, increases insulin resistance, and alters thyroid hormones. High PFC levels are associated with poor embryo quality.[10] A diet high in fiber and folate is associated with lower PFC levels, making your dietary choices even more impactful.[11] PFCs can be passed through the placenta.[12]

PFCs are used in many industries and leach into the water and soil. The main source of PFC exposure is diet, including fast-food wrapping and packaging, paper plates, and Teflon.

### SOURCES OF PFCs

| | |
|---|---|
| Teflon or nonstick surfaces | Textiles |
| Food packaging | Pesticides |
| Paper plates | Industrial surfactants and emulsifiers |
| Fast-food wrapping | |
| Firefighting foams | Contaminated drinking water |

Tips to reduce PFC exposure:

- Cook on stainless steel or cast iron (not Teflon or nonstick).
- Limit use of paper plates.
- Limit fast food and takeout.
- Don't eat microwave popcorn.
- Remove food from packaging prior to heating.
- Don't use stain protectors.
- Use a water filter (either granular activated carbon [GAC] or reverse osmosis [RO] technology).

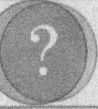 **Common Questions**

**Do essential oils cause hormone disruption?**

Two essential oils that function as EDCs are lavender and tea tree oil. Both compounds have estrogen-like properties that can impact hormonal development and health. Young boys with regular exposure to lavender and tree tea oil developed gynecomastia (breast development).[13] Premature breast development in young girls was also seen with lavender use.[14] Stopping the essential oils reversed the findings. I recommend no lavender or tea tree oil products in your house.

## OTHER TOXINS THAT HIJACK YOUR HORMONES

We are exposed to other toxins besides EDCs, especially via:

1. Heavy metals
2. Environmental contaminants
3. Toxic behaviors

### Heavy Metals

#### Mercury
Mercury is a toxic metal to all organisms. It is often used in thermometers and fluorescent lights, and it is a by-product of coal and other industries. For example, methylmercury is a waste product that accumulates in water and fish. Mercury can pass through the placenta and cause brain damage to a fetus. High mercury levels are associated with unexplained infertility and poor pregnancy outcomes.[15]

Mercury exposure largely comes from fish consumption.

## SOURCES OF MERCURY

Thermometers

Fluorescent lights

Large fish
- King mackerel
- Shark
- Swordfish
- Marlin
- Orange roughy
- Tilefish
- Tuna

Tips to reduce mercury exposure:

- Prioritize seafood with a lower mercury level (shrimp, salmon, pollock, and catfish).
- Do not eat more than three servings of seafood per week.
- Avoid large fish high in mercury.

## Lead

Lead is found in many consumer and home products, like old paint, pipes, old toys, and certain kinds of pottery. Lead is associated with impaired brain development, lower IQ, stunted growth, and puberty delay. Pregnant women should avoid lead, as it can cross the placenta and impact the baby's brain development before birth. Lead can also cause infertility, pregnancy loss, abnormal ovulation, and a decrease in sperm count.[16]

Lead often enters the body through our food or water, or by breathing in contaminated air. Older houses especially remain a potential source for lead exposure. A healthy diet including vitamin C, iron, and calcium is protective and can block lead absorption.[17]

**SOURCES OF LEAD**

| | |
|---|---|
| Old paint dust | Ceramics |
| Contaminated soil and drinking water | Foreign cosmetics (kohl) |
| | Mexican candy (tamarind) |
| Pottery | Occupations (auto repair, mining, construction) |
| Old toys | |
| Pipes | |

Tips to reduce lead exposure:

- Avoid lead-based industries.
- Repaint homes built before 1978, including trim.
- Hire professionals for any renovation of older homes.
- If there is concern about lead in paint or dust, use a wet cloth or mop; do not sweep.
- Avoid imported cosmetics.
- Test your drinking water if you are in a high-risk area.
- Avoid handling antique pottery, ceramics, and toys.
- Remove shoes when entering the house.
- Include iron, vitamin C, and calcium in your diet.

## Cadmium

Cadmium is a heavy metal used in rechargeable batteries, plastics, and paint. It is an endocrine disrupter that causes irregular cycles, infertility, and lower sperm counts. In IVF cycles, high cadmium exposure can result in poor fertilization and implantation rates.[18] It can also accumulate in the placenta, blocking progesterone and altering gene expression, leading to pregnancy loss and poor pregnancy outcomes.

Cadmium is typically a waste product that can contaminate soil and food. Outside of smoking, most exposure comes from your diet. Vitamins A, C, E, and selenium may be protective against cadmium absorption.[19]

| SOURCES OF CADMIUM | |
|---|---|
| Tobacco smoke | Wheat |
| Shellfish | Leafy vegetables |
| Organ meats | Potatoes |
| Rice | Celery |

Tips to reduce cadmium exposure:

- Don't smoke.

- Buy organic root vegetables (potatoes, celery, carrots).

- Avoid organ meat.

 *Common Questions*

**Is it safe for me to use tap water?**

Many people think that bottled water is safer than tap water, but bottled water is often a source for EDCs and other toxins, especially if kept in the heat during distribution or storage. In the USA, tap water is more tightly regulated by the EPA than bottled water. Bottled water can actually contain more contaminants than tap water. In addition, a large proportion of bottled water is actually tap water put in a plastic bottle!

I recommend using a filter with your tap water. My family and I have a reverse osmosis filter. Beware that some common plastic filters may not properly filter out heavy metals or may pose an additional risk due to plastic and aluminum components. Also, remember to never use hot tap water for drinking or cooking, as this can leach lead and other heavy metals into the water. Instead, use cold or room temperature water and then heat by boiling.

## Environmental Contaminants

### Air Pollution

Air pollution is a major threat to global health. It is a combination of human-made and natural substances. Industrial sources include exhaust, fumes from manufacturing natural gas, and coal mining. Natural sources include wildfire smoke, natural gases, and volcano emissions.

As a carcinogen, air pollution causes oxidative stress and inflammation in your cells. Living in an area with high levels of air pollution increases the risk for miscarriage, preterm birth, stillbirth, and autism.[20]

You can't always control where you live, but you should know a way to check the ozone quality of your area and modify your behavior on days with poor air quality. In the USA, the EPA runs the site AirNow (airnow.gov), which allows you to see air quality based on zip code.

Tips to decrease air pollution exposure:

- Decrease outdoor activities on high air pollution days.
- Try to avoid travel during rush hour or heavy traffic.
- Use a high-efficiency particulate air (HEPA) filter inside your home.

### Microplastics

Plastics hold an additional risk beyond EDCs, as they are composed of micro-sized particles that can accumulate inside our body. Microplastics can deposit in the reproductive and endocrine organs, causing inflammation and interfering with all aspects of the reproductive system. In the ovaries, microplastics can destroy normal ovarian tissue, causing fibrosis and leading to abnormal ovulation and hormone production, as well as early ovarian failure.[21] These small particles can even pass through the placenta and change gene expression of the fetus.[22]

Microplastics are well integrated into our world, making complete removal unrealistic. However, decreasing plastic exposure where you can, especially in ingestible sources, is essential to decrease plastic accumulation.

## SOURCES OF MICROPLASTICS

| | |
|---|---|
| Drinks in plastic bottles | Plastic cutting boards |
| Plastic food storage containers | Synthetic fabrics |
| Processed meat | Tea bags (often composed of 25 percent plastic even if marketed as paper!) |
| Processed foods | |
| Food packaging | |

Tips to decrease microplastic exposure:

- Remove all plastic that you can from your kitchen.
- Don't microwave any plastic.
- Wash any plastic by hand.
- Drink filtered tap water.
- Avoid drinking hot beverages in takeaway cups.
- Reduce single-use plastic (e.g., straws).
- Choose natural fibers over synthetic.
- Use laundry balls in the dryer and air-dry clothes.
- Avoid microbeads in cosmetic products (like exfoliating cleansers).
- Limit seafood (it accumulates plastics from the ocean).
- Choose loose-leaf tea over tea bags.
- Change your cutting board to a wooden or non-plastic one.
- Vacuum and dust frequently (to clean microplastics shed from fabrics).

## Pesticides

Pesticides and insecticides are commonly used in the food industry and in homes, so much so that more than 90 percent of Americans have detectable levels of pesticides in their blood.[23] Many people are exposed to constant low doses of pesticides every day, so it is important not to increase exposure. Pesticides are associated with neurotoxicity and degenerative brain disease. Populations with high pesticide use have lower pregnancy rates, lower live birth rates, and increased miscarriage rates.[24]

Pesticides enter the body via direct contact, air, or food contamination. Make sure to wash all fruits and vegetables and consider buying organic, especially the foods with the highest risk of contamination, called the "dirty dozen": strawberries; spinach; kale, collard, and mustard greens; grapes; peaches; pears; nectarines; apples; bell and hot peppers; cherries; blueberries; and green beans. If you do not have access to organic produce, please continue to buy produce and wash it well. Do not avoid fruits and vegetables because of fear of pesticides—simply change your produce-cleaning habits.

| SOURCES OF PESTICIDES |
| --- |
| Bug spray or bug bombs |
| Flea and tick medication/baths |
| Working in agriculture |
| Produce with high pesticide residue ("dirty dozen") |

Tips to decrease pesticide exposure:

- Wash all fruits and vegetables.
- Consider organic for fruits and vegetables, especially for the dirty dozen.
- Remove shoes before entering the house.
- Avoid using pesticides or insecticides at home, including flea baths/dips and bug bombs or sprays.

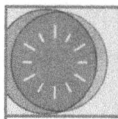 *Top Tip*

**The best way to wash fruits and vegetables**

Per the FDA, most people are not cleaning their produce correctly! The best way to clean produce:

1. Wash your hands with hand soap and water for twenty seconds.
2. Rub produce while running it under cool water for at least ten seconds.
3. For delicate produce, use a colander to run water over and rinse.
4. For firm produce, use a soft bristled vegetable brush to scrub.
5. Dry produce off with a paper towel or clean cloth.
6. Always rinse onions before peeling and chopping.
7. Always remove outermost leaves on heads of lettuce before using.

## Toxic Behaviors

### Smoking

Smoking is known to harm fertility, yet almost 20 percent of adults currently smoke. Cigarette smoke contains toxins and causes inflammation and tissue damage. Women who smoke lose eggs and go into menopause one to four years earlier than their peers.[25] Smoking also increases the risk of miscarriage, decreases sperm counts, and decreases egg quality.[26]

Smoking is transgenerational, meaning you can pass on some of the cellular damage issues to your children, even with secondhand smoke.[27] The sooner you stop smoking the better.

### Vaping

Vaping and e-cigarettes contain toxins such as heavy metals, nicotine, and volatile organic compounds. Vaping can result in hypothalamic inflammation, impaired hormone production, and infertility. Just like cigarettes, e-cigarettes can cause damage that can be passed on to a growing fetus, impacting health and future fertility.[28] Although vaping is not as well studied as cigarettes, it is clearly not a safe alternative to smoking.

## Cannabis

Cannabis interferes with hormonal function and the HPO axis. Women who use cannabis have a higher rate of anovulation and abnormal hormones, as well as a 40 percent decrease in fertility rates.[29] Marijuana use in the year prior to egg retrieval was associated with 25 percent fewer eggs retrieved at IVF and 28 percent fewer eggs fertilized.[30] Pregnancy loss is higher when either partner uses cannabis.[31]

Sperm counts, testicular size, and testosterone levels all decrease in men who use marijuana.[32] Cannabis also clearly impacts gamete development, embryo quality, and pregnancy outcomes. A key cannabis ingredient, delta-9-tetrahydrocannabinol (THC), crosses the placenta. Most edibles have more THC than previously studied, meaning the impact may be even greater than recognized.

Many people falsely believe that cannabis is a safer option than smoking or alcohol. However, cannabis in all forms appears to significantly impact reproductive hormone production and is associated with infertility. Cannabis use is one of the most common modifiable factors I see in clinical practice. There is no safe level of cannabis for your fertility.

## Alcohol

My biggest piece of advice: Just because something is common does not mean it is safe. Alcohol is popular and integrated into our society. Some people will drink and it will have minimal impact on their health, but at the end of the day, alcohol is inflammatory.[33] No amount of alcohol is safe in pregnancy.

Alcohol is metabolized directly into an inflammatory toxin, which increases intestinal permeability and chronic inflammation.[34] Drinking alcohol also increases the risk of anovulation.[35] Women who drink three drinks a week have a significantly decreased chance of conceiving.[36] IVF outcomes and live birth rates are lower if either partner drinks *at all* the month before or during IVF.[37,38]

If you stop drinking, you will decrease your inflammatory burden and improve your hormones. If you are going through fertility treatments, I recommend no alcohol. The impact of alcohol may be more profound in the luteal phase, so don't drink in the luteal phase if you have infertility.

## Caffeine

Caffeine is present in many foods and beverages and appears to increase infertility, with pregnancy loss seen at high intake levels.[39] Coffee itself may alter hormone production more than other caffeine sources.[40] Pregnancy recommendations are to limit caffeine intake to less than 200 mg a day.[41] Be mindful of caffeinated sources that also include high levels of added sugar.

Many people say one to two cups of coffee a day is fine, but this does not mean huge cups of coffee. Coffee brewed at home often has a lower caffeine level than one cup from a coffee retailer like Starbucks. One shot of espresso has 75 mg caffeine. A latte may be a safer option than brewed coffee. Starbucks does have caffeine content for all their beverages listed on their website.

I recommend you stay under 200 mg of caffeine a day, limit caffeine consumption to the morning, and beware of added toxins that can be associated with caffeine, such as added sugar or plastic exposure.

### AVERAGE CAFFEINE CONTENT PER SOURCE

| Caffeinated Food and Beverage | Average Caffeine (mg) |
|---|---|
| Coffee—brewed, drip (8 oz) | 137 |
| Coffee—instant (8 oz) | 76 |
| Coffee—Starbucks (8 oz) | 200 |
| Coffee—decaf (8 oz) | 25 |
| Espresso (1 shot) | 75 |
| Tea—brewed (8 oz) | 48 |
| Tea—instant (8 oz) | 36 |
| Chai (8 oz) | 45 |
| Soda (12 oz) | 37 |
| Hot cocoa (12 oz) | 12 |
| Chocolate milk (8 oz) | 8 |
| Dark chocolate (1.45 oz) | 30 |
| Milk chocolate (1.55 oz) | 11 |

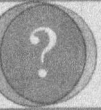 **Common Questions**

**Is heat toxic to sperm?**

The testes are suspended in the scrotum in order to allow for proper sperm development. Since the scrotum is outside the body and typically 4°F (2°C) cooler than the rest of the body, increased scrotal temperature can damage the sperm's DNA and decrease sperm production.[42] Sitting in hot water (baths or a hot tub) three times a month or more decreases fertility.[43] Although sauna use, seat warmers, and laptops on the lap have not definitively been associated with decreased fertility, they have all been shown to impair proper sperm production, especially with increased exposure to multiple heat sources.[44,45,46] Exposure to occasional heat is likely insignificant, but increased scrotal temperature can impair testicular function and decrease testosterone, sperm, and fertility. Intense exercise and increased scrotal temperature impair sperm production.[47] Excess heat should be limited if trying to conceive.

## REMOVING TOXINS FROM YOUR DAILY LIFE

Your hormones are a delicate communication system that can be altered by EDCs, toxins, and inflammation. No matter your stage of life, reducing your toxic exposure is important. But it's especially important if you are trying to conceive. Often, we don't even realize how habitual some of these exposures are, such as buying the same shampoo or using the same water bottle.

It can be easy to feel overwhelmed when trying to reduce exposure to toxins. You can't avoid *everything*, and I know that it is expensive and often not realistic to buy all new products. My recommendation is to start making progressive change. Evaluate your day and determine where the hidden toxins are and how you can start eliminating. Look especially at your:

1. Food
2. Kitchen

3. Home

4. Products

5. Behaviors

## Food

As we've been learning, anything you eat or drink can disrupt gut health and have a direct toxin effect. Changing your food habits results in the biggest bang for your buck. In general, whole foods decrease toxin exposure significantly. Although food delivery and takeout are convenient options, healthy food can be in unhealthy packaging, so cooking at home is always the safest option.

Here are some tips:

- Buy local or organic when you can, especially the dirty dozen and root vegetables.
- Always wash fruits and vegetables.
- Eat fewer processed foods, fast foods, and canned or prepackaged food.
- Reduce takeout; eat at home more.
- If you are getting takeout, remove the food from to-go containers and transfer it into glass or other dishes.
- Avoid microwave popcorn.
- Eat no more than three servings of seafood per week.
- Avoid high-mercury-level fish and prioritize seafood with a lower mercury level (shrimp, salmon, pollock, and catfish).
- Limit animal meats (which accumulate toxins) and do not eat organ meats.
- Include iron, vitamin C, and calcium in your diet.
- Choose loose-leaf tea over tea bags.
- Test your drinking water for lead if you are in a high-risk area.

- Use a water filter (either granular activated carbon [GAC] or reverse osmosis [RO] technology).

## Kitchen

The kitchen is the easiest place to make meaningful change to your toxin risk. Choosing good food is important, but the pots, pans, and packages you use impact every bite you eat. Many of the suggested changes require you to purchase new cookware or products, but you can change one at a time.

Other tips:

- Use glass, porcelain, or stainless steel for beverages.
- Stop using plastic for drinks or food storage.
- Hot drinks should not touch plastic (think about coffee!).
- Remove plastics.
- Don't microwave plastics.
- Avoid use of plastics #3 and #7.
- Choose a wooden or non-plastic cutting board.
- Consider French press or pour-over coffee over a traditional coffee maker.
- Cook on stainless steel or cast iron (not Teflon or nonstick).
- Limit your use of paper plates.
- Decrease consumption of packaged drinks in plastic bottles, including water.

## Home

Your house and your home products can be sources of hidden toxins. If you live in an older home, you may have additional risks that you need to consider. Fresh air can be great to help rid your home of toxic fumes. If the air quality is good, open up your windows, get a screen on your back door, and see if you can be exposed to the outside and the fresh air. Please do not smoke or allow anyone to smoke in your home.

Other things to be mindful of:

- Avoid air fresheners.
- Remove shoes when entering the house.
- Don't use stain protectors on fabric.
- Limit exposure to varnishes and paints.
- Use a HEPA filter inside the home.
- Choose natural fibers over synthetic.
- Use laundry balls in the dryer and air-dry clothes when you can.
- Vacuum and dust frequently to remove microplastics.
- Avoid using pesticides or insecticides at home, including flea baths/dips and bug bombs or sprays.
- Repaint homes built before 1978, including trim.
- Hire professionals for any renovation of older homes.
- If there is concern about lead in paint or dust, use a wet cloth or mop; do not sweep.
- Avoid handling antique pottery, ceramics, and toys.

## Products

The hardest change for me to make was choosing different personal products. I think everyone can relate to finding a product that works and being hesitant to change it, but your skin is a large area for potential exposure. The products you use daily are potential toxin sources, but not all labels make it clear what is "good" and what is "bad."

The product table on the following page lists ingredients to avoid when selecting products. The Environmental Working Group has evaluated many products, so you can look up a product you love and are unsure about. You can search their website (ewg.org) to understand the potential risk.

## PERSONAL PRODUCT LIST OF TOXIC INGREDIENTS TO AVOID

| Ingredients | Product |
| --- | --- |
| Butylated hydroxyanisole (BHA) | Makeup |
| Formaldehyde | Nail hardeners, hair straighteners |
| 1,4-Dioxane | Shampoo, body wash, soap, lotion |
| Parabens | Makeup, moisturizer, hair products, shaving cream, lotion |
| Phthalates | Perfume, hair spray, soap, shampoo, moisturizer, nail polish |
| Toluene | Nail polish, salon-level hair products |
| Triclosan | Toothpaste |
| Sodium lauryl sulfate and sodium laureth sulfate (SLS/SLES) | Toothpaste, soap, shampoo, bath products, moisturizer |
| Diethanolamine (DEA) | Moisturizer, sunscreen, soap, cleanser, shampoo |
| Isobutane | Aerosol products (hair spray, sunscreen) |
| Polyethylene glycols (PEGs) | Lotion, shampoo, conditioner, soap, toothpaste, makeup |

Other tips:

- Review products and avoid hidden toxic ingredients.
- Avoid imported cosmetics.
- Avoid microbeads in cosmetic products (like exfoliating cleansers).
- Look for phthalate-free and formaldehyde-free nail polish.
- Choose fragrance-free products.

## Behaviors

In your everyday life you may be exposed to situational toxins that you should try to avoid. One surprising finding is that thermal paper contains toxins. Every receipt you touch is a toxic exposure. Decline receipts, have them emailed, and don't print airline tickets. If you must handle receipts regularly, use gloves.

Keep in mind:

- Avoid strong chemicals in detergents, paints, varnishes, or glues.
- Decline thermal receipts or airline tickets (if you work in that industry, wear gloves).
- Decrease outdoor activities on high air pollution days.
- Try to avoid travel during rush hour or heavy traffic.
- Avoid smoking, vaping, and cannabis.
- Limit alcohol to less than two drinks per week (none is best).
- Limit coffee to one cup per day.
- Limit direct heat to the scrotum.

* * *

Morgan was shocked that her failed IVF cycle could be due to her husband's nightly cannabis habit. So many of her friends who smoke had no problem getting pregnant! In addition to stopping marijuana, Morgan and her husband reviewed other toxic behaviors and made changes where they could. They started eating healthier, swapped out toxic products in their kitchen, and started cooking more at home. After three months, we decided to proceed with another cycle. This time, they had four euploid embryos—a vastly different result after eliminating toxins. Morgan is now reminding her friends that just because something is common doesn't mean it is harmless.

It is easy to get caught up in an all-or-nothing mentality when discussing eliminating toxins and changing behavior, but don't fall into that trap.

Every single choice, every single change, is an opportunity for you to take better care of yourself, to improve your hormones, and to optimize your fertility. Make the decision right now to choose one thing you can do to reduce your toxin burden. You do not need to be perfect all the time, but you do need to start putting your own health first.

### Facts to Remember

- Even one change to limit toxic exposures can be impactful.
- Eat fewer processed foods and cook at home as much as you can.
- Limit plastic food and beverage containers; never heat plastic.
- Use stainless steel or glass drinkware.
- Use stainless steel and cast-iron cookware rather than nonstick.
- Evaluate all cleaning products and stain removers.
- Limit fragrance in products.
- Review your personal products and swap out any with toxic ingredients.
- Avoid alcohol, smoking, vaping, and cannabis.

PART IV

# THE FERTILITY FORMULA ROAD MAP

# A Guide to Optimizing Your Fertility

Your hormones are the basic building blocks of your body. Now that you understand how they are influenced by the world around you, it is time to evaluate your day-to-day life and how you can integrate these principles into your daily living.

One of the biggest issues I see with my patients is a persistent "all-or-nothing" mentality. Any single change you make is for the positive. Your goal is to craft a healthier life and to understand the impact of each choice you make on your future fertility.

The information presented in this guide is a supplement to the rest of the book. If you came here first, please know that I believe change starts with education. If you don't know the "why" behind these lifestyle recommendations, you are less likely to understand the impact and importance of your choices. This information has already been covered, but it is condensed here for easier implementation and reference.

You should prioritize your hormones, gut health, and fertility regardless of whether you are trying to conceive. My goal is for you to understand what happens throughout your cycle and to be empowered to make the right choices for yourself. This is not just a plan to get pregnant, although it will help you get pregnant. It is a plan to optimize your fertility—and your overall health.

## TWELVE WEEKS OF HORMONE BALANCING

We begin with the Fertility Formula Road Map—my plan for healthy hormones. I'll take you through twelve weeks of a progressive, anti-inflammatory lifestyle. The core of the program is plant-based nutrition, optimizing the world around you, and decreasing inflammation. Although the following guidelines are structured like rules, remember that life happens. But every choice you make has the opportunity to benefit your health.

### Reduce Stress

You need at least twenty to thirty minutes a day dedicated to an activity that helps you lower your cortisol. It doesn't have to be all at once. In fact, you can divide it up equally throughout your day in whatever way works best for you.

Stress reduction requires active thought, planning, and behavior change. I think the most important practice for reducing your stress is setting boundaries and saying no to things that feel more like obligation than opportunity. Pick one activity for stress reduction and plan time for it. My favorite time to reduce stress is in the morning, before my kids wake up. This allows me to start the day in a better mood and mindset—and makes me a better and less stressed mom, friend, and doctor.

Options for stress reduction:

- Mindfulness
- Meditation
- Yoga
- Therapy
- Journaling
- Time outside
- Acupuncture

- Stretching
- Quality time with others
- Napping

## *Daily checklist for change:*

- ☐ Don't look at your phone for the first thirty minutes of the day.
- ☐ Practice five minutes of journaling in the morning.
    - Write down three things you are grateful for.
    - Brain dump for the rest of the time.
    - End with one goal for the day.
- ☐ Walk outside for ten minutes at some point in the day.
- ☐ Don't consume caffeine after 11 a.m., and drink only one cup of coffee a day.
- ☐ Practice five minutes of meditation before bed.
    - If the practice of meditation is new to you, you can go to nataliecrawfordmd.com/meditate for my free "5 Minute Guided Calming Meditation to Reduce Cortisol and Stress."

## Prioritize Sleep

Lack of consistent sleep leads to inflammation and stress, inability to heal, and immune susceptibility. Sleep is the single most impactful change you can make for your hormones, but it is often the first thing we sacrifice. To get the sleep you need, you have to take proactive steps to prioritize your body's healing time.

Recommendations to improve sleep:

- Set a schedule. Your body likes routine. Try to go to bed and wake up at the same time.

- Set a goal of seven to nine hours of sleep at night.
- Limit exposure to electronics in the evening.
- Don't charge your phone by your bed.
- I recommend an alarm that is not your phone and that changes your environment with light and sound (I love my Hatch).
- Make your room dark. I love my sleep mask (highly recommend).
- Consider nighttime meditation. Even five minutes while lying in your bed can be helpful. Use a meditation app if needed.
- Stop eating two hours before bed.
- Consider taking melatonin each night.

## *Daily checklist for change:*

- ☐ Avoid screens one hour before bed.
- ☐ Upon waking, open the curtains or go outside to see morning light.
- ☐ Set a consistent time to go to bed and wake up (which will ideally give you eight hours of sleep).
  - Wake-up time: _____ a.m.
  - Sleep time: _____ p.m.
- ☐ Keep your room dark and cool, and consider getting a sleep mask.
- ☐ Make a new place to charge your phone away from your bed.
- ☐ Create a wind-down routine. My suggestion:
  - Consider taking low-dose melatonin (no more than 3 mg) thirty minutes before bed.
  - Darken the room; have only one lamp on (no screens).
  - Consider light yoga or stretching before bed (I like a downward dog, upward dog, child's pose series, but do whatever your body needs).

- Do a five-minute meditation (you can do the same one as yesterday).
- Turn on a sound machine, use an eye mask, and get in bed.

## Exercise Consistently

Your goal is to build strength to optimize your hormones. In addition to muscle mass, exercise helps to build improved balance, core strength, and flexibility that will help you transition through different life stages. Work to incorporate exercise every day, but if you miss a day, just keep going. Allow your body time to rest if you need it.

My favorite blend of exercise includes strength training, yoga, and a moderate-vigorous activity of choice (hiking is a current personal favorite). For me, knowing what to do each day removes one barrier to success. Instead of trying to figure out a game plan, you know that on Monday, you do upper-body strength training. Your job is to figure out when you will do it, not what to do. Of course, switch the days or create a schedule that works best for you.

### HORMONE-BALANCING EXERCISE PLAN

| Day of the Week | Suggested Activity |
| --- | --- |
| Monday | Strength training (arms/chest focus) |
| Tuesday | Moderate activity (hiking, brisk walking, low-impact cycling) |
| Wednesday | Strength training (legs/glutes focus) |
| Thursday | Pilates or yoga (vinyasa, focus on strength) |
| Friday | Strength training (full-body focus) |
| Saturday | Moderate-vigorous activity (hiking, jogging, cycling) |
| Sunday | Yoga (hatha, focus on flexibility) |

If you already lift weights, continue to do so and work on progressively lifting heavier to challenge your skeletal muscles. You do not need to lift lighter if you are trying to conceive or pregnant.

I know that strength training can be overwhelming if it is new to you. Here are some of my suggestions for easy, go-to workouts for upper body, lower body, and full body. These utilize body weight and both 5 lb. and 10 lb. dumbbells, but they can be modified according to your ability. The goal here is to learn to move your body and not be afraid to lift weights.

The goal is to do ten reps of each exercise for each round. Start with two rounds, with the goal of working up to three. Start with lighter weight and then increase once you can easily get through the set. There are many amazing exercise options, but this can be a starting place if you are unsure where to begin. To see these exercises demonstrated by Dr Shannon Ritchey, physical therapist and founder of Evlo Fitness, go to nataliecrawfordmd.com/strength for instructional videos.

### *Upper body:*

- Shoulder abductions
- Kickstand rows
- Bicep curls
- Skull crushers
- Narrow presses
- Push-ups

### *Lower body:*

- Sissy squats
- Prone hamstring curls
- Reverse lunges
- Standing calf raises with weights
- Glute bridges
- Clamshells

## Full body:

- Bulgarian split squats
- Chest presses
- Reverse lunges
- Push-ups
- Glute bridges
- Ball crunches

## Daily checklist for change:

- ☐ Get at least twenty minutes of movement a day (consider walking, yoga, strength training).
- ☐ Give yourself permission to choose whatever works for your body.
- ☐ Schedule a time to make your movement happen, and commit to it now.
  - Movement time: _____
  - Movement type: _____
- ☐ Increase time on your feet.
  - Stand every hour during the day to avoid long periods of sitting.
  - Track your steps and try to get ten thousand steps a day.
  - Take the stairs when you can.
- ☐ Stretch before and after your movement. Stretching is important to avoid injury and also to improve flexibility.

## Eat an Anti-Inflammatory Diet

Inflammation damages the intestinal lining, so your health and fertility depend on maintaining a healthy gut. Most of us have to start by healing the damage chronic inflammation has caused to our gut health by stopping the influx of inflammatory substances and replacing them with healthy alternatives.

**HORMONE-BALANCING PLAN BASIC PRINCIPLES**

| Encourage | Avoid |
| --- | --- |
| Fruits | Sugar |
| Vegetables | Alcohol |
| Complex grains | Processed foods |
| Fiber | Refined carbohydrates |
| Healthy fats | Fried food |
| Plant-based protein | Processed meat |
| Vitamin D | Red meat* |
| Vitamin B12 | Dairy* |
| Omega-3 fatty acids | Gluten* |

*May be resumed after elimination

In chapter 9, we reviewed each food group in detail to discuss how nutrients can help our fertility and hormone health and how certain foods can actually cause more harm. A summary of fertility-friendly recommendations for each food group is provided in the table on the next page. Remember that there is no perfect diet for everyone, but your goal is to find a healthier way of living and establish a new relationship with food.

## HORMONE-BALANCING FOOD GROUP RECOMMENDATIONS

| Food Group | Recommendations |
|---|---|
| Fruits and veggies | - 2 servings of fruits/vegetables at every meal<br>- Goal 25 g of fiber a day<br>- Eat the rainbow; aim for a variety<br>- Buy organic when you can; wash all produce completely |
| Protein | - Incorporate plant-based protein into every meal; soy is fine; encourage lentils, beans, and other fiber-rich protein sources<br>- Aim for 50–70 g of protein a day<br>- Meatless Monday (no animal meat on Monday); max one serving of animal meat a day on the other days of the week<br>- Up to 3 servings of fish per week<br>- Limit red meat to once per week at most<br>- Animal meat should be sustainable<br>- Eggs are neutral, potentially beneficial in plant-based diets |
| Fat | - Incorporate dietary sources of omega-3 fatty acids<br>- Encourage unsaturated fats from whole foods (avocado, olives, olive oil, nuts, seeds, fish) over trans fats |
| Carbohydrates | - Eliminate gluten for 8 weeks, then add back in as per program<br>- Include complex, low–glycemic index carbohydrates that are high in fiber over high-glycemic refined carbohydrates and processed foods |
| Dairy | - Eliminate dairy for at least 4 weeks, then add back in as per program and limit to once per day<br>- If you do consume dairy, choose full-fat products |
| Sugar | - Limit added sugars; prioritize real sugars—honey, maple syrup, and dates—when needed over artificial sweeteners or high-fructose corn syrup |

## Top Foods for Hormonal Health

Adding fiber and nutrient-rich foods to your diet not only decreases inflammation but can also improve gut health and help eliminate toxins. Below is my list of favorite hormone-supporting foods to consider incorporating into your diet. Review and add foods that you do not normally consume, and allow yourself to try new things.

*Cruciferous vegetables* **(rich in sulforaphane, which supports liver health and estrogen metabolism)**

- Broccoli
- Cauliflower
- Brussels sprouts
- Cabbage
- Kale

*Allium vegetables* **(support liver function and boost glutathione, an antioxidant)**

- Garlic
- Onions
- Leeks
- Shallots

*Leafy greens* **(rich in fiber and chlorophyll, which may help bind and remove toxins)**

- Spinach
- Arugula
- Swiss chard
- Parsley
- Cilantro

*Citrus fruits* (vitamin C in citrus boosts glutathione [antioxidant] and liver function)

- Lemons
- Oranges
- Grapefruit
- Limes

*Berries* (rich in antioxidants, which combat oxidative stress)

- Blueberries
- Strawberries
- Raspberries
- Blackberries

*Healthy fats* (support hormone production and fat-soluble toxin elimination)

- Avocado
- Extra virgin olive oil
- Chia seeds
- Hemp seeds
- Walnuts

*Fiber-rich foods* (help eliminate toxins via the gut and improve gut permeability and the gut microbiome)

- Flaxseed
- Oats
- Lentils
- Beans

- Apples
- Artichokes

*Natural inflammation detox enhancers*
- Turmeric
- Ginger
- Green tea
- Seaweed
- Beets
- Fermented foods
- Warm water with lemon in the morning

Approach the next twelve weeks as an investment in yourself. Your new focus is leaning in and learning to listen to your body so you understand what your inflammation signals are and how to avoid them. Over the twelve weeks, you will start with an elimination phase, followed by adding back, and then maintenance. I view this as time to really get to know your body and optimize your health. Dietary change is an essential step in the Fertility Formula.

PHASE 1: GUT REST AND ELIMINATION

*Weeks 1–4*
- Fruits and vegetables: one to two servings at every meal, eat the rainbow.
- Protein: meatless Monday, then limit animal meat servings to once per day (no red meat).
- Fat: no trans fats.
- Carbs: recommend complex carbs, avoid refined carbohydrates.
- Dairy: no dairy.
- Sugar: no added sugar or processed foods.

- Other: no alcohol, smoking, or marijuana; limit coffee to one cup a day before 11 a.m.

## PHASE 2: ADD BACK DAIRY TRIAL

### *Weeks 5–8*

- Can add back red meat once per week if desired.
- Can add back dairy once per day for two weeks. If you notice inflammatory symptoms, remove dairy for weeks seven to eight. If you do not have any symptoms or gut problems, you can continue once per day.

## PHASE 3: GLUTEN TOLERANCE TEST

### *Weeks 9–12*

- Can continue red meat once per week if desired.
- Can continue dairy once per day if tolerated.
- Can add back in gluten once per day for two weeks. If you notice inflammatory symptoms, remove gluten for weeks eleven to twelve. If you do not have any symptoms or gut problems, you can continue once per day.

## PHASE 4: MAINTENANCE

### *Weeks 12+*

- Can continue red meat once per week.
- Can continue dairy and/or gluten if tolerated.
- Can add back celebration foods on special occasions, as long as there is no inflammatory response based on previous testing.

## Daily checklist for change:

- ☐ Start the day with breakfast, goal 20 g of protein (I love a smoothie).
- ☐ Eat at least six different fruits/vegetables throughout the day.
- ☐ Goal 25 g of fiber a day.
  - High-fiber fruits: raspberries, blackberries, pears, apples
  - High-fiber veggies: green peas, brussels sprouts, sweet potato, broccoli, avocado
- ☐ Include one serving of omega-3 fatty acids (1 oz. of walnuts is an easy snack).
- ☐ No added sugar or sugary drinks.
- ☐ Eliminate ultra-processed foods.
- ☐ Avoid grazing if you are not hungry; think each time before you eat.
- ☐ Look at the "Top Foods for Hormonal Health" food list and add one different food from the list each day. Be adventurous and challenge yourself to try something new.

## Reduce Toxins

Your hormones are a delicate communication system that can be altered by EDCs and inflammation. No matter your stage of life, reducing your toxic exposures is important. It can be easy to feel overwhelmed looking at each toxin individually and trying to figure out what to do, because you can't avoid everything. My recommendation is to start making progressive change to your exposures.

**Fertility Formula Toxin Exposure Self-Assessment**
We have grown up in a world full of toxins, exposed at such frequent intervals that we don't even really think about them. Assessing your current exposure level is the start to learning about how you can optimize your fertility.

Answer Yes or No to the following questions to get an idea of your current environmental toxin exposure level.

## FERTILITY FORMULA TOXIN EXPOSURE SELF-ASSESSMENT

| | Yes | No |
|---|---|---|
| **Personal Care Products** | | |
| I use lotions, perfumes, or hair products that list "fragrance" on the label. | | |
| I use sunscreen that is not labeled "mineral-based" or does not contain zinc oxide. | | |
| I use deodorant that contains aluminum. | | |
| I use nail polish that does not say "phthalate-free" or "formaldehyde-free." | | |
| My cosmetics contain parabens, phthalates, or triclosan (or I have not checked my cosmetic labels). | | |
| **Kitchen and Food Storage** | | |
| I store or heat food in plastic containers or "steamable" microwave bags. | | |
| I use nonstick (Teflon) cookware. | | |
| I use plastic kitchen tools (strainer) or plastic plates or cups. | | |
| I get take-out food regularly (more than once a week). | | |
| I use a traditional drip coffee maker. | | |
| **Food and Water** | | |
| I do not purchase organic produce. | | |
| I eat fast food at least once per week. | | |
| I don't use a water filter at home. | | |
| I consume processed food or soda at least once per week. | | |

|  | Yes | No |
|---|---|---|
| I eat seafood more than three times per week. | | |
| **Home and Cleaning** | | |
| I use air fresheners, scented candles, or plug-ins. | | |
| I use conventional cleaning products (not labeled "nontoxic"). | | |
| I use synthetic fabric softeners or dryer sheets. | | |
| I do not remove my shoes at home. | | |
| I do not dust and vacuum weekly. | | |
| **Behaviors and Habits** | | |
| I touch thermal receipts weekly (from stores, ATMs, airline tickets). | | |
| I am exposed to smoke, vaping, or cannabis at least once per week. | | |
| I drink more than 2 alcoholic drinks per week. | | |
| I drink more than 1 cup of coffee a day. | | |
| I live in a home built before 1978 and am not certain if all lead paint has been removed or covered (including trim). | | |

### SELF-ASSESSMENT SCORING:

Tally up all of your Yes answers. Each Yes is one point.

**0–6 points** → *Low Exposure:* You are doing a great job of decreasing your exposure to daily toxins. Continue to reinforce good habits and keep up the good work.

**7–13 points** → *Moderate Exposure:* You are doing well, but you could benefit from a few key lifestyle swaps to optimize your health.

**14+ points** → *High Exposure:* Your daily environment contains environmental toxins that are causing inflammation and likely impacting your fertility and hormone health. You need to evaluate how you can decrease toxin levels.

## Eliminating Toxin Exposures

You have many small encounters each day that can result in toxic exposures. It can be difficult to look at all the changes you should make and know where to start. Look at the chart below, review immediate changes you can make, and cross them out. After that, we will approach gradual changes that can be made over the next twelve weeks.

### WAYS TO REDUCE ENVIRONMENTAL TOXIN EXPOSURE

| | |
|---|---|
| Food | • Buy local or organic when you can, especially the dirty dozen. |
| | • Always wash fruits and vegetables. |
| | • Eat fewer processed foods, fast foods, and canned or prepackaged foods. |
| | • Reduce takeout; eat at home more. |
| | • Avoid microwave popcorn. |
| | • Consume no more than 3 servings of seafood per week. |
| | • Avoid high-mercury-level fish; prioritize seafood with a lower mercury level (shrimp, salmon, pollock, and catfish). |
| | • Limit animal meats, and do not eat organ meats. |
| | • Include iron, vitamin C, and calcium in your diet. |
| | • Choose loose-leaf tea over tea bags. |
| | • Test your drinking water for lead if you live in a high-risk area. |
| | • Use a water filter (either granular activated carbon [GAC] or reverse osmosis [RO] technology). |

| | |
|---|---|
| Kitchen | - Use glass, porcelain, or stainless steel for beverages.
- Stop using plastic for drinks or food storage.
- Hot drinks should not touch plastic (think about coffee!).
- Don't microwave plastics.
- Avoid plastics #3 and #7.
- Choose a wooden or non-plastic cutting board.
- If getting takeout, remove food from to-go containers and transfer into glass or other dishes.
- Consider French press or pour-over coffee over a traditional coffee maker.
- Cook on stainless steel or cast iron (not Teflon or nonstick).
- Limit your use of paper plates.
- Decrease your consumption of packaged drinks in plastic bottles, including water. |
| Home | - Avoid air fresheners.
- Remove shoes when entering the house.
- Don't use stain protectors on fabric.
- Limit exposure to varnishes and paints.
- Use a HEPA filter inside your home.
- Choose natural fibers over synthetic.
- Use laundry balls in the dryer and air-dry clothes when you can.
- Vacuum and dust frequently.
- Avoid using pesticides or insecticides at home, including flea baths/dips and bug bombs or sprays.
- Repaint homes built before 1978, including trim.
- Hire professionals for any renovation of older homes.
- If there is concern for lead in paint or dust, use a wet cloth or mop; do not sweep.
- Avoid handling antique pottery, ceramics, and toys. |

| | |
|---|---|
| Products | • Review products and avoid hidden toxic ingredients.<br>• Avoid imported cosmetics.<br>• Avoid microbeads in cosmetic products (like exfoliating cleansers).<br>• Look for phthalate-free and formaldehyde-free nail polish.<br>• Choose fragrance-free products. |
| Behaviors | • Avoid strong chemicals in detergents, paints, varnishes, or glues.<br>• Avoid handling thermal paper.<br>• Decrease outdoor activities on high air pollution days.<br>• Try to avoid travel during rush hour or heavy traffic.<br>• Avoid smoking, vaping, and cannabis.<br>• Limit alcohol to less than 2 drinks per week (none is best).<br>• Limit coffee to one cup per day.<br>• Limit direct heat to the scrotum. |

Next, take the next twelve weeks to create gradual changes.

PHASE 1: FOOD AND KITCHEN INTERVENTION

## Weeks 1–4

I think the kitchen is the easiest place to make meaningful change to your toxin risk. Choosing good food is important, but the pots, pans, and packages you use impact every bite you eat. Many of the recommended changes require you to purchase new cookware or products, but you can start by changing one at a time. This is where I started my own journey to decrease inflammation.

- Review the list of food toxins and see what changes to make. Many toxins will be reduced by following the diet recommendations.
- Look through your kitchen and immediately remove any plastic you can. You do not need a complete kitchen right away, but start to make a list of products that will benefit you most so that you can buy them when you're able to.

- My recommendations for important products: glass containers for meal prep, stainless steel water bottles and cookware, wooden cutting board (get a new one, start fresh), and a pour-over coffee maker or French press.

## What do I need to eliminate from my pantry?

You need to spend time looking through your pantry and refrigerator and removing food with toxins to donate to a food bank or shelter. If you are not in a position to purchase new food immediately, you can note which foods need to be replaced with better options once you have eaten them. In both scenarios, understanding what is harmful and stopping repetitive behavior is key.

- Prepackaged snacks and processed foods
- Microwave popcorn
- Artificial sweetener and nonnutritive sweetener
- Deli meats and processed meats
- Animal organ meats
- High-toxin seafood (king mackerel, shark, swordfish, marlin, orange roughy, tilefish, tuna)
- Soda and sweetened beverages

## What foods should I begin to purchase, or how should I change my approach to meals?

Changing your eating habits is one of the hardest things to do. Even though I believe the single biggest change you can make for your body is improving the food you eat, I am often told that it feels too difficult. I completely understand this, but I want you to start by focusing on food to decrease toxins, and then we will work to make daily anti-inflammatory choices.

- Buy organic when you can, but especially for the dirty dozen and root vegetables.

- Always wash fruits and vegetables after purchasing before putting them away (so that you can easily grab and eat).
- Work to cook more at home and meal prep; decrease takeout.
- If you order out, remove food from the take-out containers immediately.
- Limit seafood to no more than three times a week; prioritize seafood with lower mercury levels.
- Use natural sweeteners, such as honey and maple syrup.
- Switch to loose-leaf tea instead of tea bags.
- Include iron, vitamin C, and calcium in your diet.
- Incorporate foods high in fiber and antioxidants to support hormone health:
    - Broccoli
    - Berries
    - Beets
    - Lemons
    - Leafy greens
    - Lentils
    - Flaxseeds
    - Garlic
    - Turmeric
    - Green tea

## What do I need to eliminate from my kitchen?

Dedicate a day to opening up cabinets, and get a big box for donations. Changing products in your kitchen requires you to think about your habits. Everything on this list needs to be removed. We can make do with less and curate a small list of products to purchase once you have the funds.

- All plastic storage containers for food (Tupperware, etc.)
- All plastic cups or paper plates
- Plastic water bottles
- Any plastic plates or serving dishes
- Plastic spatulas or utensils
- Plastic cutting boards
- Nonstick cookware and baking sheets
- Plastic bowls, strainers, etc.
- Plastic food wrap
- Aluminum foil for cooking (at high temperatures it can leach chemicals)

*What should I purchase when I am ready?*

I keep an ongoing list on my phone's Notes app or an Amazon wish list for things like this. Then, at the holidays or when I have saved up money, I know exactly what I want to purchase to make our kitchen safer.

- Glass food storage containers
- Stainless steel drinkware
- Stainless steel mixing bowl
- Stainless steel strainer
- Wooden or silicone kitchen tools
- Wooden cutting board
- French press or pour-over coffee maker
- Stainless steel or cast-iron cookware
- Parchment paper for cooking
- Hot beverages (coffee, tea) should only be consumed from glass, ceramic, or stainless steel mugs (even paper to-go cups are often lined

with plastic and chemicals, so bring a mug with you and switch your coffee into it immediately if ordering to-go)

## *What do I need to do to improve my water safety?*

I recommend using a filter with your tap water. We have a reverse osmosis filter. Beware that some common plastic filters may not properly filter out heavy metals or may pose an additional risk due to the plastic and aluminum components. Remember to never use hot tap water for drinking or cooking, as this can leach lead and other heavy metals into the water. Instead, use cold or room temperature water and then heat by boiling.

- Go to the Environmental Working Group database (ewg.org/tapwater) to evaluate what is in your tap water.

- Get a water filter. I recommend either granular activated carbon (GAC) or reverse osmosis (RO) technology (on the EWG site listed above, you can see which filters will remove the toxins in your drinking water).

- Test your drinking water for heavy metals if you live in a high-risk area or you use well water (the EPA website offers options for well water testing, or you can independently test your water with a water testing kit, which you can get at mytapscore.com).

- Reduce consumption of bottled water as much as possible.

- Do not use hot water for cooking or cleaning produce.

PHASE 2: HOME AND PRODUCT EVALUATION

## *Weeks 5–8*

Your household exposures and your home products present sources of toxins that you are exposed to every day. These toxic exposures may be in the form of an older home, the products you use in your home, or your personal products. It can take time to go through these products and to make changes. Start with awareness of what behaviors you can modify (such as opening windows to improve air quality and prohibiting smoking in your home). Pay attention to your personal care products. When you run out of a product, take the time to research a safer alternative to try.

- Throw out home goods you don't need (like air fresheners). Consider getting laundry balls when you are out of dryer sheets.

- Review the ingredients on all your beauty and bath products. Decide which ones need to be replaced after they run out. Learn how to look at the labels on personal products (reviewed in chapter 10).

- Make a list of alternative products to purchase when you can.

## What do I need to eliminate from my home?

Inside our home, we are constantly touching and sitting on products that impact our toxin exposure. Start by removing home goods that increase your risk.

- Throw out air fresheners, incense, and candles that are not natural.
- Stop using fabric stain protectors or flame retardants.
- Throw out dryer sheets.
- Avoid using flea baths/dips and bug bombs or sprays.
- Do not use scented trash bags.
- Remove couches and furniture made before 2013 (when you can).

## What should I change to decrease toxins in my home?

Purchasing new products can be expensive, but often your daily behavior and choices can make a huge impact in your home. Look through this list and make a plan for what you need to purchase next and how you can set your home up to be more toxin-free with your actions.

- Purchase a HEPA filter to improve air quality in your home.
- Remove shoes when entering the home. Make a dedicated shoe space by the front door or your most frequent home entry site.
- Vacuum and dust weekly.
- Buy laundry balls for the dryer or air-dry clothes.
- Always use an exhaust fan when cooking on a gas stove.

- Search the Environmental Working Group Guide to Healthy Cleaning database (ewg.org/cleaners) for your current cleaning products and make swaps for safer alternatives.
- If you like candles, find natural wax options instead of paraffin.
- Open your windows when you can, especially to off-gas new products (mattresses, rugs, furniture, etc.).
- Choose natural fibers for clothing and furniture whenever possible.
- Iron or steam clean clothes instead of dry-cleaning.
- Purchase green plants to fill your home and improve air quality.

## *What personal products do I need to remove?*

You can look at the product table below to see ingredients to avoid when selecting products. The Environmental Working Group has evaluated many products, and you can search for them on their site (ewg.org) to understand the potential risk of products you love and are unsure about. Any products with the following ingredients should be discarded or at least replaced with a safer alternative once they are used.

**PERSONAL PRODUCT TOXIC INGREDIENT LIST TO AVOID**

| Ingredient | Product | Label Listing |
|---|---|---|
| Butylated hydroxyanisole (BHA) | Makeup | "Butylated hydroxyanisole," BHA, E320 |
| Formaldehyde | Nail hardeners, hair straighteners | "Formaldehyde," "Methylene glycol" |
| 1,4-Dioxane | Shampoo, body wash, soap, lotion | Avoid ethoxylated terms: -oxynol, -eth, polysorbate, polyethylene glycol (PEG) |
| Parabens | Makeup, moisturizer, hair products, shaving cream, lotion | Methyl/ethyl/propyl/butyl/isobutyl-paraben |

| Ingredient | Product | Label Listing |
|---|---|---|
| Phthalates | Perfume, hairspray, soap, shampoo, moisturizer, nail polish | "fragrance/parfum"; diethyl phthalate (DEP) |
| Toluene | Nail polish, salon-level hair products | "Toluene" |
| Triclosan | Toothpaste | "Triclosan" (and "Triclocarban") |
| Sodium lauryl sulfate and sodium laureth sulfate (SLS/SLES) | Toothpaste, soap, shampoo, bath products, moisturizer | SLS, SLES, "laureth-" |
| Diethanolamine (DEA) | Moisturizer, sunscreen, soap, cleanser, shampoo | DEA, cocamide DEA, lauramide DEA |
| Isobutane | Aerosol products (hair spray, sunscreen) | "Isobutane," "butane," "propane" |

*How can I reduce toxins in my personal products?*

Remember that each time you change out a product, you are making progress. It may take time to find alternative options that you like. The best place to start is with the products you use daily, as these will have the biggest impact.

- Review products and remove/replace those with toxic ingredients. Research safe alternatives on the EWG site (ewg.org/skindeep).
- Simplify your routine. You most likely do not need as many products as you have.
- Avoid imported cosmetics.
- Avoid microbeads in cosmetic products (like exfoliating cleansers).
- Look for phthalate-free and formaldehyde-free nail polish. Bring your own nail polish to the salon.
- Choose fragrance-free products (look specifically for fragrance-free, not unscented).

- Choose mineral sunscreen whenever possible (with zinc oxide or titanium dioxide). Chemical sunscreens are better than no sunscreen at all, though, because sunburns increase the risk of melanoma and skin cancer.
- Look for menstrual products made from 100 percent cotton or consider a silicone menstrual cup.
- Stop using aerosolized products, as they increase exposure through both inhalation and skin absorption.

## *Label-Reading Guide*

Refer to this table if you are trying to decide whether a product is safe to use. Remember that many "greenwashing" terms exist—meaning the brand uses a word without meaning that gives the appearance of safety. Always remember to look at the ingredients.

| Category | Avoid | Look for Instead | Watch Out For |
|---|---|---|---|
| Personal Care | Fragrance | Fragrance-free | "Natural fragrance" |
| | Phthalates | Certified organic | "Unscented" |
| | Parabens | EWG verified | "Dermatologist tested" |
| | Triclosan | Made safe | |
| | Formaldehyde | Jojoba or coconut oil | |
| | PEGs | | |
| | SLS/SLES | | |
| Cleaning Products | Fragrance | Vinegar | "Plant-derived" |
| | Ammonia | Baking soda | "Eco-friendly" (without verification) |
| | Chlorine bleach | Castile soap | |
| | Quats | Essential oils | |
| | 2-butoxyethanol | Plant-based surfactants | |

| Category | Avoid | Look for Instead | Watch Out For |
|---|---|---|---|
| Food | Artificial sweeteners<br>Food dyes<br>BHT, BHA<br>Sunflower oil<br>Soybean oil<br>BPA-lined cans | USDA organic<br>Non-GMO Project verified<br>BPA-free packaging label | "Clean" (without details)<br>"Natural flavor" |

*Smart Shopper Tips:*

- Don't trust the front label alone; always look at the ingredients.
- Use EWG or the Think Dirty app to research products.
- Less is more, and simple ingredients are better.

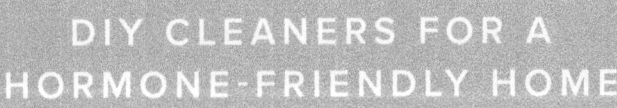

# DIY CLEANERS FOR A HORMONE-FRIENDLY HOME

If you are feeling crafty, try making your own home cleaners so you know exactly what is in them.

## All-Purpose Citrus Cleaner

**INGREDIENTS:**

1 cup white vinegar

1 cup filtered water

2 tbsp lemon juice

1 lemon peel

**INSTRUCTIONS:**

Combine all ingredients in a glass bottle.

Shake to combine before using.

## Mirror and Glass Spray

**INGREDIENTS:**

- 1 cup white vinegar
- 1 cup filtered water
- 1 tbsp rubbing alcohol
- Optional: 5 drops peppermint essential oil

**INSTRUCTIONS:**

Combine all ingredients in a glass bottle.

Shake to combine before using.

## Kitchen Counter Cleaner

**INGREDIENTS:**

- 3 cups filtered water
- 1 cup rubbing alcohol
- 1 tbsp dish soap
- Optional: 10 drops essential oil (I like peppermint)

**INSTRUCTIONS:**

Combine all ingredients in a glass bottle.

Shake to combine before using.

## PHASE 3: BEHAVIOR CHANGE

### Weeks 9–12

In your everyday life you may be exposed to situational toxins that you should try to avoid. Some of these toxins you may be aware of, and others may surprise you, but now you know the importance of taking charge of what you can.

You can't always control where you live, but you should know a way to check the ozone quality of your area and modify your behavior on days with poor air quality. The EPA runs airnow.gov, which will allow you to see the air quality based on US zip code.

### *How can I reduce toxins by changing my behaviors?*

Daily toxins sneak in through the air outside, during our commute, and from the choices we make each day. Changing behavior is important if you want to optimize hormone health.

- Avoid strong chemicals in detergents, paints, varnishes, or glues.
- Decline thermal receipts or airline tickets (if you work in that industry, wear gloves); ask for a digital copy instead.
- Decrease outdoor activities on high air pollution days.
- Have your car AC set to recycle air instead of bringing in outside air.
- Try to avoid travel during rush hour or heavy traffic.
- Avoid smoking, vaping, and cannabis.
- Limit alcohol to less than two drinks per week (none is best).
- Limit coffee to one cup per day.
- Limit direct heat to the scrotum.

## PHASE 4: MAINTENANCE

### Weeks 12+

At this point, you know how to limit toxins to the best of your ability. Encourage others and educate them about the importance of toxin avoidance and how to make changes.

## *Daily checklist for change:*

- ☐ Drink at least eight cups of filtered water a day.
- ☐ Use a stainless steel or glass water bottle, not plastic.
- ☐ Go to the Environmental Working Group database (ewg.org/tapwater) to evaluate what is in your tap water.
- ☐ Get a water filter. I recommend granular activated carbon (GAC) or reverse osmosis (RO) technology (at the EWG site listed above, you can see which filters will remove the toxins in your drinking water).
- ☐ Limit caffeine to one drink a day.
- ☐ Limit alcohol (none is best).
- ☐ Start your morning with 12 oz. of filtered tap water before you have coffee or tea. My favorite is a glass of hot water, one slice of lemon, and a pinch of sea salt first thing in the morning.
- ☐ Get rid of all plastic or nonstick cookware in your kitchen that you absolutely do not need. Make a list of what to replace when you can. Remember that you don't need a pot of every size.
- ☐ If you do not have one, purchase a stainless steel or glass water bottle. No more plastic for drinking water.
- ☐ Read the labels on your three most used personal care products and make a plan to replace any that include harmful toxins. Review the Label-Reading Guide for help.
- ☐ Open your windows for fifteen minutes a day while you are in your house.
- ☐ Remove a toxic cleaning product and replace it with a safe alternative. Consider making one of my favorite DIY cleaning products.

## SUPPLEMENT YOUR DIET

Supplements can be helpful to optimize nutritional needs. Please always discuss any supplements with your doctor and listen to their recommendations. Some supplements can interact with medications or may not be indicated in your personal case. Always pay attention to the dosing.

These are my recommendations for everyone to consider:

- Folic acid (400 mcg daily)—needed for cell division
- Vitamin D (1,000 IU daily)—cell growth, inflammation repair, and calcium absorption (bone health)
- Omega-3 fatty acids (300 mg daily)—important in cell health and decreasing inflammation
- Magnesium (250 mg daily)—for estrogen metabolism, insulin sensitivity, decreasing inflammation

In an ideal world, all your nutrients would come from food. Look at your diet and think about where you may be deficient and what may benefit you. In addition to the recommendations above, other supplements may be helpful, depending on your specific medical situation or diagnosis. Review this guide with your physician to see if these supplements can benefit you.

**FERTILITY**

| Supplement | Daily Dose | How It Helps |
|---|---|---|
| CoQ10 | 600 mg | antioxidant used in growth and repair stages |
| Zinc | 30 mg | follicular development and ovulation |
| Melatonin | 3 mg | antioxidant, decreases inflammation, improves egg quality |

## PCOS

| Supplement | Daily Dose | How It Helps |
|---|---|---|
| CoQ10 | 600 mg | antioxidant used in growth and repair stages |
| Zinc | 30 mg | improves glucose uptake and utilization, antioxidant decreasing inflammation |
| Inositol | 1 g | improves how insulin is utilized by the cells, improves insulin sensitivity |
| N-acetylcysteine (NAC) | 1 g | antioxidant, improves DNA damage, also improves insulin sensitivity |
| Melatonin | 3 mg | antioxidant, decreases inflammation, improves egg quality and progesterone production |

## ENDOMETRIOSIS

| Supplement | Daily Dose | How It Helps |
|---|---|---|
| CoQ10 | 600 mg | antioxidant used in growth and repair stages |
| Vitamin C | 1,000 mg | improves pain and inflammatory markers |
| Vitamin E | 800 IU | antioxidant and anticoagulant, may improve blood flow and egg quality |
| Zinc | 30 mg | improves glucose uptake and utilization, antioxidant decreasing inflammation |
| N-acetylcysteine (NAC) | 1 g | antioxidant, improves DNA damage, also improves insulin sensitivity |
| Melatonin | 3 mg | antioxidant, decreases inflammation, important for circadian rhythm and sleep |

## LOW OVARIAN RESERVE

| Supplement | Daily Dose | How It Helps |
|---|---|---|
| Omega-3 fatty acids | 300 mg | important in cell health and decreasing inflammation |
| CoQ10 | 600 mg | antioxidant used in growth and repair stages |
| Vitamin C | 1,000 mg | antioxidant, improves pain and inflammatory markers |
| Vitamin E | 800 IU | antioxidant and anticoagulant, may improve blood flow and egg quality |
| Zinc | 30 mg | important for insulin metabolism and androgen production, can aid in improving libido |
| N-acetylcysteine (NAC) | 1 g | antioxidant, improves DNA damage, also improves insulin sensitivity |
| DHEA | 75 mg | precursor hormone to estrogen and testosterone, may help with low ovarian reserve |
| Melatonin | 3 mg | antioxidant, decreases inflammation, important for circadian rhythm and sleep |

## SHORT LUTEAL PHASE

| Supplement | Daily Dose | How It Helps |
|---|---|---|
| CoQ10 | 600 mg | antioxidant used in growth and repair stages |
| Vitamin C | 1,000 mg | antioxidant, improves pain and inflammatory markers |
| Vitamin E | 800 IU | antioxidant and anticoagulant, may improve blood flow |
| Melatonin | 3 mg | antioxidant, decreases inflammation, important for circadian rhythm and sleep |

## THIN UTERINE LINING

| Supplement | Daily Dose | How It Helps |
| --- | --- | --- |
| Vitamin C | 1,000 mg | antioxidant, improves pain and inflammatory markers |
| Vitamin E | 800 IU | antioxidant and anticoagulant, may improve blood flow |
| Melatonin | 3 mg | antioxidant, decreases inflammation, important for circadian rhythm and sleep |

## UNEXPLAINED INFERTILITY

| Supplement | Daily Dose | How It Helps |
| --- | --- | --- |
| CoQ10 | 600 mg | antioxidant used in growth and repair stages |
| N-acetylcysteine (NAC) | 1 g | antioxidant, improves DNA damage, improves insulin sensitivity |
| Vitamin C | 1,000 mg | antioxidant, improves pain and inflammatory markers |
| Vitamin E | 800 IU | antioxidant and anticoagulant, may improve blood flow |
| Melatonin | 3 mg | antioxidant, decreases inflammation, important for circadian rhythm and sleep |

## POOR EGG QUALITY

| Supplement | Daily Dose | How It Helps |
| --- | --- | --- |
| CoQ10 | 600 mg | antioxidant used in growth and repair stages |
| N-acetylcysteine (NAC) | 1 g | antioxidant, improves DNA damage, improves insulin sensitivity |

| Supplement | Daily Dose | How It Helps |
|---|---|---|
| Vitamin C | 1,000 mg | antioxidant, improves pain and inflammatory markers |
| Vitamin E | 800 IU | antioxidant and anticoagulant, may improve blood flow |
| Melatonin | 3 mg | antioxidant, decreases inflammation, important for circadian rhythm and sleep |

## PMS

| Supplement | Daily Dose | How It Helps |
|---|---|---|
| CoQ10 | 600 mg | antioxidant used in growth and repair stages |
| Vitamin C | 1,000 mg | improves pain and inflammatory markers |
| Vitamin E | 800 IU | antioxidant and anticoagulant, may improve blood flow and egg quality |
| N-acetylcysteine (NAC) | 1 g | antioxidant, improves DNA damage, improves insulin sensitivity |
| Melatonin | 3 mg | antioxidant, decreases inflammation, important for circadian rhythm and sleep |

## POOR SPERM QUALITY

| Supplement | Daily Dose | How It Helps |
|---|---|---|
| Zinc | 66 mg | important in sperm formation |
| CoQ10 | 400 mg | antioxidant, helps with motility, concentration |
| Selenium | 200 mcg | antioxidant, protects against DNA damage |
| N-acetylcysteine (NAC) | 600 mg | antioxidant, improves DNA damage, improves insulin sensitivity |

| Supplement | Daily Dose | How It Helps |
|---|---|---|
| Vitamin C | 1,000 mg | antioxidant, improves all sperm counts |
| Vitamin E | 400 IU | antioxidant, improves motility |
| L-arginine | 1,000 mg | helps stabilize sperm, improves sperm DNA and concentration |
| L-carnitine | 3 g | improves motility |

## HORMONE-HEALTHY HABIT TRACKER

I'm guilty of loving checkboxes and to-do lists. A list can keep me on track and helps hold me accountable. You may not have the same affinity for lists that I do, but in case you do, this is for you. After following the seven-day plan to reset your hormones and decrease inflammation, you need to keep up the good work and make hormone-friendly habits a part of your daily life. I created this hormone habit tracker as a way for you to see how small changes can add up to a huge lifestyle improvement.

*Sleep:* **Get at least seven hours of sleep at night.**
*Tip:* Get a sleep mask and a sound machine.

*Fiber:* **Eat 25 g of fiber a day.**
*Tip:* Review the high-fiber food list.

*Food:* **Do not eat processed foods or foods with added sugar.**
*Tip:* Remember to try to cook at home and meal prep.

*Water:* **Drink eight glasses of filtered water a day.**
*Tip:* Get a water filter.

*Caffeine:* **Drink no more than one cup per day.**

*Tip:* Replace additional (or all) coffee with green tea.

*Toxins:* **No alcohol, cannabis, smoking, or vaping.**

*Tip:* Sparkling water, ice, and lemon is a great substitute for alcohol.

*Move:* **Move your body at least twenty minutes a day.**

*Tip:* Prioritize strength training during the week.

*Stress:* **Practice five minutes of meditation a day.**

*Tip:* Go to nataliecrawfordmd.com/meditate for my free "5 Minute Guided Calming Meditation to Reduce Cortisol and Stress."

## THE FERTILITY FORMULA HORMONE-HEALTHY HABIT TRACKER

| Day | Sleep | Fiber | Food | Water | Caffeine | Toxins | Move | Stress |
|---|---|---|---|---|---|---|---|---|
| Day 1 | | | | | | | | |
| Day 2 | | | | | | | | |
| Day 3 | | | | | | | | |
| Day 4 | | | | | | | | |
| Day 5 | | | | | | | | |
| Day 6 | | | | | | | | |
| Day 7 | | | | | | | | |

# THE ULTIMATE CYCLE GUIDE

Understanding your cycle allows you to detect early changes in cycle patterns that can impact your current and future fertility. In addition, learning to track your cycle will allow you to know when your body is in your follicular or luteal phase and give you the opportunity to tailor your lifestyle to your different needs in each cycle phase. Cycle tracking and cycle syncing allow you to harness your hormones and feel your absolute best. It's important to note that these principles are all based on the normal hormone changes of each month. If you are on hormonal contraception, you can't track or sync your cycle because you do not have hormone changes. This doesn't mean you need to stop your contraception, but come back to this guide once you do so that you can master your cycle.

## Cycle Tracking Cheat Sheet

Tracking your cycle is capturing the hormonal change indicating ovulation. Understanding the basics of the menstrual cycle will help you detect small and subtle changes and decide which cycle tracking method is best for you. Remember that prior to ovulation, your body is in the follicular phase, when you are growing a follicle and making estrogen. After ovulation, you are in the luteal phase, when your body is making progesterone from a corpus luteum. Knowing how to detect ovulation accurately is the first step to cycle tracking.

### Simple Calendar Method
Ovulation day = average cycle length - 14 days

### Basal Body Temperature (BBT)
Ovulation = in the three days prior to first temp elevation of at least 0.4°F (temperature remains elevated for at least three days)
BBT tracking steps:

1. You need a thermometer that can measure to 1/10 of a degree.
2. Take your temperature at the same time every morning, before getting out of bed or engaging in any other activity (even before checking your cell phone).
3. Get BBT charting paper or create your own. Record your temperature.
4. After ten days of tracking, mark your coverline 0.1°F above the highest value.
5. Ovulation occurs between the nadir and crossing the coverline.
6. Confirm ovulation by checking BBT and confirming three days above the coverline.

## Cervical Mucus Monitoring (CMM)

Ovulation day = last day of Type 4 cervical mucus (egg white, sticky, stretchy)

Your cervical mucus starts to increase in volume and stickiness five to six days prior to ovulation. Type 4 cervical mucus is seen with peak estrogen around ovulation.

**CERVICAL MUCUS MONITORING**

| Cervical Mucus Type | Sensation | Mucus Properties |
|---|---|---|
| Type 1 | dry, rough | no secretions |
| Type 2 | damp, smooth | no secretions |
| Type 3 | damp, smooth | thick, creamy, and whitish; sticky |
| Type 4 | wet, slippery | transparent and stretchy or elastic; "egg white" |

CMM tracking steps:

1. Wipe with toilet paper PRIOR to using the restroom and then inspect the paper.
2. Some women will want to separate their labial lips before wiping in order to capture the mucus on toilet paper (everyone has different anatomy).
3. How does your vulva feel? (dry, damp, wet)
4. How does the toilet paper feel as you wipe? (rough, smooth, slippery)
5. How does the mucus look? (no secretions, thick and creamy, stretchy and elastic)

## Cervical Position

As your estrogen rises, your cervix changes from firm and closed to softer and open by the time of ovulation. After ovulation, the cervix changes back to a non-fertile state. Within twenty-four hours of progesterone production, the cervix will return back to a low and firm position.

**CERVICAL POSITION AND FERTILITY**

| Cycle Phase | Cervical Position | Cervical Texture | Cervical Opening |
| --- | --- | --- | --- |
| Not fertile | low | firm | closed |
| Fertile window | midway | medium | partial opening |
| Peak fertility | high | soft | open |

Cervical position tracking steps:

1. Insert a finger into your vagina and feel for your cervix.
2. Keep your nails short, insert your middle finger (as it is longer), and try to check at the same time every day.
3. I think it is easiest to check your cervical position by elevating one leg on the side of the tub or a shower seat when you are in the shower.

### Ovulation Predictor Kit (OPK)

Ovulation day = day after a positive OPK (day after LH surge)

OPKs are urine LH-detection strips that need to be used daily in order to detect the first surge of LH. The best time to test is between 10 a.m. and 2 p.m. Ovulation is the day after a positive OPK.

### Cycle Syncing 101

Cycle syncing is the understanding that your body has different needs in each phase of your cycle. It makes sense that you will have different metabolic needs when you have hormonal highs versus hormonal lows. I love the idea of looking at your life and trying to synchronize your lifestyle with the different phase of the cycles, and cycle syncing can help you be more aware of your cycle phase and help you feel your best regardless of whether you are trying to conceive. You do not have to cycle sync, but it can be a great way to listen to your body and adjust as needed.

**CYCLE SYNCING SUMMARY**

| Cycle Phase | Diet | Exercise | Energy |
| --- | --- | --- | --- |
| Menses | Avoid inflammatory foods. Increase fruits and vegetables, foods with omega-3 fatty acids like eggs, seafood, walnuts, flaxseed, chia seeds, edamame, seaweed, and leafy greens. Plant-based iron and protein sources: spinach, kale, broccoli, tofu, lentils, and beans. Season with turmeric, cinnamon, curry, cayenne, and garlic. | Low-inflammatory movement. Walks, slow yoga, resistance training. Listen to your body. | Fatigue is common. Allow yourself more time to complete tasks and try to avoid huge projects. Take a nap. |

| Cycle Phase | Diet | Exercise | Energy |
|---|---|---|---|
| Follicular phase | Nutrient-dense fruits and veggies to support egg growth, especially those high in fiber. Add carrots, broccoli, cauliflower, brussels sprouts, sweet potatoes, green beans, and avocados. Vitamin E and B foods: berries, mango, kiwi, oranges, bananas, apples, avocados, nuts, chia seeds, hemp seeds, quinoa. | Better glucose usage and aerobic performance. Excellent time for heavier weights, HIIT training, and long runs. Try for a personal best; you can build more muscle. | Your best energy, focus, and mental clarity. Complete big projects. Set creative goals and plans. Load your to-do list here. |
| Luteal phase | Increase caloric requirements and healthy fats. Add brown rice, quinoa, lentils, sweet potatoes, broccoli, figs, sunflower seeds, dark chocolate, avocados, olives, olive oil, and nuts. Increase water and avoid alcohol. | Moderate activity, strength training, sustained movement. Pilates, yoga, stretching, low-intensity zone 2 training. | Lower concentration and easily fatigued. Complete your most important task first thing in the day. |

By now, you know that your fertility is not a matter of chance but a net sum of the choices you make each day. The Fertility Formula is your guide to take charge of your fertility by optimizing your hormones and reproductive health. I want you to remember:

- **Fertility is a marker of your health and matters long before you want to conceive.** Understanding your body, menstrual cycle, and hormones is the first step to taking charge of your fertility.

- **Your hormones and fertility are influenced by your lifestyle and the world around you.** Chronic inflammation is toxic for your fertility.

- **You have more control over your fertility than you have been told.** Prioritizing lifestyle choices that work together to decrease inflammation can improve your health and fertility.

PART V

# THE FERTILITY FORMULA RECIPES

# Eating Your Way to Better Fertility

Welcome to the food that my family eats. When I first decided to make big changes to my diet, I had no idea what to eat to decrease inflammation. I found it easiest to start simple by structuring my day with breakfast, lunch, one to two snacks, and dinner. I plan out our weekly meals each Sunday. This allows us to get groceries, prep lunch and dinner needs before the craziness of the week, and reduce bad choices due to lack of options. Allowing yourself to fall into a calorie deficiency during the day is a huge culprit for nighttime binges—so don't put yourself in that position.

Examples of breakfast, lunch, and snack options appear in the following table, and my favorite recipes are included. I have an omnivore husband who eats 100 percent plant-based in our house without complaint. These meals are filling, simple, healthy, and delicious. For balance, he gets whatever he wants if we order or go out, but we don't cook meat in the house. This one change alone has also lowered his cholesterol (without medication) and allows us to know we are providing nutritious meals for our family.

## WHOLE-FOOD MEAL BASICS

| Breakfast | Lunch | Snacks |
|---|---|---|
| Fruit | Salads | Fruit |
| Granola | Grain bowls | Nuts |
| Nuts | Bean or avocado tacos | Roasted chickpeas |
| Smoothies | Veggie sushi | Hummus with veggies/pretzels |
| Avocado toast | Veggie sandwiches (cucumber, hummus, avocado, tomato, carrots) | Guacamole with veggies or chips |
| Oatmeal | | |
| Tofu scramble | | |
| Overnight oats | Veggie soup | Trail mix (make your own with Rice Chex, nuts, fruit) |
| Breakfast tacos | Baked potato or sweet potato | Kale chips |
| | Pasta salad | Apples and almond butter |

Be open to recipes and foods that you haven't before and allow yourself the opportunity to try some of our favorite recipes.

# Roasted Cauliflower Tacos

*Serves 4*

INGREDIENTS:

8 corn tortillas

1 cup cherry tomatoes

1–2 avocados

1 can black beans

½ sweet onion

Handful of fresh spinach

1 head of cauliflower

Salt & pepper

Avocado oil

**DIRECTIONS:**

Preheat oven to 350°F/180°C.

Cut and wash cauliflower, place on a baking sheet, sprinkle salt on top.

Cook for 20–30 minutes until cauliflower begins to brown.

While cauliflower is cooking: Chop onion and sauté in a pan with avocado oil until soft, then remove.

Drain and rinse black beans, put in same pan used for onion, and cook on low. Add salt and pepper to taste.

Cut avocado and tomato, sprinkle with salt.

*To serve:*

Place all fillings in a tortilla, top with spinach and salsa if you desire.

You can omit cauliflower or substitute with butternut squash (we usually buy precut), baked sweet potato, or roasted broccoli.

# Veggie Stir-Fry

*Serves 4*

**INGREDIENTS:**

- Brown rice
- 1 bag carrot chips
- 1 head of broccoli
- ½ sweet onion
- Teriyaki sauce
- Salt & pepper
- Sesame seeds
- Avocado oil

**DIRECTIONS:**

Preheat oven to 350°F/180°C.

Cut and wash the broccoli, place on a baking sheet, sprinkle salt on top.

Cook for 20–30 minutes broccoli begins to brown.

While broccoli is cooking: Boil water and cook rice according to instructions.

Cut onion into 1-inch pieces and sauté in a pan with avocado oil until soft (then remove). Place carrots in the same pan and sauté carrots on medium until soft, add salt.

*To serve:*

Place all veggies (onion, carrots, broccoli) in a bowl and coat with teriyaki sauce. Place veggies on top of rice to serve. Add sesame seeds if desired.

Frequent substitutes include sweet-and-sour sauce or peanut sauce instead of teriyaki. Instead of carrots and broccoli, sometimes we substitute sugar snap peas, cauliflower, edamame, or Broccolini (a kid favorite).

You could also sauté peppers (yellow/orange/red) with the onion or add tofu.

# Tahini Kale Salad

*Serves 4*

**INGREDIENTS:**

- 1 bunch of kale
- 1 can chickpeas
- 2 avocados
- 1 cup blueberries
- 2 lemons
- Extra virgin olive oil
- 2 tbsp tahini
- 1 tsp maple syrup
- Salt & pepper
- Hemp seeds

**DIRECTIONS:**

Preheat oven to 350°F/180°C.

Rinse the chickpeas, coat heavily with salt while slightly damp, and place on a baking sheet. Cook for 20 minutes, until crispy on the outside.

While chickpeas are cooking: Rinse and dry kale, separate leaves from stalks.

Chop kale into small pieces and place in a bowl. Coat with juice of 1 lemon and 1 tbsp of extra virgin olive oil. Massage with hands until soft.

Make tahini dressing: Add 2 tbsp tahini, 1 tsp maple syrup, juice of one lemon, and 2 tbsp water to a bowl and whisk. Add more water to desired consistency.

Cut avocado and top with salt and pepper to taste. Rinse blueberries.

*To serve:*

Place chickpeas, avocado, and blueberries on top of the chopped kale; top with hemp seeds if desired.

Frequent substitutes include whatever fruits and vegetables we have around.

You can also add salad dressing.

Trader Joe's Everything but the Bagel seasoning is also delicious on this.

You can add tofu or any other additional protein source.

Make extra roasted chickpeas for snacks (one of my kids' favorites).

# BBQ Chickpeas with Roasted Broccoli & Sweet Potatoes

*Serves 4*

**INGREDIENTS:**

- 4 large sweet potatoes
- 1 head of broccoli
- 1 can chickpeas
- BBQ sauce (Franklin Barbecue Original is our favorite)
- Salt
- Avocado oil

**DIRECTIONS:**

Preheat oven to 350°F/180°C.

Wash sweet potatoes. Poke a few holes with a fork and then coat skin with avocado oil and salt. Wrap each potato with foil and place in oven 2 hours prior to serving (may need longer if larger).

Cut and wash the broccoli, and rinse the chickpeas; coat both with salt and place on a baking sheet.

Cook broccoli and chickpeas for 20 minutes until broccoli is browned and chickpeas are crispy on the outside.

Remove from oven.

Place chickpeas in a bowl, coat with BBQ sauce, and mix.

*To serve:*

Cut sweet potatoes lengthwise and then add roasted broccoli and chickpeas to the inside. Top with extra BBQ sauce if desired.

BBQ lentils or tofu are great substitutes. You can buy raw lentils and cook them according to package directions. Coat with BBQ sauce after they are cooked.

# Natalie's Christmas Spaghetti

*Serves 8–10*

**INGREDIENTS:**

16 oz. (approx 450g) spaghetti (we use gluten-free, but any will work)

1 jar pasta sauce (I like Rao's Sensitive Marinara Sauce)

2 cans diced tomatoes

½ sweet onion

4–6 cloves garlic

Extra virgin olive oil

Salt

Sugar

**DIRECTIONS:**

Boil water and cook entire package of spaghetti, drain, and set aside.

Chop onion and garlic and sauté in a large pot on medium heat with extra virgin olive oil until soft, then remove. I like to use the same pot I cooked the spaghetti in.

Add pasta sauce and diced tomatoes to the pot, bring to a simmer. Add salt and sugar (trust me, this is the secret ingredient). The goal taste is just the tiniest bit sweet.

Add noodles back to the pot and stir together.

Place in a casserole dish, cover, and refrigerate. You can serve immediately, but this allows the sauce to soak into the noodles and is tastier (also easier for holidays!).

*To serve:*

Heat oven to 350°F/180°C.

Cook for 35 minutes covered with foil until warm in the center.

You can always sauté and add other veggies. In the past, I've added chopped yellow squash, courgette, mushrooms, and more.

We make this for special occasions, because I can make it ahead and then serve. Christmas spaghetti, lake spaghetti, beach spaghetti, and more.

# Butternut Squash Curry Soup

*Serves 4*

**INGREDIENTS:**

- 2 cups chopped butternut squash
- 2 shallots, chopped
- 1 tsp avocado oil
- 1 block of tofu
- 1 tsp cinnamon
- 2 tbsp maple syrup
- 2 cups vegetable broth

1 tbsp curry

1 can coconut milk

2 cups chopped kale

Salt

**DIRECTIONS:**

Preheat oven to 400°F/200°C

Add butternut squash and shallots to baking sheet, drizzle with avocado oil and salt. Bake for 20 minutes.

Drain block of tofu, press between paper towels to remove excess moisture. Chop tofu, place on baking sheet lined with parchment paper, cover with salt, and bake for 20 minutes.

To a large pot, add cooked butternut squash and shallot. Then add curry, cinnamon, maple syrup, 1 tsp salt, vegetable broth, and coconut milk. Blend.

Bring to a boil, then cover and reduce heat to medium for 10 minutes.

Change to low heat, add cooked tofu and kale, cover, and cook for 20 minutes.

*To serve:*

Stir, dish to bowl.

If desired, top with toasted pepitas.

# Sweet Potato Chickpea Curry

*Serves 4*

**INGREDIENTS:**

1 small sweet onion

4 cloves garlic

1 tsp curry

1 tsp garam masala

1 tsp cinnamon

1 tsp coriander

1 tsp turmeric

2 tsp salt

2 cans diced tomatoes

1 can coconut milk

2 cans drained chickpeas

3 medium sweet potatoes (peeled and chopped)

Agave

1 head of cauliflower

1 block of tofu

1 cup uncooked brown rice

Extra virgin olive oil

**DIRECTIONS:**

Preheat oven to 350°F/180°C.

Chop cauliflower, add to a baking sheet lined with parchment paper, lightly cover with extra virgin olive oil and salt.

Drain block of tofu, chop, and add to baking sheet with cauliflower. Cover with salt, put in oven for 20 minutes, then set aside.

Chop sweet onion and garlic, then sauté on medium with extra virgin olive oil until soft.

Add curry, garam masala, cinnamon, coriander, turmeric, and salt to the onion and garlic.

Next, add diced tomatoes, coconut milk, drained chickpeas, sweet potatoes.

Bring to a boil, then cover, reduce heat, and simmer for 30 minutes. Add agave and salt to taste.

*To serve:*

Add roasted cauliflower, tofu, and rice to the pot. Scoop and serve.

Baking the sweet potatoes first can make them easier to chop and cuts down on cooking time later.

You can add everything to a Crock-Pot except the cauliflower, rice, and tofu (just add those before serving).

## Carrot & Lentil Gnocchi

*Serves 4*

**INGREDIENTS:**

- 1 cup red lentils
- 2 packages gnocchi
- 1 bag shredded carrots
- ½ sweet onion
- 6 cloves garlic
- 1 cup cashews
- 1 jar marinara sauce
- ¼ cup nutritional yeast
- ¼ cup water
- Salt
- Extra virgin olive oil

**DIRECTIONS:**

Preheat oven to 400°F/200°C.

Soak cashews in hot water.

Cook red lentils per package instructions, set aside.

Cook gnocchi, set aside.

Chop sweet onion and garlic, cook in pan on medium heat with extra virgin olive oil until soft, then add shredded carrots.

Cook on medium until carrots are soft (10–12 minutes), add salt.

While cooking, add drained cashews, jar of marinara, water, salt, and nutritional yeast to food processor or blender. Blend until smooth.

Once carrots are soft, add lentils, gnocchi, and sauce to the pot and stir on low.

*To serve:*

Mix together on low heat, remove, and serve.

# Broccoli & Peanut Tofu

*Serves 2*

**INGREDIENTS:**

- 1 block of tofu
- 2 crowns of broccoli
- 1 cup dried quinoa
- Avocado oil

**SAUCE:**

- 4 large tbsp peanut butter
- 2 tbsp coconut aminos
- 1 tbsp maple syrup
- 1 lemon juiced
- Water (for mixing)

**DIRECTIONS:**

Preheat oven to 400°F/200°C.

Cook 1 cup quinoa per package instructions.

Drain block of tofu, press between paper towels to remove excess moisture, then cut into blocks, cover with salt, and place on parchment paper–lined baking sheet in oven for 20 minutes.

Cut up broccoli, toss in avocado oil and salt, and roast for 20–25 minutes.

Make sauce: Mix peanut butter, coconut aminos, maple syrup, and lemon juice. Add water to thin and mix sauce.

*To serve:*

Combine all ingredients to enjoy.

You can use any veggies instead of or in addition to the broccoli.

Brown rice works as a quinoa substitute.

# Tunnel Pasta (My Kids' Favorite)

*Serves 4*

**INGREDIENTS:**

- 3 courgettes
- 1 cup cashews
- 1 package rigatoni (penne is a substitute)
- 4 tbsp nutritional yeast
- 1 jar marinara sauce
- Avocado oil
- Salt

**DIRECTIONS:**

Preheat oven to 350°F/180°C.

Chop courgettes, toss with avocado oil and salt, place on parchment paper, and bake for 20 minutes.

Boil water. Take 1 cup of boiling water and soak cashews. To the remaining water, add pasta, boil until cooked.

Add cashews (and water) to blender with nutritional yeast, salt, and marinara. Blend. Add additional water as needed to get desired consistency.

Drain pasta and then put back in pot. Add cooked courgettes and sauce to pasta, heat over low.

*To serve:*

Stir and serve.

# Three-Bean Chili

*Serves 6–8*

### INGREDIENTS:

- 1 can kidney beans
- 1 can black beans
- 1 can pinto beans
- 2 cans diced tomato
- 1 can tomato sauce
- 1 can corn
- 1 bag shredded carrots
- ½ sweet onion
- 4–6 cloves garlic
- Avocado oil
- Chili seasoning of choice
- Salt
- 1 head of cauliflower

### DIRECTIONS:

Heat oven to 400°F/200°C.

Chop cauliflower and place on parchment paper–lined baking sheet, toss with avocado oil and salt. Bake for 20 minutes until lightly browned.

Chop onion and garlic and add to large pot with avocado oil. Cook on medium until onion is soft.

Add shredded carrots and sauté for 10 minutes over medium.

Drain 3 cans of beans and can of corn, add to pot.

Add diced tomatoes and tomato sauce, season as desired, and bring to a boil.

Reduce to simmer and cover for 20 minutes.

*To serve:*

Scoop chili over cauliflower and serve.

I love to serve over a baked potato.

# Pasta and Courgette Tofu Marinara

*Serves 4*

**INGREDIENTS:**

- 2 courgettes
- 1 block of tofu
- 1 jar of marinara sauce
- 1 package of pasta (any shape)
- 3 tbsp nutritional yeast
- Salt
- Avocado oil

**DIRECTIONS:**

Heat oven to 350°F/180°C.

Cut the courgettes and toss in avocado oil and salt, place on parchment paper–lined baking sheet, and cook for 20 minutes.

Boil water and add pasta, cook until soft. Drain and set aside.

Drain tofu, then crumble and add to a large pot. Cook for 5 minutes, add salt and then 1 jar of marinara.

Let simmer for 10 minutes.

Add pasta and courgettes, stir over low for a few minutes.

*To serve:*

Add salt to taste and sprinkle with nutritional yeast.

I like to serve this over chickpea pasta, but any will work.

You can also change up the vegetable for variety. Green peas work nicely.

# Pasta Salad

*Serves 4*

**INGREDIENTS:**

- 1 box pasta (penne or fusilli)
- 2 cucumbers, peeled
- 1 bag shredded carrots
- 1 container microgreens (optional)
- 1 carton cherry tomatoes
- 1 block of tofu

**DRESSING:**

- ¼ cup red wine vinegar
- ¾ cup extra virgin olive oil
- 1 tsp garlic powder
- 1 tsp dried Italian herb seasoning
- 1 tsp lemon juice
- ½ tsp salt
- ½ tsp pepper

**DIRECTIONS:**

Heat oven to 400°F/200°C.

Drain and press tofu on paper towels, cut into small blocks, place on parchment paper, cover with salt, cook for 20 minutes.

Make Italian dressing by combining the dressing ingredients in a small bowl and mixing. Chop tomatoes and cucumbers.

Boil water and cook pasta according to package, drain.

In a large bowl, combine pasta, cooked tofu, tomatoes, cucumbers, carrots, and microgreens. Add dressing and mix.

Add salt to taste.

*To serve:*

Refrigerate and serve.

I like to add cooked chickpeas (drain and add salt, cook along with tofu).

We make a batch of this at the beach or lake and keep in the fridge for easy lunches. Also a favorite for weekly lunch meal prepping.

## Minestrone Soup

*Serves 8*

### INGREDIENTS:

- ½ sweet onion
- 6 cloves garlic
- 1 bag carrots
- 12 oz. green beans
- 2 courgettes
- 2 cans beans (I use white and kidney, but any will work)
- 2 tbsp sugar or agave
- 2 tbsp nutritional yeast
- 2 tsp oregano
- 2 tsp basil
- 2 cans fire-roasted diced tomatoes
- 6 cups vegetable broth
- 1 package small-shape pasta (fusilli, elbows, etc.)
- 6 oz. bag baby spinach
- Extra virgin olive oil

### DIRECTIONS:

Bring water to a boil, cook pasta according to package instructions. Drain and set aside.

In same large pot, chop onion and garlic, sauté in extra virgin olive oil on medium.

Chop and add carrots and green beans, add salt.

Cook 10 minutes on medium/high.

Chop courgettes and add.

Drain and add beans.

Add sugar, nutritional yeast, oregano, basil, fire-roasted diced tomatoes, and vegetable broth; bring to boil, then cover and reduce to a simmer for 30 minutes.

Add pasta and baby spinach, keep on low for 10 minutes.

*To serve:*

Stir and serve.

You can also precook the pasta, then add everything else to a Crock-Pot during the day. Add the pasta and spinach in the last 10–20 minutes before serving.

Any veggies can be added; clean out the fridge and add them.

On New Year's Day, we use black-eyed peas for good luck.

# Sweet Potato Bowl with Cashew Curry Sauce

*Serves 4*

**INGREDIENTS:**

- 3–4 sweet potatoes
- 1 cup brussels sprouts
- 1 tbsp avocado oil
- Salt
- 1 block of tofu
- 1 cup uncooked brown rice

**CASHEW CURRY SAUCE:**

- 1 cup cashews
- 1 tsp avocado oil
- 4 cloves garlic
- 5 tbsp nutritional yeast
- 1 tsp curry
- 1½ cups almond milk
- Salt

**DIRECTIONS:**

Heat oven to 400°F/200°C.

Soak cashews in water.

Chop sweet potatoes and brussels sprouts, toss with avocado oil and salt, place on parchment paper–lined baking sheet, and put in oven for 30 minutes.

Drain tofu and chop, top with salt (no oil needed), place on a separate baking sheet lined with parchment paper, and add to the oven to cook for 20 minutes.

Wrap garlic cloves in foil with 1 tsp avocado oil and add to the oven for 20 minutes.

Cook brown rice as per instructions, set aside.

Make cashew curry sauce: Add roasted garlic, cashews (with water), nutritional yeast, curry, salt, and almond milk to a blender. Blend until smooth. Transfer to a small pan and heat on the stove until bubbling, stir, and take off heat.

*To serve:*

Top rice with brussels sprouts, sweet potatoes, and tofu and top with curry sauce.

You can use quinoa instead of brown rice.

You can substitute with broccoli or another available vegetable.

# Black Bean Taco Bowl

*Serves 4*

**INGREDIENTS:**

- Butternut squash
- 1 head of cauliflower
- ½ sweet onion
- Brown rice
- 1 can black beans
- Spinach, mixed greens, or romaine
- 1 cup cherry tomatoes
- 2 avocados
- Salsa
- Avocado oil
- Salt

**DIRECTIONS:**

Preheat oven to 350°F/180°C.

Chop butternut squash, cauliflower, and sweet onion. Place on parchment paper–lined baking sheet, drizzle with avocado oil, and add salt. Cook for 20–30 minutes until brown.

Cook brown rice per instructions.

Drain a can of black beans and then heat on stove, add salt and stir.

Chop greens, avocados, and tomatoes.

*To serve:*

Add rice, greens, and veggies to a bowl, top with salsa, and serve.

You can substitute quinoa for brown rice.

You can also place in corn tortillas for a black bean taco.

We do a version of this weekly.

## SIMPLE SIDES

# Baked Tofu

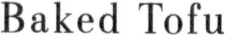

**INGREDIENTS:**

1 block of extra-firm tofu

Salt

**DIRECTIONS:**

Heat oven to 400°F/200°C.

Drain tofu and press out extra liquid with paper towels.

Chop tofu: Cut block in half in each dimension (including splitting the thickness), then make additional cuts to get the desired block size (1 block makes 48 pieces for me, but you can decide what works for you).

Place chopped tofu on parchment paper–lined baking sheet (parchment paper helps prevent it from sticking to the pan or foil—this is important).

Cover with salt (I prefer sea salt), no oil needed.

Bake for 20 minutes.

# Green Beans

**INGREDIENTS:**

- Fresh regular or French green beans
- Vegan or regular butter
- Salt

**DIRECTIONS:**

Boil water and then place green beans in a steamer and cover.

Cook 3–5 minutes.

Add 1 tbsp butter and let melt, top with salt.

## Roasted Broccoli

INGREDIENTS:

- 1 head of broccoli
- Avocado oil
- Salt

DIRECTIONS:

Preheat oven to 350°F/180°C.

Cut and wash broccoli, place on a parchment paper–lined baking sheet, drizzle with avocado oil, sprinkle salt on top.

Cook for 20–30 minutes until browned.

## Roasted Cauliflower

INGREDIENTS:

- 1 head of cauliflower
- Avocado oil
- Salt

DIRECTIONS:

Preheat oven to 350°F/180°C.

Cut and wash cauliflower, place on parchment paper–lined baking sheet, drizzle with avocado oil, sprinkle salt on top.

Cook for 20–30 minutes until browned.

## Roasted Carrots

**INGREDIENTS:**

1 bag baby carrots

Salt

**DIRECTIONS:**

Boil water and then place carrots in a steamer and cover.

Cook 3–5 minutes, then remove.

Preheat oven to 350°F/180°C.

Coat tender carrots with salt and place on a parchment paper–lined baking sheet.

Cook for 20–30 minutes until soft.

## Sugar Snap Peas

**INGREDIENTS:**

Sugar snap peas

Vegan or regular butter

Salt

**DIRECTIONS:**

Boil water, then place peas in a steamer and cover.

Cook 3–5 minutes.

Add 1 tbsp butter and let melt, top with salt.

## Roasted Okra (My Favorite)

**INGREDIENTS:**

Okra

Avocado oil

Salt

**DIRECTIONS:**

Preheat oven to 350°F/180°C.

Rinse and cut okra into ½-inch pieces. Toss with avocado oil and salt.

Place on parchment paper–lined baking sheet.

Cook for 20–30 minutes until brown on the outside.

---

# THANKSGIVING AND HOLIDAY

## Green Bean Casserole

*Serves 8–10*

**INGREDIENTS:**

- 3 lbs. green beans
- ½ cup sliced almonds
- ½ stick vegan butter
- Extra virgin olive oil
- 2 sweet onions
- 2 tbsp fresh thyme
- Salt
- Pepper

**DIRECTIONS:**

Cut onion into extremely thin slices.

Rinse green beans.

Fill large skillet or pot with water and bring to a boil.

Add green beans and cook for 5 minutes.

Drain water (green beans will still be crunchy) and run beans under cold water, set aside.

Add ½ stick vegan butter and 4 tbsp extra virgin olive oil to the skillet, melt butter on medium.

Add onions to butter and oil, season with salt, and stir occasionally until caramelized (about 20 minutes).

Add thyme and mix.

Add green beans and stir completely.

Transfer to a casserole dish.

Top with sliced almonds.

Place in oven on warm until ready to serve.

*To serve:*

I usually make this earlier in the day and then keep in the oven on warm until serving.

Avoid overcooking the green beans initially in order to keep them crispy if you also want to prepare this dish ahead of time.

Fan favorite to replace traditional green bean casserole.

# Cornbread-and-Herb Stuffing

*Serves 8–10*

**INGREDIENTS:**

- 2 boxes cornbread stuffing mix (I use gluten-free)
- Muffin cups
- 2 tbsp fresh sage
- 2 tbsp fresh parsley
- 2 tbsp fresh rosemary
- 1 stick vegan or regular butter
- 3 cups veggie broth
- 1 sweet onion
- 1 tbsp flax or 1 egg
- Salt

**DIRECTIONS:**

Cook the cornbread as muffins according to the package instructions (make 2 trays, cook until golden and a little crispy). I usually make these the day before.

Heat oven to 375°F/190°C.

Chop onion, sage, rosemary, parsley.

Heat a large pan over medium and melt the butter, sauté onion and herbs until soft. Remove from heat to cool.

If using flax instead of egg: Combine 1 tbsp flax with 3 tbsp water, mix aggressively. Set flax mixture aside for 3–5 minutes.

Crumble the cornbread into big chucks in another bowl.

Add onion and herbs, mix.

Add salt, veggie broth, and egg (or flax) and mix well.

Rub vegan butter on casserole dish, then add stuffing.

Cook at 375°F/180°C. for 45 minutes, then can keep at warm until serving.

*To serve:*

The night before, I chop everything (onion, herbs) and make the muffins.

Assemble everything else on the morning of serving; cook, then keep in warmer.

You may not need all the muffins depending on the size of your casserole dish—judge appropriately.

# Homemade Cranberry Sauce

*Serves 8–10*

**INGREDIENTS:**

- 12 oz. fresh cranberries
- ½ cup orange juice
- ⅔ cup sugar
- ¼ tsp cinnamon
- ¼ tsp salt

**DIRECTIONS:**

Combine all ingredients in a saucepan and simmer on medium for 15–20 minutes while stirring. Remove from heat and refrigerate until serving.

# Acknowledgments

This book would not exist without the team of people who supported me and my passion along the way. I started writing this book in 2018. I was years into working as a fertility doctor, seeing women ask the same questions time after time. After experiencing my own infertility, I knew how it felt to be on the other side of the exam table and told there was nothing you could do. After finding an agent, writing a proposal, and going on submission—I was told there was no market for a fertility book. This was a topic too depressing for anyone to choose to read.

I quietly shelved this project, but I did not give up. You now hold this book in your hands because my wonderful agents Mia Vitale and Sarah Passick at Park, Fine & Brower believed in it completely. I'll always thank Dr Karen Tang for insisting I meet with Mia, and since the time of our first meeting, Mia has advocated for this book. To my incredible editor, Nina Rodríguez-Marty, and the team at Penguin Life, your vision and guidance have been essential in shaping the book into what it is today. Thank you for making *The Fertility Formula* possible. To Steven Bartlett and Holly Whitaker at Ebury and Flight Books, thank you for believing in me. And a huge thanks to Dr Shannon Ritchey, physical therapist and founder of Evlo fitness, for her input and demonstrations of exercises included in Part IV; and to Toni Weschler, author of *Taking Charge of Your Fertility*, for her insights and edits in chapter 5.

To my husband, Jason, thank you doesn't feel appropriate for everything you have done—and continue to do—for me. From helping out at home to listening to me through every chapter and supporting every dream (this book and beyond), I love you and thank you. To my children, Campbell and Rhett, I hope this book is a tangible representation that you should never give up on your dreams. Thank you for being proud of me, cheering me on, and giving me grace for the moments I was less present in order to write and edit.

To my parents, Steve and Nancy Minns, thank you for believing in me when I said I wanted to become a doctor and supporting me completely. Needless to say, I wouldn't be where I am without you. To my sisters, Emily Chambers and Megan King, thanks for always keeping me grounded and reminding me why this work is so important. To my mother-in-law, Dorothy Crawford, thank you for always being willing to help out in any way—it doesn't go unnoticed. To Brittany Crawford and Nikki Velebil, your faith in me as not only your sister-in-law but also as your own fertility doctor means more than you know.

All the art you see in this book was created by Kayla Cavagnaro, who has been working behind the scenes for me since 2020. Kayla, thank you for supporting me, my work, and this book so passionately. To the women who inspire me daily, my cofounders at Pinnacle, Dr Pamela Mehta and Dr Rupa Wong—thank you for pushing me outside my comfort zone and through the process of opening a practice. You can't be it if you can't see it. To Emily Whitlock, thank you for helping me spread my message to the world every day on all the platforms.

To Dr Amanda Skillern: I love you, Louise—thanks for letting me be your Thelma. From driving off the cliff to being doubted by everyone every step of the way, cheers to us. I'll forever bet on us. Being your partner is the highlight of my professional life. Huge thanks to the Fora Fertility family—especially the team who have kept our dream alive, Rikki, Mel, Hannah, Savannah, Lindsey, Emily, Hank, Ruth, Jenn, and Lexi. And to every patient who has trusted me with your journey, you make being a fertility doctor worth it.

For my Austin crew, Kristi, Gayle, Lisa, and Amanda, I'm so lucky to have you. From brainstorming book ideas way back when to celebrating the book deal and all the moments in between, thank you for always being there. To my Austin lady docs, and especially Dr Amanda Horton and Dr Brooke Stubbs, there are not enough words for what it means to have friends like you. To Krisli, my roomie and best friend since the seventh grade, I love you. I know you think this social media world is crazy, but thank you for supporting me endlessly. To the rest of the KDDC, Jenny, Katie, and Jess—thank you for loving me as I am for all this time. To Dr Sarah Wakefield and Dr Kyler Silver, I wouldn't have survived medical school or residency without you.

To my fertility colleagues who supported me when others thought it was crazy to be on social media, thank you. To the OGs—Dr Lora Shahine, Dr Serena Chen, Dr Roohi Jeelani, and Dr Stephanie Gustin—I love you and am honored to be in your circle. To Dr Mary Claire Haver, who has given me honest advice without hesitation, I aspire to lift others as you do. To the Parkland OB-GYN residency program, especially Dr Lisa Halvorson, thank you for embracing me in the lab. To the UNC Fertility team when I was there—Dr Anne Steiner, Dr Steve Young, Dr Marc Fritz, Dr Jenny Mersereau, Dr Matt Coward, Dr Emily Evans-Hoeker, Dr Tolga Mesen, Dr Heather Hoff, and Dr Brianna Schumacher—thank you for supporting me then and now, and for pushing me to ask questions, do the research, and find answers. I'm the clinician I am today because of you.

To the worst club with the best members, the infertility community who rallied behind me from day one, this book exists because of you. Despite every no and being told there was no market for a fertility book—your support of me online and in real life mattered. You were tangible proof to the publishing world that women want to learn about their fertility, and I'll forever be thankful that you helped this dream come true. This book is for us.

APPENDIX

# Navigating Your Fertility Appointments

One of the hardest parts of infertility is understanding how to advocate for yourself at the doctor's office and knowing what questions to ask. I want you to feel prepared for each visit and stage of the journey, from the moment you make a fertility consult all the way through treatment. Here are my recommended questions to ask and tips for how to prepare for your fertility appointments.

## WHAT TO EXPECT AT YOUR FIRST FERTILITY APPOINTMENT

Walking into a fertility clinic is not something planned by most women. As a fertility doctor I know that when we don't plan for something, we are not prepared. I want you to know what might be in store for you or your friends and family members when it comes to this first visit.

Infertility does not discriminate, and I am a firm believer that each couple needs a full evaluation. Infertility is not a woman's disease but a couple's disease. If you have a partner, you both need a complete evaluation.

First, you need to decide which clinic to see. There are many different ways to choose a fertility clinic and many factors to consider, but I think these are the two best ways to find a clinic:

1. Ask your OB-GYN who they recommend. Many OB-GYNs may start the initial testing and workup.
2. Ask your friends if they know anyone who has needed to see a fertility doctor. Odds are someone in your friend circle has intimate experience with infertility.

## Scheduling an Appointment

Below are questions you may want to consider when choosing a fertility clinic or deciding where to go for your evaluation. Reminder: You are your best advocate. Ask questions. If something does not feel right at a clinic, find a different one. These questions don't have a "right" answer, but they help you set expectations.

### *Who are you going to see?*

- Do you get to request a doctor, or does the clinic randomly assign you to someone?
- Will your clinic have you see a doctor or another provider first?

### *What is the first appointment structure?*

- Is your first consultation in person or via telemedicine?
- If it is in person, will blood work and an ultrasound be done? Ask about parking and give yourself plenty of time.
- If the meeting is via telemedicine, can your partner (if applicable) join if you are in different locations?
- Are there multiple locations, and if so, are you assigned to one location? If the location is assigned, make sure it is the one you want.
- How long will the first appointment last?
- Do you have paperwork to complete ahead of time?

## *Who do you see for what?*

- Who will you see for ultrasounds or procedures?
- Does your clinic have a "doctor of the day" model, or will you always see your doctor?
- If you always see your doctor, what happens when they are out of town?
- Do you have an assigned nurse?

## *How does the clinic communicate with patients?*

- What is the preferred method of communication? Portal? Email? Phone calls?
- Can you speak directly with your nurse?
- Can you send your doctor a message?
- Do you get results immediately, or do you have to wait for a visit?

## *Where is the lab?*

- Is the IVF lab at a different location?
- Is the IVF lab owned by a different entity than your clinic?
- Where will your eggs, embryos, or sperm be stored?
- Who covers the weekends if a weekend procedure is needed?

## *What is the financial structure?*

- Do you pay for things individually?
- Is there a package price for treatments?

- Is there a dedicated financial staff member?
- Are prices different on the weekend or with different doctors?
- What is the storage cost for eggs, embryos, or sperm?

## Preparing for Your Visit

I prepare for every single patient I see prior to their appointment. I review the medical history forms, any blood work we have, and any prior medical records. One of the biggest challenges I face is being asked a question and not having all the information. You are paying money for your fertility doctor's time and expertise. You should leave the visit with a clear idea of your next steps and a game plan, which will likely be a follow-up visit once all testing has been completed.

### *Do they have your prior medical records?*

- Did you complete a medical record release of information (ROI) form? This is required for clinics to send medical records to each other.
- If you completed an ROI, has the clinic received your records? Clinics have thirty days to send records (though this may vary from state to state). This means you want to fill out your ROI immediately, especially if you have done testing or treatment at another clinic.
- Do you have a copy of your records? If yes, get them to the clinic in advance. Ask if they want them emailed or uploaded into a system.

### *Is there an online medical history to complete?*

- Please fill out all medical history paperwork to the best of your ability.
- If you have had any fertility testing or treatment, include all the details you have.
- If you have a partner, make sure they complete their medical history as well.

## *Are you ready to share your story?*

- Think through your story and be ready to give the highlights. Make sure to share your goals with your fertility doctor.
- How long have you been trying? How did you prevent pregnancy before this?
- Have you been tracking? Are your cycles regular?
- Any difficulties with intercourse?
- Any prior pregnancies or pregnancy losses?
- Any abdominal surgeries or procedures on your uterus or cervix?
- Any known medical problems for you or your partner?
- Any medical problems in your family?
- Any other concerning symptoms?

## *What should you ask during your visit?*

- What are my next steps?
- How can I talk to someone from the financial team about my options?
- Who can I reach out to with questions?
- How do I find out any results?

## WHAT SHOULD YOU ASK BEFORE STARTING FERTILITY TREATMENTS?

I see a lot of patients for second opinion consults. One consistent source of frustration is a lack of understanding why a treatment is recommended or what the expected outcome should be. It is important to know what to ask before starting a cycle and also during your monitoring visits so that you can be your best advocate.

## Questions to Ask Before Ovulation Induction or IUI

- What medication are we using?
- Are there side effects I should be aware of?
- What is my goal number of follicles?
- What number of follicles will result in a canceled cycle?
- How will we monitor for a response? Ultrasound? OPK?
- Will I use a trigger shot?
- How will intercourse or IUI be timed?
- Will IUI samples be collected at home or in the office?
- What will the IUI process be like?
- Are there recommendations or restrictions after IUI?
- How many cycles will we be doing before we need to move on to more aggressive treatment?
- What is the success rate per cycle based on my scenario?

## Questions to Ask Before IVF

### *What should you know before starting a cycle?*

- Is my ovarian reserve normal for my age?
- How many eggs do we expect from one IVF cycle?
- How many embryos might we expect if all things are average?
- Should we do genetic testing?
- If we want __ number of kids, how does that change the plan?
- How often are monitoring visits?
- Who does the monitoring visits?
- How long will I wait at monitoring visits?

- How will I find out the plan after monitoring? Who will contact me and how?
- Why are we choosing this protocol?
- What are the side effects from this protocol?
- How long will the entire process take if everything goes as expected?
- What is the expected rate of progression through culture (fertilized number to blast)?
- How is sperm collected (if applicable)? At home? Lab?
- Who does the retrieval?
- What should I expect on retrieval day? Anesthesia?
- What should I do after retrieval? Are there restrictions? What are my next steps?
- Who communicates embryo results?

### *What should you be asking during your monitoring visits?*

- How many follicles are growing?
- Is this consistent with my AFC?
- Are these results in line with what we are expecting?
- How many mature eggs are we expecting based on this (ultrasound on trigger day or close to trigger day)?

## Questions to Ask Before Embryo Transfer

### *What should you know before starting a cycle?*

- Who does the embryo transfer?
- Who does the monitoring ultrasounds?
- Do you recommend valium on transfer day?

- What blood work will we follow at monitoring?
- When do we check hCG levels?
- Do I need suppression first, like birth control pills or Lupron?
- What is the timeline for this protocol?
- Do I get to choose which embryo (sex)?
- How many embryos will we transfer?
- What is the expected rate of success based on my scenario?
- What testing will be done prior to transfer? Saline sonogram? Hysteroscopy?
- Do we need any additional testing based on _____ (pregnancy loss, endometriosis, etc.)?
- What embryo transfer protocol do you recommend?
- Why is this the best protocol for me?
- What are the expected side effects of this protocol?
- What happens on transfer day?
- Can I have a support person in the room?

## *What should you be asking during your monitoring visits?*

- What are we looking for today?
- Is the lining trilaminar?
- What is my endometrial thickness?
- Are we checking labs today? If so, what are we looking for?
- Does anything we see today change my plan?

# WHAT SHOULD YOU DO AFTER A FAILED CYCLE?

It can be devastating when a treatment cycle ends without the outcome we were hoping for. A failed cycle can be many different things—you didn't get any eggs at retrieval, you had no blastocysts develop, there were no euploid embryos, or your embryo transfer failed. Sometimes a failed cycle may not be surprising, even if it is disappointing, and sometimes a failed cycle can be shocking. My first piece of advice is to allow yourself space to grieve. After this, consider setting up a WTF visit with your doctor to review the game plan. Sometimes we need to change the protocol or make adjustments, and other times the cycle protocol did exactly what it should—we just need to give it another go. Remember that even with a genetically normal embryo, highest live birth rates are around 65 percent, which means that not every euploid embryo will implant.

## Questions to Ask After a Failed IVF Cycle:

- How many follicles did we measure about 14 mm on the last monitoring day?
- Did we get as many mature eggs as we were expecting?
- Do you think another protocol could help improve the number of mature eggs?
- Should we consider a different dose of medication? A different suppression option?
- If maturity was low, what could we do to improve this? Change the mature follicle range? Change the trigger type? Change the trigger time?
- What was the fertilization rate? Was this expected?
- If fertilization was low, is there anything we can do to improve this? Change to ICSI? Anything abnormal with the sperm on retrieval day?
- How many embryos reached the blastocyst stage? Was this what we expected?

- If the blast rate was low, when did development stop? Does this information change our next cycle game plan?
- If no blasts developed, were there any concerning signs for a male factor? Should we consider a sperm DNA fragmentation?
- Did the lab have any notes on fragmentation, abnormal cleavage, or any egg/sperm/embryo quality concerns?
- If PGT was used, did we have the expected number or euploid embryos based on my age?
- If euploid rate was low, is there anything we can do to try to improve egg or sperm quality? Are there any protocol changes that could help? Should we consider adding on human growth hormone?
- What protocol changes do you recommend for the next cycle (if any)?

## Questions to Ask After a Failed Embryo Transfer:

- How did my lining look at the last monitoring visit? What was the thickness? Was it trilaminar?
- Was there any fluid in the lining or evidence of a uterine niche?
- What was my peak lining thickness in my IVF cycle? If this is much different than your FET lining, should we try another protocol or different medications? What about adding vaginal estradiol or Viagra?
- What was my estrogen level at monitoring (if checked)? Was this in the optimal range? Should we make any changes based on this?
- What was my progesterone level (if checked)? Was this in the optimal range? Should we make any changes based on this?
- When was my last uterine cavity evaluation? If it was not in the last six months, should we repeat this (saline-infused sonogram or hysteroscopy) prior to the next transfer?
- When was the last time I had labs checked for thyroid, prolactin, and HbA1c (or fasting insulin)? If these were not in the last six months, can they be repeated?

- Have we ruled out a hydrosalpinx?

- Is there any concern for possible adenomyosis or endometriosis? What would be the optimal protocol if there was (would we make any cycle changes)? What about if there are signs of recurrent implantation failure? Should we consider a protocol with suppression to decrease inflammation (Lupron, Lupron and letrozole, or Orilissa)?

- Should we consider evaluating for chronic endometritis (with an endometrial biopsy or hysteroscopy) or empirically treating with antibiotics?

- Are there any additional medications we should add to our treatment plan that are low risk and may help, such as steroids, baby aspirin, antibiotics?

- Will we make any changes if the next transfer fails?

- What protocol changes do you expect for the next cycle (if any)?

Reminder: You are your best advocate. Ask questions. If something does not feel right, listen to your gut. You are now prepared to take an active role in your fertility journey.

# Notes

**CHAPTER 1**

1. Stentz NC, Griffith KA, Perkins E, Jones RD, Jagsi R. Fertility and childbearing among American female physicians. *J Womens Health (Larchmt)*. 2016 Oct;25(10):1059–65.
2. Weiss G, Goldsmith LT, Taylor RN, Bellet D, Taylor HS. Inflammation in reproductive disorders. *Reprod Sci*. 2009 Feb;16(2):216–29.
3. Ameho S, Klutstein M. The effect of chronic inflammation on female fertility. *Reproduction*. 2025 Mar 3;169(4):e240197. doi: 10.1530/REP-24-0197. PMID: 39932461; PMCID: PMC11896653.
4. Pisarska MD. Fertility status and overall health. *Semin Reprod Med*. 2017 May;35(3):203–4.
5. Cox CM, Thoma ME, Tchangalova N, Mburu G, Bornstein MJ, Johnson CL, Kiarie J. Infertility prevalence and the methods of estimation from 1990 to 2021: a systematic review and meta-analysis. *Hum Reprod Open*. 2022 Nov 12;2022(4):hoac051.
6. Centers for Disease Control and Prevention. Women's reproductive health. https://www.cdc.gov/reproductive-health/women-health/index.html. Published May 15, 2024.
7. World Health Organization. Infertility prevalence estimates, 1990–2021. Geneva: World Health Organization; 2023. License: CC BY-NY-SA3.0 IGO. https://www.who.int/publications/i/item/978920068315.
8. Guttmacher AF. Factors affecting normal expectancy of conception. *JAMA*. 1956;161:855.
9. Centers for Disease Control and Prevention. National public health action plan for the detection, prevention, and management of infertility. June 2014. https://www.cdc.gov/reproductive-health/media/pdfs/infertility/DRH-NAP-Final-508.pdf.
10. Nugent CN, Chandra A. Infertility and impaired fecundity in women and men in the United States, 2015–2019. *Natl Health Stat Report*. 2024 Apr;202:1–19.
11. Malesza IJ, Malesza M, Walkowiak J, Mussin N, Walkowiak D, Aringazina R, Bartkowiak-Wieczorek J, Mądry E. High-fat, Western-style diet, systemic inflammation, and gut microbiota: a narrative review. *Cells*. 2021 Nov 14;10(11):3164.
12. Bishop B, Webber WS, Atif SM, Ley A, Pankratz KA, Kostelecky R, Colgan SP, Dinarello CA, Zhang W, Li S. Micro- and nano-plastics induce inflammation and cell death in human cells. *Front Immunol*. 2025 Mar 31;16:1528502.
13. Gouin JP, Glaser R, Malarkey WB, Beversdorf D, Kiecolt-Glaser J. Chronic stress, daily stressors, and circulating inflammatory markers. *Health Psychol*. 2012 Mar;31(2):264–68.
14. Devine K, Mumford SL, Wu M, DeCherney AH, Hill MJ, Propst A. Diminished ovarian reserve in the United States assisted reproductive technology population: diagnostic trends among 181,536 cycles from the Society for Assisted Reproductive Technology Clinic Outcomes Reporting System. *Fertil Steril*. 2015 Sep;104(3):612–19.e3.

15. Rasmark Roepke E, Matthiesen L, Rylance R, Christiansen OB. Is the incidence of recurrent pregnancy loss increasing? A retrospective register-based study in Sweden. *Acta Obstet Gynecol Scand.* 2017 Nov;96(11):1365–72.
16. Travison TG, Araujo AB, O'Donnell AB, Kupelian V, McKinlay JB. A population-level decline in serum testosterone levels in American men. *J Clin Endocrinol Metab.* 2007 Jan;92(1):196–202.
17. Levine H, Jørgensen N, Martino-Andrade A, Mendiola J, Weksler-Derri D, Mindlis I, Pinotti R, Swan SH. Temporal trends in sperm count: a systematic review and meta-regression analysis. *Hum Reprod Update.* 2017 Nov 1;23(6):646–59.
18. Boots CE, Jungheim ES. Inflammation and human ovarian follicular dynamics. *Semin Reprod Med.* 2015;33(4):270–75.
19. Amini MA, Karimi M, Talebi SS, Piri H, Karimi J. The association of oxidative stress and reactive oxygen species modulator 1 (ROMO1) with infertility: a mini review. *Chonnam Med J.* 2022 Sep;58(3):91–95.
20. Tomioka RB, Ferreira GRV, Aikawa NE, Maciel GAR, Serafini PC, Sallum AM, Campos LMA, Goldestein-Schainberg C, Bonfá E, Silva CA. Non-steroidal anti-inflammatory drug induces luteinized unruptured follicle syndrome in young female juvenile idiopathic arthritis patients. *Clin Rheumatol.* 2018 Oct;37(10):2869–73.
21. Mendonça LL, Khamashta MA, Nelson-Piercy C, Hunt BJ, Hughes GR. Non-steroidal anti-inflammatory drugs as a possible cause for reversible infertility. *Rheumatology (Oxford).* 2000 Aug;39(8):880–82.
22. Li H, Meng Y, He S, Tan X, Zhang Y, Zhang X, Wang L, Zheng W. Macrophages. Chronic inflammation, and insulin resistance. *Cells.* 2022 Sep 26;11(19):3001.
23. Martínez-Montoro JI, Damas-Fuentes M, Fernández-García JC, Tinahones FJ. Role of the gut microbiome in beta cell and adipose tissue crosstalk: a review. *Front Endocrinol (Lausanne).* 2022 May 12;13:869951.
24. Lei R, Chen S, Li W. Advances in the study of the correlation between insulin resistance and infertility. *Front Endocrinol (Lausanne).* 2024 Jan 26;15:1288326.
25. Craig LB, Ke RW, Kutteh WH. Increased prevalence of insulin resistance in women with a history of recurrent pregnancy loss. *Fertil Steril.* 2002 Sep;78(3):487–90.
26. Pisetsky DS. Pathogenesis of autoimmune disease. *Nat Rev Nephrol.* 2023 Aug;19(8):509–24.
27. Moulton VR. Sex hormones in acquired immunity and autoimmune disease. *Front Immunol.* 2018 Oct 4;9:2279.
28. Gleicher N, Weiner R, Vietzke M. The impact of abnormal autoimmune function on reproduction: maternal and fetal consequences. *J Autoimmun.* 2006 Nov;27(3):161–65.
29. Nelson JL, Koepsell TD, Dugowson CE, Voigt LF, Daling JR, Hansen JA. Fecundity before disease onset in women with rheumatoid arthritis. *Arthritis Rheum.* 1993 Jan;36:7–14.
30. Dinse GE, Parks CG, Weinberg CR, Co CA, Wilkerson J, Zeldin DC, Chan EKL, Miller FW. Increasing prevalence of antinuclear antibodies in the United States. *Arthritis Rheum.* 2022 Dec;74(12):2032–41.
31. World Health Organization. Infertility. https://www.who.int/news-room/fact-sheets/detail/infertility. Published May 22, 2024.
32. Murugappan G, Li S, Lathi RB, Baker VL, Eisenberg ML. Increased risk of incident chronic medical conditions in infertile women: analysis of US claims data. *Am J Obstet Gynecol.* 2019 May;220(5):473.e1–473.e14.
33. Huttler A, Murugappan G, Stentz NC, Cedars MI. Reproduction as a window to future health in women. *Fertil Steril.* 2023 Sep;120(3 Pt 1):421–28.
34. Stentz NC, Koelper N, Barnhart KT, Sammel MD, Senapati S. Infertility and mortality. *Am J Obstet Gynecol.* 2020 Mar;222(3):251.e1–251.e10.
35. Wang YX, Farland LV, Wang S, Gaskins AJ, Wang L, Rich-Edwards JW, Tamimi R, Missmer SA, Chavarro JE. Association of infertility with premature mortality among US women: prospective cohort study. *Lancet Reg Health Am.* 2022 Mar;7:100122.
36. Murugappan G, Li S, Lathi RB, Baker VL, Eisenberg ML. Risk of cancer in infertile women: analysis of US claims data. *Hum Reprod.* 2019 May 1;34(5):894–902.
37. Gleason JL, Shenassa ED, Thoma ME. Self-reported infertility, metabolic dysfunction, and cardiovascular events: a cross-sectional analysis among US women. *Fertil Steril.* 2019 Jan;111(1):138–46.

## CHAPTER 2

1. Turnbull AV, Rivier CL. Regulation of the hypothalamic-pituitary-adrenal axis by cytokines: actions and mechanisms of action. *Physiol Rev.* 1999 Jan;79(1):1–71.
2. Yeung EH, Zhang C, Mumford SL, Ye A, Trevisan M, Chen L, Browne RW, Wactawski-Wende J, Schisterman EF. Longitudinal study of insulin resistance and sex hormones over the menstrual cycle: the BioCycle Study. *J Clin Endocrinol Metab.* 2010 Dec;95(12):5435–42.
3. Gaskins AJ, Wilchesky M, Mumford SL, Whitcomb BW, Browne RW, Wactawski-Wende J, Perkins NJ, Schisterman EF. Endogenous reproductive hormones and C-reactive protein across the menstrual cycle: the BioCycle Study. *Am J Epidemiol.* 2012 Mar 1;175(5):423–31.
4. Mukamal KJ, Muller JE, Maclure M, Sherwood JB, Mittleman MA. Variation in the risk of onset of acute myocardial infarction during the menstrual cycle. *Am J Cardiol.* 2002 Jul 1;90(1):49–51.
5. Harris BS, Steiner AZ, Faurot KR, Long A, Jukic AM. Systemic inflammation and menstrual cycle length in a prospective cohort study. *Am J Obstet Gynecol.* 2023 Feb;228(2):215.e1-215.e17.
6. Gaskins AJ, Wilchesky M, Mumford SL, Whitcomb BW, Browne RW, Wactawski-Wende J, Perkins NJ, Schisterman EF. Endogenous reproductive hormones and C-reactive protein across the menstrual cycle: the BioCycle Study. *Am J Epidemiol.* 2012 Mar 1;175(5):423–31.
7. McGlade EA, Miyamoto A, Winuthayanon W. Progesterone and inflammatory response in the oviduct during physiological and pathological conditions. *Cells.* 2022 Mar 23;11(7):1075. doi: 10.3390/cells11071075. PMID: 35406639; PMCID: PMC8997425.
8. Motomura K, Miller D, Galaz J, Liu TN, Romero R, Gomez-Lopez N. The effects of progesterone on immune cellular function at the maternal-fetal interface and in maternal circulation. *J Steroid Biochem Mol Biol.* 2023 May;229:106254.
9. Filicori M, Butler JP, Crowley WF Jr. Neuroendocrine regulation of the corpus luteum in the human. Evidence for pulsatile progesterone secretion. *J Clin Invest.* 1984;73:1638–47.
10. Skiba MA, Bell RJ, Islam RM, Handelsman DJ, Desai R, Davis SR. Androgens during the reproductive years: what is normal for women? *J Clin Endocrinol Metab.* 2019 Nov 1;104(11):5382–92.
11. Gaskins AJ, Wilchesky M, Mumford SL, Whitcomb BW, Browne RW, Wactawski-Wende J, Perkins NJ, Schisterman EF. Endogenous reproductive hormones and C-reactive protein across the menstrual cycle: the BioCycle Study. *Am J Epidemiol.* 2012 Mar 1;175(5):423–31.
12. Zhao H, Zhang J, Cheng X, Nie X, He B. Insulin resistance in polycystic ovary syndrome across various tissues: an updated review of pathogenesis, evaluation, and treatment. *J Ovarian Res.* 2023 Jan 11;16(1):9.
13. Lei R, Chen S, Li W. Advances in the study of the correlation between insulin resistance and infertility. *Front Endocrinol (Lausanne).* 2024 Jan 26;15:1288326.
14. Li D, Radulescu A, Shrestha RT, Root M, Karger AB, Killeen AA, Hodges JS, Fan SL, Ferguson A, Garg U, Sokoll LJ, Burmeister LA. Association of biotin ingestion with performance of hormone and nonhormone assays in healthy adults. *JAMA.* 2017 Sep 26;318(12):1150–60.
15. Young JR, Jaffe RB. Strength-duration characteristics of estrogen effects on gonadotropin response to gonadotropin-releasing hormone in women. II. Effects of varying concentrations of estradiol. *J Clin Endocrinol Metab.* 1976;42(3):432–42.
16. Harris BS, Steiner AZ, Faurot KR, Long A, Jukic AM. Systemic inflammation and menstrual cycle length in a prospective cohort study. *Am J Obstet Gynecol.* 2023 Feb;228(2):215.e1-215.e17.
17. Najmabadi S, Schliep KC, Simonsen SE, Porucznik CA, Egger MJ, Stanford JB. Menstrual bleeding, cycle length, and follicular and luteal phase lengths in women without known subfertility: a pooled analysis of three cohorts. *Paediatr Perinat Epidemiol.* 2020 May;34(3):318–27.

## CHAPTER 3

1. Doxsey M, Patel K, Faschan K, Reyes L. Assessing student and physician fertility awareness utilizing the Fertility and Infertility Treatment Knowledge Score (FIT-KS). *Cureus.* 2024 Sep 26;16(9):e70244.

2. Nugent CN, Chandra A. Infertility and impaired fecundity in women and men in the United States, 2015–2019. *Natl Health Stat Report.* 2024 Apr;202:1–19.
3. Stein A. A woman's age, childbearing, and childrearing. *Am J Epidemiol.* 1985;121:327–42.
4. Baker TG. A quantitative and cytological study of germ cells in human ovaries. *Pro R Soc Lond B Biol Sci.* 1963;158:417–33.
5. Faddy MJ, Gosden RG. A model conforming the decline in follicle numbers to the age of menopause in women. *Hum Reprod.* 1996 Jul;11(7):1484–46.
6. Block E. Quantitative and morphologic investigations of the follicular system in women; variations at different ages. *Acta Anat (Basel).* 1952;14:108–23.
7. Zeng Y, Wang C, Yang C, Shan X, Meng XQ, Zhang M. Unveiling the role of chronic inflammation in ovarian aging: insights into mechanisms and clinical implications. *Hum Reprod.* 2024 Aug 1;39(8):1599–1607.
8. Zhu Q, Li Y, Ma J, Ma H, Liang X. Potential factors result in diminished ovarian reserve: a comprehensive review. *J Ovarian Res.* 2023 Oct 25;16(1):208.
9. Shalom-Paz E, Weill S, Ginzberg Y, Khatib N, Anabusi S, Klorin G, Sabo E, Beloosesky R. IUGR induced by maternal chronic inflammation: long-term effect on offspring's ovaries in rat model—a preliminary report. *J Endocrinol Invest.* 2017;40:1125–31.
10. Cramer DW, Xu H, Harlow BL. Family history as a predictor of early menopause. *Fertil Steril.* 1995 Oct;64(4):740–45.
11. Practice Committee of the American Society for Reproductive Medicine. Testing and interpreting measures of ovarian reserve: a committee opinion. *Fertil Steril.* 2020 Dec;114(6):1151–57.
12. Nelson SM, Davis SR, Kalantaridou S, Lumsden MA, Panay N, Anderson RA. Anti-Müllerian hormone for the diagnosis and prediction of menopause: a systematic review. *Hum Reprod Update.* 2023 May 2;29(3):327–46.
13. American College of Obstetricians and Gynecologists. ACOG Committee opinion no. 773 summary: the use of antimüllerian hormone in women not seeking fertility care. *Obstet Gynecol.* 2019 Apr;133(4):840–41.
14. Scheffer GJ, Broekmans FJ, Dorland M, Habbema JD, Looman CW, te Velde ER. Antral follicle counts by transvaginal ultrasonography are related to age in women with proven natural fertility. *Fertil Steril.* 1999;72:845–51.
15. Cedars MI. Evaluation of female fertility—AMH and ovarian reserve testing. *J Clin Endocrinol Metab.* 2022 May 17;107(6):1510–19.
16. Hendricks DJ, Mol BW, Bancsi LF, Te Velde ER, Broekmans FJ. Antral follicle count in the prediction of poor ovarian response and pregnancy after in vitro fertilization: a meta-analysis and comparison with basal follicle-stimulating hormone level. *Fertil Steril.* 2005;83:191–301.
17. Broekmans FJ, Faddy MJ, Scheffer G, te Velde ER. Antral follicle counts are related to age at natural fertility loss and age at menopause. *Menopause.* 2004 Nov–Dec;11(6 Pt 1):607–14.
18. Rosen MP, Johnstone E, Addauan-Andersen C, Cedars MI. A lower antral follicle count is associated with infertility. *Fertil Steril.* 2011 May;95(6):1950–54, 1954.e1.
19. Klein NA, Battaglia DE, Fujimoto VY, Davis GS, Bremner WJ, Soules MR. Reproductive aging: accelerated ovarian follicular development associated with a monotropic follicle-stimulating hormone rise in normal older women. *J Clin Endocrinol Metab.* 1996;81:1038–45.
20. Burger HG, Dudley EC, Hopper JL, Groome N, Guthrie JR, Green A, Dennerstein L. Prospectively measured levels of serum follicle-stimulating hormone, estradiol, and the dimeric inhibins during the menopausal transition in a population-based cohort of women. *J Clin Endocrinol Metab.* 1999 Nov;84(11):4025–30.
21. Biniasch M, Laubender RP, Hund M, Buck K, De Geyter C. Intra- and inter-cycle variability of anti-Müllerian hormone (AMH) levels in healthy women during non-consecutive menstrual cycles: the BICYCLE study. *Clin Chem Lab Med.* 2021 Oct 29;60(4):597–605.
22. Melado L, Lawrenz B, Sibal J, Abu E, Coughlan C, Navarro AT, Fatemi HM. Antimüllerian hormone during natural cycle presents significant intra and intercycle variations when measured with fully automated assay. *Front Endocrinol (Lausanne).* 2018 Nov 27;9:686.
23. Tal R, Seifer DB. Ovarian reserve testing: a user's guide. *Am J Obstet Gynecol.* 2017 Aug;217(2):129–40.
24. Lie Fong S, Visser JA, Welt CK, et al. Serum anti-müllerian hormone levels in healthy females: a nomogram ranging from infancy to adulthood. *J Clin Endocrinol Metab.* 2012;97:4650–55.

25. Steiner AZ, Pritchard D, Stanczyk FZ, Kesner JS, Meadows JW, Herring AH, Baird DD. Association between biomarkers of ovarian reserve and infertility among older women of reproductive age. *JAMA.* 2017;318:1367-76.
26. Harris BS, Jukic AM, Truong T, Nagle CT, Erkanli A, Steiner AZ. Markers of ovarian reserve as predictors of future fertility. *Fertil Steril.* 2023 Jan;119(1):99-106.
27. Nelson SM, Shaw M, Ewing BJ, McLean K, Vechery A, Briggs SF. Antimüllerian hormone levels are associated with time to pregnancy in a cohort study of 3,150 women. *Fertil Steril.* 2024 Dec;122(6):1114-23.
28. Hariton E, Shirazi TN, Douglas NC, Hershlag A, Briggs SF. Anti-müllerian hormone levels among contraceptive users: evidence from a cross-sectional cohort of 27,125 individuals. *Am J Obstet Gynecol.* 2021 Nov;225(5):515.e1-515.e10.
29. Landersoe SK, Birch Petersen K, Sørensen AL, Larsen EC, Martinussen T, Lunding SA, Kroman MS, Nielsen HS, Nyboe Andersen A. Ovarian reserve markers after discontinuing long-term use of combined oral contraceptives. *Reprod Biomed Online.* 2020 Jan;40(1):176-86.
30. Hassold T, Chiu D. Maternal age-specific rates of numerical chromosomal abnormalities with specific reference to trisomy. *Hum Genet.* 1985;70:11-17.
31. Morimoto A, Rose RD, Smith KM, Dinh DT, Umehara T, Winstanley YE, Shibahara H, Russell DL, Robker RL. Granulosa cell metabolism at ovulation correlates with oocyte competence and is disrupted by obesity and aging. *Hum Reprod.* 2024 Sep 1;39(9):2053-66.
32. Wang H, Zhang Y, Fang X, Kwak-Kim J, Wu L. Insulin resistance adversely affect IVF outcomes in lean women without PCOS. *Front Endocrinol (Lausanne).* 2021 Sep 6;12:734638.
33. Li F, Qi JJ, Li LX, Yan TF. Impact of insulin resistance on IVF/ICSI outcomes in women with polycystic ovary syndrome: A systematic review and meta-analysis. *Eur J Obstet Gynecol Reprod Biol.* 2024 Aug;299:54-61.
34. Zhang Y, Li T, Wang Y, Yu Y. Key glycometabolism during oocyte maturation and early embryonic development. *Reproduction.* 2025 Feb 4;169(3):e240275.
35. Pacella L, Zander-Fox DL, Armstrong DT, Lane M. Women with reduced ovarian reserve or advanced maternal age have an altered follicular environment. *Fertil Steril.* 2012 Oct;98(4):986-94.e1-2.
36. Liu Y, Han M, Li X, Wang H, Ma M, Zhang S, Guo Y, Wang S, Wang Y, Duan N, Xu B, Yin J, Yao Y. Age-related changes in the mitochondria of human mural granulosa cells. *Hum Reprod.* 2017 Dec 1;32(12):2465-73.
37. Steiner AZ, Jukic AM. Impact of female age and nulligravidity on fecundity in an older reproductive age cohort. *Fertil Steril.* 2016;105(6):1584-88.
38. Magnus MC, Wilcox AJ, Morken NH, Weinberg CR, Håberg SE. Role of maternal age and pregnancy history in risk of miscarriage: prospective register based study. *BMJ.* 2019 Mar 20;364:l869.
39. Minasi MG, Colasante A, Riccio T, Ruberti A, Casciani V, Scarselli F, Spinella F, Fiorentino F, Varricchio MT, Greco E, et al. Correlation between aneuploidy, standard morphology evaluation and morphokinetic development in 1730 biopsied blastocysts: a consecutive case series study. *Hum Reprod.* 2016;31:2245-54.
40. Steiner AZ, Jukic AM. Impact of female age and nulligravidity on fecundity in an older reproductive age cohort. *Fertil Steril.* 2016;105(6):1584-88.
41. Habbema JD, Eijkemans MJ, Leridon H, te Velde ER. Realizing a desired family size: when should couples start? *Hum Reprod.* 2015 Sep;30(9):2215-21.
42. Gougeon A. Regulation of ovarian follicular development in primates: facts and hypotheses. *Endocr Rev.* 1996; 17:121-55.
43. Sasaki H, Hamatani T, Kamijo S, et al. Impact of oxidative stress on age-associated decline in oocyte developmental competence. *Front Endocrinol (Lausanne).* 2019;10:811.
44. Cil AP, Bang K, Oktay K. Age specific probability of live birth with oocyte cryopreservation: an individual patient data meta-analysis. *Fertil Steril.* 2013;100:492-99.
45. Mesen TB, Mersereau JE, Kane JB, Steiner AZ. Optimal timing for elective egg freezing. *Fertil Steril.* 2015 Jun;103(6):1551-6.e1-4.

## CHAPTER 4

1. Harris BS, Steiner AZ, Faurot KR, Long A, Jukic AM. Systemic inflammation and menstrual cycle length in a prospective cohort study. *Am J Obstet Gynecol.* 2023 Feb;228(2):215.e1-215.e17.

2. Zeng Y, Wang C, Yang C, Shan X, Meng XQ, Zhang M. Unveiling the role of chronic inflammation in ovarian aging: insights into mechanisms and clinical implications. *Human Reprod.* 2024 Aug 1;39(8):1599–1607.
3. Aboeldalyl S, James C, Seyam E, Ibrahim EM, Shawki HE, Amer S. The role of chronic inflammation in polycystic ovarian syndrome—a systematic review and meta-analysis. *Int J Mol Sci.* 2021 Mar 8;22(5):2734.
4. Ameho S, Klutstein M. The effect of chronic inflammation on female fertility. *Reproduction.* 2025 Mar 3;169(4):e240197.
5. Brundu B, Loucks TL, Adler LJ, Cameron JL, Berga SL. Increased cortisol in the cerebrospinal fluid of women with functional hypothalamic amenorrhea. *J Clin Endocrinol Metab.* 2006 Apr;91(4):1561–65.
6. Schury MP, Adigun R. Sheehan syndrome. StatPearls. Updated Sep 4, 2023. https://www.ncbi.nlm.nih.gov/books/NBK459166/.
7. Vekemans M. Postpartum contraception: the lactational amenorrhea method. *Eur J Contracept Reprod Health Care.* 1997 Jun;2(2):105–11.
8. Molitoris J. Breast-feeding during pregnancy and the risk of miscarriage. *Perspect Sex Reprod Health.* 2019 Sep;51(3):153–63.
9. Sheehan MT. Biochemical testing of the thyroid: TSH is the best and, oftentimes, only test needed—a review for primary care. *Clin Med Res.* 2016 Jun;14(2):83–92.
10. Dosiou C. Thyroid and fertility: recent advances. *Thyroid.* 2020 Apr;30(4):479–86.
11. Krassas GE, Poppe K, Glinoer D. Thyroid function and human reproductive health. *Endocr Rev.* 2010 Oct;31(5):702–55.
12. Krassas GE, Poppe K, Glinoer D. Thyroid function and human reproductive health. *Endocr Rev.* 2010 Oct;31(5):702–55.
13. Chaker L, Bianco AC, Jonklaas J, Peeters RP. Hypothyroidism. *Lancet.* 2017 Sep 23;390(10101):1550–62.
14. Antonelli A, Ferrari SM, Corrado A, Di Domenicantonio A, Fallahi P. Autoimmune thyroid disorders. *Autoimmun Rev.* 2015 Feb;14(2):174–80.
15. Tingi E, Syed AA, Kyriacou A, Mastorakos G, Kyriacou A. Benign thyroid disease in pregnancy: a state of the art review. *J Clin Transl Endocrinol.* 2016 Nov 23;6:37–49.
16. Alexander EK, Pearce EN, Brent GA, Brown RS, Chen H, Dosiou C, Grobman WA, Laurberg P, Lazarus JH, Mandel SJ, Peeters RP, Sullivan S. 2017 Guidelines of the American Thyroid Association for the diagnosis and management of thyroid disease during pregnancy and the postpartum. *Thyroid.* 2017 Mar;27(3):315–89.
17. De Groot L, Abalovich M, Alexander EK, Amino N, Barbour L, Cobin RH, Eastman CJ, Lazarus JH, Luton D, Mandel SJ, Mestman J, Rovet J, Sullivan S. Management of thyroid dysfunction during pregnancy and postpartum: an Endocrine Society clinical practice guideline. *J Clin Endocrinol Metab.* 2012 Aug;97(8):2543–65.
18. De Leo S, Lee SY, Braverman LE. Hyperthyroidism. *Lancet.* 2016 Aug 27;388(10047):906–18.
19. ESHRE, ASRM, CREWHIRL, and IMS Guideline Group on POI. Premature ovarian insufficiency (POI). POI Guideline 2024. 2024:43. https://www.asrm.org/practice-guidance/practice-committee-documents/evidence-based-guideline-premature-ovarian-insufficiency--2024.
20. Sullivan SD, Sarrel PM, Nelson LM. Hormone replacement therapy in young women with primary ovarian insufficiency and early menopause. *Fertil Steril.* 2016 Dec;106(7):1588–99.
21. Ishizuka B. Current understanding of the etiology, symptomatology, and treatment options in premature ovarian insufficiency (POI). *Front Endocrinol (Lausanne).* 2021 Feb 25;12:626924.
22. Huang Y, Hu C, Ye H, Luo R, Fu X, Li X, Huang J, Chen W, Zheng Y. Inflamm-Aging: a new mechanism affecting premature ovarian insufficiency. *J Immunol Res.* 2019 Jan 2;2019:8069898.
23. Bachelot A, Nicolas C, Bidet M, Dulon J, Leban M, Golmard JL, et al. Long-term outcome of ovarian function in women with intermittent premature ovarian insufficiency. *Clin Endocrinol (Oxf).* 2017;86:223–28.
24. Teede H, Deeks A, Moran L. Polycystic ovary syndrome: a complex condition with psychological, reproductive and metabolic manifestations that impacts on health across the lifespan. *BMC Med.* 2010;8:41.
25. Ovalle F, Azziz R. Insulin resistance, polycystic ovary syndrome, and type 2 diabetes mellitus. *Fertil Steril.* 2002 Jun;77(6):1095–105.

26. Zhao H, Zhang J, Cheng X, Nie X, He B. Insulin resistance in polycystic ovary syndrome across various tissues: an updated review of pathogenesis, evaluation, and treatment. *J Ovarian Res.* 2023;16(1):9.
27. Teede HJ, Tay CT, Laven J, Dokras A, Moran LJ, Piltonen TT, Costello MF, Boivin J, Redman LM, Boyle JA, Norman RJ, Mousa A, Joham AE; International PCOS Network. Recommendations from the 2023 international evidence-based guideline for the assessment and management of polycystic ovary syndrome. *Fertil Steril.* 2023 Oct;120(4):767–93.
28. Adeva-Andany MM, González-Lucán M, Fernández-Fernández C, Carneiro-Freire N, Seco-Filgueira M, Pedre-Piñeiro AM. Effect of diet composition on insulin sensitivity in humans. *Clin Nutr ESPEN.* 2019 Oct;33:29–38.
29. Legro RS, Barnhart HX, Schlaff WD, Carr BR, Diamond MP, Carson SA, Steinkampf MP, Coutifaris C, McGovern PG, Cataldo NA, Gosman GG, Nestler JE, Giudice LC, Leppert PC, Myers ER; Cooperative Multicenter Reproductive Medicine Network. Clomiphene, metformin, or both for infertility in the polycystic ovary syndrome. *N Engl J Med.* 2007 Feb 8;356(6):551–66.
30. Sharpe A, Morley LC, Tang T, Norman RJ, Balen AH. Metformin for ovulation induction (excluding gonadotrophins) in women with polycystic ovary syndrome. *Cochrane Database of Syst Rev.* 2019 Dec 17;12(12):CD013505.
31. Unfer V, Nestler JE, Kamenov ZA, Prapas N, Facchinetti F. Effects of Inositol(s) in women with PCOS: a systematic review of randomized controlled trials. *Int J Endocrinol.* 2016;2016:1849162.
32. Bahri Khomami M, Shorakae S, Hashemi S, et al. Systematic review and meta-analysis of pregnancy outcomes in women with polycystic ovary syndrome. *Nat Commun.* 2024 Jul 4;15(1):5591.
33. Dreisler E, Stampe Sorensen S, Ibsen PH, Lose G. Prevalence of endometrial polyps and abnormal uterine bleeding in a Danish population aged 20–74 years. *Ultrasound Obstet Gynecol.* 2009 Jan;33(1):102–8.
34. Stamatellos I, Apostolides A, Stamatopoulos P, Bontis J. Pregnancy rates after hysteroscopic polypectomy depending on the size or number of the polyps. *Arch Gynecol Obstet.* 2008 May;277(5):395–99.
35. Al Chami A, Saridogan E. Endometrial polyps and subfertility. *J Obstet Gynaecol India.* 2017 Feb;67(1):9–14.
36. Kalampokas T, Tzanakaki D, Konidaris S, Iavazzo C, Kalampokas E, Gregoriou O. Endometrial polyps and their relationship in the pregnancy rates of patients undergoing intrauterine insemination. *Clin Exp Obstet Gynecol.* 2012;39(3):299–302.
37. Gu J, Sun Q, Qi Y, et al. The effect of chronic endometritis and treatment on patients with unexplained infertility. *BMC Women's Health.* 2023;23:345.
38. Volodarsky-Perel A, Badeghiesh A, Shrem G, Steiner N, Tulandi T. Chronic endometritis in fertile and infertile women who underwent hysteroscopic polypectomy. *J Minim Invasive Gynecol.* 2020 Jul–Aug;27(5):1112–118.
39. Hanstede MM, van der Meij E, Goedemans L, Emanuel MH. Results of centralized Asherman surgery, 2003–2013. *Fertil Steril.* 2015 Dec;104(6):1561–8.e1.
40. *Heavy Menstrual Bleeding: Assessment and Management.* London: National Institute for Health and Care Excellence (NICE); 2021 May 24.
41. Vannuccini S, Petraglia F, Carmona F, Calaf J, Chapron C. The modern management of uterine fibroids-related abnormal uterine bleeding. *Fertil Steril.* 2024 Jul;122(1):20–30.
42. Practice Committee of the American Society for Reproductive Medicine. Removal of myomas in asymptomatic patients to improve fertility and/or reduce miscarriage rate: a guideline. *Fertil Steril.* 2017 Sep;108(3):416–25.
43. Nirgianakis K, Kalaitzopoulos DR, Schwartz ASK, Spaanderman M, Kramer BW, Mueller MD, Mueller M. Fertility, pregnancy and neonatal outcomes of patients with adenomyosis: a systematic review and meta-analysis. *Reprod. Biomed. Online.* 2021;42:185–206.
44. Borghese G, Doglioli M, Orsini B, Raffone A, Neola D, Travaglino A, Rovero G, del Forno S, de Meis L, Locci M, et al. Progression of adenomyosis: rate and associated factors. *Int. J. Gynecol. Obstet.* 2024 Oct;167(1).
45. Ge L, Li Y, Zhou J, Zhao X, Chen X, Wang W, Li Z, Ge P, Cui L. Effect of different treatment protocols on in vitro fertilisation/intracytoplasmic sperm injection (IVF/ICSI) outcomes in adenomyosis women: a systematic review and meta-analysis. *BMJ Open.* 2024 Jul 18;14(7):e077025.

46. Kim H, Frisch EH, Falcone T. From diagnosis to fertility: optimizing treatment of adenomyosis for reproductive health. *J Clin Med.* 2024 Aug 21;13(16):4926.
47. Ghai V, Jan H, Shakir F, Haines P, Kent A. Diagnostic delay for superficial and deep endometriosis in the United Kingdom. *J Obstet Gynaecol.* 2020 Jan;40(1):83–89.
48. Leone Roberti Maggiore U, Chiappa V, Ceccaroni M, Roviglione G, Savelli L, Ferrero S, Raspagliesi F, Spanò Bascio L. Epidemiology of infertility in women with endometriosis. *Best Pract Res Clin Obstet Gynaecol.* 2024 Feb;92:102454.
49. Mohammed Rasheed HA, Hamid P. Inflammation to infertility: panoramic view on endometriosis. *Cureus.* 2020 Nov 16;12(11):e11516.
50. Lee D, Kim SK, Lee JR, Jee BC. Management of endometriosis-related infertility: considerations and treatment options. *Clin Exp Reprod Med.* 2020 Mar;47(1):1–11.
51. Seyhan A, Ata B, Uncu G. The impact of endometriosis and its treatment on ovarian reserve. *Semin Reprod Med.* 2015 Nov;33(6):422–28.
52. Uncu G, Kasapoglu I, Ozerkan K, Seyhan A, Oral Yilmaztepe A, Ata B. Prospective assessment of the impact of endometriomas and their removal on ovarian reserve and determinants of the rate of decline in ovarian reserve. *Hum Reprod.* 2013 Aug;28(8):2140–45.
53. Monsanto SP, Edwards AK, Zhou J, Nagarkatti P, Nagarkatti M, Young SL, Lessey BA, Tayade C. Surgical removal of endometriotic lesions alters local and systemic proinflammatory cytokines in endometriosis patients. *Fertil Steril.* 2016 Apr;105(4):968-977.e5.
54. Leonardi M, Gibbons T, Armour M, Wang R, Glanville E, Hodgson R, Cave AE, Ong J, Tong YYF, Jacobson TZ, Mol BW, Johnson NP, Condous G. When to do surgery and when not to do surgery for endometriosis: a systematic review and meta-analysis. *J Minim Invasive Gynecol.* 2020 Feb;27(2):390–407.e3.
55. Uncu G, Kasapoglu I, Ozerkan K, Seyhan A, Oral Yilmaztepe A, Ata B. Prospective assessment of the impact of endometriomas and their removal on ovarian reserve and determinants of the rate of decline in ovarian reserve. *Hum Reprod.* 2013 Aug;28(8):2140–55.

## CHAPTER 5

1. Choi J, Chan S, Wiebe E. Natural family planning: physicians' knowledge, attitudes, and practice. *J Obstet Gynaecol Can.* 2010 Jul;32(7):673–78.
2. Wilcox AJ, Weinberg CR, Baird DD. Timing of sexual intercourse in relation to ovulation. Effects on the probability of conception, survival of the pregnancy, and sex of the baby. *N Engl J Med.* 1995 Dec 7;333(23):1517–21.
3. Wilcox AJ, Dunson D, Baird DD. The timing of the "fertile window" in the menstrual cycle: day specific estimates from a prospective study. *BMJ.* 2000 Nov 18;321(7271):1259–62.
4. Soumpasis I, Grace B, Johnson S. Real-life insights on menstrual cycles and ovulation using big data. *Hum Reprod Open.* 2020 Apr 14;2020(2):hoaa011.
5. Johnson S, Marriott L, Zinaman M. Can apps and calendar methods predict ovulation with accuracy? *Curr Med Res Opin.* 2018 Sep;34(9):1587–94.
6. Wilcox AJ, Weinberg CR, Baird DD. Timing of sexual intercourse in relation to ovulation. Effects on the probability of conception, survival of the pregnancy, and sex of the baby. *N Engl J Med.* 1995 Dec 7;333(23):1517–21.
7. Moghissi KS. Prediction and detection of ovulation. *Fertil Steril.* 1980;34(2):89–98.
8. Bauman JE. Basal body temperature: unreliable method of ovulation detection. *Fertil Steril.* 1981 Dec;36(6):729–33.
9. de Mouzon J, Testart J, Lefevre B, Pouly JL, Frydman R. Time relationships between basal body temperature and ovulation or plasma progestins. *Fertil Steril.* 1984 Feb;41(2):254–59.
10. Marinho AO, Sailam HN, Goessens LKV, Collins WP, Rodeck CH, Campbell S. Real time pelvic ultrasonography during the periovulatory period of patients attending an artificial insemination clinic. *Fertil Steril.* 1982;37(5):633.
11. Guida M, Tommaselli GA, Palomba S, Pellicano M, Moccia G, Di Carlo C, Nappi C. Efficacy of methods for determining ovulation in a natural family planning program. *Fertil Steril.* 1999 Nov;72(5):900–904.
12. Su HW, Yi YC, Wei TY, Chang TC, Cheng CM. Detection of ovulation, a review of currently available methods. *Bioeng Transl Med.* 2017 May 16;2(3):238–46.
13. Alliende ME, Cabezón C, Figueroa H, Kottmann C. Cervicovaginal fluid changes to detect ovulation accurately. *Am J Obstet Gynecol.* 2005;193(1):71–75.

14. Najmabadi S, Schliep KC, Simonsen SE, Porucznik CA, Egger MJ, Stanford JB. Cervical mucus patterns and the fertile window in women without known subfertility: a pooled analysis of three cohorts. *Hum Reprod*. 2021 Jun 18;36(7):1784–95.
15. Scarpa B, Dunson DB, Colombo B. Cervical mucus secretions on the day of intercourse: an accurate marker of highly fertile days. *Eur J Obstet Gynecol Reprod Biol*. 2006 Mar 1;125(1): 72–78.
16. Check JH, Adelson HG, Wu CH. Improvement of cervical factor with guaifenesin. *Fertil Steril*. 1982 May;37(5):707–8.
17. Guermandi E, Vegetti W, Bianchi MM, Uglietti A, Ragni G, Crosignani P. Reliability of ovulation tests in infertile women. *Obstet Gynecol*. 2001;97(1):92–96.
18. Eichner SF, Timpe EM. Urinary-based ovulation and pregnancy: point-of-care testing. *Ann Pharmacother*. 2004 Feb;38(2):325–31.
19. McGovern PG, Myers ER, Silva S, Coutifaris C, Carson SA, Legro RS, et al. Absence of secretory endometrium after false-positive home urine luteinizing hormone testing. *Fertil Steril*. 2004;82:1273–77.
20. Practice Committees of the American Society for Reproductive Medicine and the Society for Reproductive Endocrinology and Infertility. Diagnosis and treatment of luteal phase deficiency: a committee opinion. *Fertil Steril*. 2021 Jun;115(6):1416–23.
21. Ecochard R, Leiva R, Bouchard T, et al. Use of urinary pregnanediol 3-glucuronide to confirm ovulation. *Steroids*. 2013;78(10):1035–40.
22. Arévalo M, Jennings V, Nikula M, Sinai I. Efficacy of the new TwoDay Method of family planning. *Fertil Steril*. 2004 Oct;82(4):885–92.
23. Bhargava H, Bhatia JC, Ramachandran L, Rohatgi P, Sinha A. Field trial of Billings ovulation method of natural family planning. *Contraception*. 1996 Feb;53(2):69–74.
24. Frank-Herrmann P, Heil J, Gnoth C, Toledo E, Baur S, Pyper C, Jenetzky E, Strowitzki T, Freundl G. The effectiveness of a fertility awareness based method to avoid pregnancy in relation to a couple's sexual behaviour during the fertile time: a prospective longitudinal study. *Hum Reprod*. 2007 May;22(5):1310–19.
25. Centers for Disease Control and Prevention (CDC). Contraception and birth control methods. https://www.cdc.gov/contraception/about/index.html. Published August 6, 2024. Accessed November 1, 2024.
26. Bradley SEK, Polis CB, Micks EA, Steiner MJ. Effectiveness, safety and comparative side effects. In: Cason P, Cwiak C, Edelment A, et al., eds. *Contraceptive Technology*. 22nd ed. Burlington, MA: Jones-Bartlett Learning, 2023.

### CHAPTER 6

1. American College of Obstetricians and Gynecologists. ACOG committee opinion no. 762: prepregnancy counseling. *Obstet Gynecol*. 2019 Jan;133(1):e78–e89.
2. Schummers L, Hutcheon JA, Hernandez-Diaz S, et al. Association of short interpregnancy interval with pregnancy outcomes according to maternal age. *JAMA Intern Med*. 2018;178(12):1661–70.
3. Quinn MM, Rosen MP, Allen IE, Huddleston HG, Cedars MI, Fujimoto VY. Decreased clinical pregnancy and live birth rates after short interval from delivery to subsequent assisted reproductive treatment cycle. *Hum Reprod*. 2018 Jul 1;33(7):1316–21.
4. Kangatharan C, Labram S, Bhattacharya S. Interpregnancy interval following miscarriage and adverse pregnancy outcomes: systematic review and meta-analysis. *Hum Reprod Update*. 2017 Mar 1;23(2):221–31.
5. Westhoff CL, Torgal AH, Mayeda ER, Pike MC, Stanczyk FZ. Pharmacokinetics of a combined oral contraceptive in obese and normal-weight women. *Contraception*. 2010 Jun;81(6):474–80.
6. Dinehart E, Lathi RB, Aghajanova L. Levonorgestrel IUD: is there a long-lasting effect on return to fertility? *J Assist Reprod Genet*. 2020 Jan;37(1):45–52.
7. Doll H, Vessey M, Painter R. Return of fertility in nulliparous women after discontinuation of the intrauterine device: comparison with women discontinuing other methods of contraception. *BJOG*. 2001 Mar;108(3):304–14.
8. Kaneshiro B, Aeby T. Long-term safety, efficacy, and patient acceptability of the intrauterine Copper T-380A contraceptive device. *Int J Womens Health*. 2010 Aug 9;2:211–20.

9. Girum T, Wasie A. Return of fertility after discontinuation of contraception: a systematic review and meta-analysis. *Contracept Reprod Med.* 2018 Jul 23;3:9.
10. American College of Obstetricians and Gynecologists. ACOG committee opinion no. 762: prepregnancy counseling. *Obstet Gynecol.* 2019 Jan;133(1):e78–e89.
11. American College of Obstetricians and Gynecologists. Nutrition during pregnancy. https://www.acog.org/womens-health/faqs/nutrition-during-pregnancy. Accessed November 1, 2024.
12. Gordts S, Campo R, Brosens I. Endoscopic visualization of oocyte release and oocyte retrieval in humans. *Reprod Biomed Online.* 2002;4 Suppl 3:10–3.
13. Wilcox AJ, Baird DD, Weinberg CR. Time of implantation of the conceptus and loss of pregnancy. *N Engl J Med.* 1999 Jun 10;340(23):1796–99.
14. Isaacs JD Jr, Young RA, Cowan BD. Cumulative pregnancy analysis of one-tube versus two-tube tubal anastomosis. *Fertil Steril.* 1997 Aug;68(2):217–19.
15. Wilcox AJ, Weinberg CR, Baird DD. Timing of sexual intercourse in relation to ovulation. Effects on the probability of conception, survival of the pregnancy, and sex of the baby. *N Engl J Med.* 1995 Dec 7;333(23):1517–21.
16. Practice Committee of American Society for Reproductive Medicine in collaboration with Society for Reproductive Endocrinology and Infertility. Optimizing natural fertility. *Fertil Steril.* 2008 Nov;90(5 Suppl):S1–6.
17. Stirnemann JJ, Samson A, Bernard JP, Thalabard JC. Day-specific probabilities of conception in fertile cycles resulting in spontaneous pregnancies. *Hum Reprod.* 2013 Apr;28(4): 1110–16.
18. Gibbons T, Reavey J, Georgiou EX, Becker CM. Timed intercourse for couples trying to conceive. *Cochrane Database Syst Rev.* 2023 Sep 15;9(9):CD011345.
19. Evans-Hoeker E, Pritchard DA, Long DL, Herring AH, Stanford JB, Steiner AZ. Cervical mucus monitoring prevalence and associated fecundability in women trying to conceive. *Fertil Steril.* 2013 Oct;100(4):1033–1038.e1.
20. Stanford JB, Willis SK, Hatch EE, Rothman KJ, Wise LA. Fecundability in relation to use of mobile computing apps to track the menstrual cycle. *Hum Reprod.* 2020 Oct 1;35(10):2245–52.
21. Williams M, Hill CJ, Scudamore I, Dunphy B, Cooke ID, Barratt CLR. Sperm numbers and distribution within the human fallopian tube around ovulation. *Hum Reprod.* 1993 Dec;8(12):2019.
22. Levitas E, Lunenfeld E, Weiss N, Friger M, Har-Vardi I, Koifman A, et al. Relationship between the duration of sexual abstinence and semen quality: analysis of 9,489 semen samples. *Fertil Steril.* 2005;83:1680–86.
23. Wilcox AJ, Weinberg CR, Baird DD. Timing of sexual intercourse in relation to ovulation. Effects on the probability of conception, survival of the pregnancy, and sex of the baby. *N Engl J Med.* 1995 Dec 7;333(23):1517–21.
24. Martins MV, Fernandes J, Pedro J, Barros A, Xavier P, Schmidt L, Costa ME. Effects of trying to conceive using an every-other-day strategy versus fertile window monitoring on stress: a 12-month randomized controlled trial. *Hum Reprod.* 2022 Nov 24;37(12):2845–55.
25. Shettles LB, Rorvik DM. *How to Choose the Sex of Your Baby.* New York: Doubleday, 1984.
26. Zarutskie PW, Muller CH, Magone M, Soules MR. The clinical relevance of sex selection techniques. *Fertil Steril.* 1989 Dec;52(6):891–905.
27. Wilcox AJ, Weinberg CR, Baird DD. Timing of sexual intercourse in relation to ovulation. Effects on the probability of conception, survival of the pregnancy, and sex of the baby. *N Engl J Med.* 1995 Dec 7;333(23):1517–21.
28. Practice Committee of American Society for Reproductive Medicine in collaboration with Society for Reproductive Endocrinology and Infertility. Optimizing natural fertility. *Fertil Steril.* 2008 Nov;90(5 Suppl):S1–6.
29. Agarwal SK, Coe S, Buyalos RP. The influence of uterine position on pregnancy rates with in vitro fertilization–embryo transfer. *J Assist Reprod Genet.* 1994 Jul;11(6):323–24.
30. Sandhu RS, Wong TH, Kling CA, Chohan KR. In vitro effects of coital lubricants and synthetic and natural oils on sperm motility. *Fertil Steril.* 2014 Apr;101(4):941–44.
31. Agarwal A, Deepinder F, Cocuzza M, Short RA, Evenson DP. Effect of vaginal lubricants on sperm motility and chromatin integrity: a prospective comparative study. *Fertil Steril.* 2008 Feb;89(2):375–79.
32. Tulandi T, Plouffe L Jr, McInnes RA. Effect of saliva on sperm motility and activity. *Fertil Steril.* 1982 Dec;38(6):721–23.

33. Elster AB, Lach PA, Roghmann KJ, McAnarney ER. Relationship between frequency of sexual intercourse and urinary tract infections in young women. *South Med J.* 1981 Jun;74(6):704–8.
34. Stanford JB, Hansen JL, Willis SK, Hu N, Thomas A. Peri-implantation intercourse does not lower fecundability. *Hum Reprod.* 2020 Sep 1;35(9):2107–12.
35. Barnhart KT, Guo W, Cary MS, Morse CB, Chung K, Takacs P, Senapati S, Sammel MD. Differences in serum human chorionic gonadotropin rise in early pregnancy by race and value at presentation. *Obstet Gynecol.* 2016 Sep;128(3):504–11.
36. Practice Committee of the American Society for Reproductive Medicine. Uterine septum: a guideline. *Fertil Steril.* 2016 Sep 1;106(3):530–40.

## CHAPTER 7

1. Guttmacher AF. Factors affecting normal expectancy of conception. *JAMA.* 1956;161:855.
2. Practice Committee of the American Society for Reproductive Medicine. Fertility evaluation of infertile women: a committee opinion. *Fertil Steril.* 2021 Nov;116(5):1255–65.
3. Zinaman MJ, Brown CC, Selevan SG, Clegg ED. Semen quality and human fertility: a prospective study with healthy couples. *J Androl.* 2000 Jan–Feb;21(1):145–53.
4. Keihani S, Verrilli LE, Zhang C, Presson AP, Hanson HA, Pastuszak AW, Johnstone EB, Hotaling JM. Semen parameter thresholds and time-to-conception in subfertile couples: how high is high enough? *Hum Reprod.* 2021 Jul 19;36(8):2121–33.
5. Carson SA, Kallen AN. Diagnosis and Management of Infertility: A Review. *JAMA.* 2021 Jul 6;326(1):65–76.
6. Carson SA, Kallen AN. Diagnosis and Management of Infertility: A Review. *JAMA.* 2021 Jul 6;326(1):65–76.
7. Munster K, Schmidt L, Helm P. Length and variation in the menstrual cycle—a cross-sectional study from a Danish county. *Br J Obstet Gynaecol.* 1992;99:422.
8. Practice Committee of the American Society for Reproductive Medicine. Role of tubal surgery in the era of assisted reproductive technology: a committee opinion. *Fertil Steril.* 2021 May;115(5):1143–50.
9. Zeyneloglu HB, Arici A, Olive DL. Adverse effects of hydrosalpinx on pregnancy rates after in vitro fertilization–embryo transfer. *Fertil Steril.* 1998 Sep;70(3):492–99.
10. Levine H, Jørgensen N, Martino-Andrade A, Mendiola J, Weksler-Derri D, Jolles M, Pinotti R, Swan SH. Temporal trends in sperm count: a systematic review and meta-regression analysis of samples collected globally in the 20th and 21st centuries. *Hum Reprod Update.* 2023 Mar 1;29(2):157–76.
11. Kolettis PN, Purcell ML, Parker W, Poston T, Nangia AK. Medical testosterone: an iatrogenic cause of male infertility and a growing problem. *Urology.* 2015;85:1068–73.
12. Marinaro JA. Sperm DNA fragmentation and its interaction with female factors. *Fertil Steril.* 2023 Oct;120(4):715–19.
13. Esteves SC, Roque M, Bradley CK, Garrido N. Reproductive outcomes of testicular versus ejaculated sperm for intracytoplasmic sperm injection among men with high levels of DNA fragmentation in semen: systematic review and meta-analysis. *Fertil Steril.* 2017 Sep;108(3):456–67.e1.
14. de La Rochebrochard E, Thonneau P. Paternal age > or = 40 years: an important risk factor for infertility. *Am J Obstet Gynecol.* 2003 Oct;189(4):901–5.
15. Sharma R, Agarwal A, Rohra VK, Assidi M, Abu-Elmagd M, Turki RF. Effects of increased paternal age on sperm quality, reproductive outcome and associated epigenetic risks to offspring. *Reprod Biol Endocrinol.* 2015 Apr 19;13:35.
16. de la Rochebrochard E, Thonneau P. Paternal age and maternal age are risk factors for miscarriage; results of a multicentre European study. *Hum Reprod.* 2002 Jun;17(6):1649–56.
17. Lee D, Kim SK, Lee JR, Jee BC. Management of endometriosis-related infertility: considerations and treatment options. *Clin Exp Reprod Med.* 2020 Mar;47(1):1–11.
18. Practice Committee of the American Society for Reproductive Medicine. Definitions of infertility and recurrent pregnancy loss: a committee opinion. *Fertil Steril.* 2020 Mar;113(3):533–35.
19. Practice Committee of the American Society for Reproductive Medicine. Evaluation and treatment of recurrent pregnancy loss: a committee opinion. *Fertil Steril.* 2012 Nov;98(5):1103–11.

20. Carrera M, Pérez Millan F, Alcázar JL, Alonso L, Caballero M, Carugno J, Dominguez JA, Moratalla E. Effect of hysteroscopic metroplasty on reproductive outcomes in women with septate uterus: systematic review and meta-analysis. *J Minim Invasive Gynecol.* 2022 Apr;29(4):465-75.
21. Bortoletto P, Romanski PA, Pfeifer SM. Müllerian anomalies: presentation, diagnosis, and counseling. *Obstet Gynecol.* 2024 Mar 1;143(3):369-77.
22. Singh M, Wambua S, Lee SI, et al. Autoimmune diseases and adverse pregnancy outcomes: an umbrella review. *BMC Med.* 2024;22:94.
23. Harlow AF, Wesselink AK, Hatch EE, Rothman KJ, Wise LA. Male preconception marijuana use and spontaneous abortion: a prospective cohort study. *Epidemiology.* 2021 Mar 1;32(2):239-47.
24. Coomarasamy A, Devall AJ, Brosens JJ, Quenby S, Stephenson MD, Sierra S, Christiansen OB, Small R, Brewin J, Roberts TE, Dhillon-Smith R, Harb H, Noordali H, Papadopoulou A, Eapen A, Prior M, Di Renzo GC, Hinshaw K, Mol BW, Lumsden MA, Khalaf Y, Shennan A, Goddijn M, van Wely M, Al-Memar M, Bennett P, Bourne T, Rai R, Regan L, Gallos ID. Micronized vaginal progesterone to prevent miscarriage: a critical evaluation of randomized evidence. *Am J Obstet Gynecol.* 2020 Aug;223(2):167-76.
25. Guzick DS, Sullivan MW, Adamson GD, Cedars MI, Falk RJ, Peterson EP, Steinkampf MP. Efficacy of treatment for unexplained infertility. *Fertil Steril.* 1998;70:207.
26. Franik S, Le QK, Kremer JA, Kiesel L, Farquhar C. Aromatase inhibitors (letrozole) for ovulation induction in infertile women with polycystic ovary syndrome. *Cochrane Database Syst Rev.* 2022 Sep 27;9(9):CD010287.
27. Practice Committees of the American Society for Reproductive Medicine and Society for Reproductive Endocrinology and Infertility. Use of exogenous gonadotropins for ovulation induction in anovulatory women: a committee opinion. *Fertil Steril.* 2020 Jan;113(1):66-70.
28. Franik S, Le QK, Kremer JA, Kiesel L, Farquhar C. Aromatase inhibitors (letrozole) for ovulation induction in infertile women with polycystic ovary syndrome. *Cochrane Database Syst Rev.* 2022 Sep 27;9(9):CD010287.
29. Guzick DS, Sullivan MW, Adamson GD, Cedars MI, Falk RJ, Peterson EP, Steinkampf MP. Efficacy of treatment for unexplained infertility. *Fertil Steril.* 1998;70:207.
30. Reindollar RH, Regan MM, Neumann PJ, Levine BS, Thornton KL, Alper MM, Goldman MB. A randomized clinical trial to evaluate optimal treatment for unexplained infertility: the fast track and standard treatment (FASTT) trial. *Fertil Steril.* 2010 Aug;94(3):888-99.
31. Goldman MB, Thornton KL, Ryley D, Alper MM, Fung JL, Hornstein MD, Reindollar RH. A randomized clinical trial to determine optimal infertility treatment in older couples: the Forty and Over Treatment Trial (FORT-T). *Fertil Steril.* 2014 Jun;101(6):1574-81.e1-2.
32. Legro RS, Barnhart HX, Schlaff WD, Carr BR, Diamond MP, Carson SA, Steinkampf MP, Coutifaris C, McGovern PG, Cataldo NA, Gosman GG, Nestler JE, Giudice LC, Leppert PC, Myers ER; Cooperative Multicenter Reproductive Medicine Network. Clomiphene, metformin, or both for infertility in the polycystic ovary syndrome. *N Engl J Med.* 2007 Feb 8;356(6):551-66.
33. Sharpe A, Morley LC, Tang T, Norman RJ, Balen AH. Metformin for ovulation induction (excluding gonadotrophins) in women with polycystic ovary syndrome. *Cochrane Database of Syst Rev.* 2019 Dec 17;12(12):CD013505.
34. Muthigi A, Jahandideh S, Bishop LA, Naeemi FK, Shipley SK, O'Brien JE, Shin PR, Devine K, Tanrikut C. Clarifying the relationship between total motile sperm counts and intrauterine insemination pregnancy rates. *Fertil Steril.* 2021 Jun;115(6):1454-60.
35. Stanhiser J, Mersereau JE, Dock D, Boylan C, Caprell H, Coward RM, Berger DS, Fritz M. Sperm morphology from the actual inseminated sample does not predict clinical pregnancy following intrauterine insemination. *F S Rep.* 2020 Dec 9;2(1):16-21.
36. Grigoriou O, Pantos K, Makrakis E, Hassiakos D, Konidaris S, Creatsas G. Impact of isolated teratozoospermia on the outcome of intrauterine insemination. *Fertil Steril.* 2005 Mar;83(3):773-75.
37. Reindollar RH, Regan MM, Neumann PJ, Levine BS, Thornton KL, Alper MM, Goldman MB. A randomized clinical trial to evaluate optimal treatment for unexplained infertility: the fast track and standard treatment (FASTT) trial. *Fertil Steril.* 2010 Aug;94(3):888-99.
38. Guzick DS, Carson SA, Coutifaris C, Overstreet JW, Factor-Litvak P, Steinkampf MP, et al. Efficacy of superovulation and intrauterine insemination in the treatment of infertility. National Cooperative Reproductive Medicine Network. *N Engl J Med.* 1999;340:177-83.

39. van Rijswijk J, Caanen MR, Mijatovic V, Vergouw CG, van de Ven PM, Lambalk CB, Schats R. Immobilization or mobilization after IUI: an RCT. *Hum Reprod.* 2017 Nov 1;32(11):2218–24.
40. Minasi MG, Colasante A, Riccio T, Ruberti A, Casciani V, Scarselli F, Spinella F, Fiorentino F, Varricchio MT, Greco E, et al. Correlation between aneuploidy, standard morphology evaluation and morphokinetic development in 1730 biopsied blastocysts: a consecutive case series study. *Hum Reprod.* 2016;31:2245–54.
41. Practice Committees of the American Society for Reproductive Medicine and the Society for Assisted Reproductive Technology. The use of preimplantation genetic testing for aneuploidy: a committee opinion. *Fertil Steril.* 2024 Sep;122(3):421–34.
42. Franasiak JM, Forman EJ, Hong KH, Werner MD, Upham KM, Treff NR, Scott RT Jr. The nature of aneuploidy with increasing age of the female partner: a review of 15,169 consecutive trophectoderm biopsies evaluated with comprehensive chromosomal screening. *Fertil Steril.* 2014 Mar;101(3):656–63.e1.
43. Martel RA, Lee MB, Schadwell A, Siavoshi M, Kwan L, Miller J, Leonard C, Roman RA, Armstrong A, Kroener L. Aneuploidy rates and likelihood of obtaining a usable embryo for transfer among in vitro fertilization cycles using preimplantation genetic testing for monogenic disorders and aneuploidy compared with in vitro fertilization cycles using preimplantation genetic testing for aneuploidy alone. *Fertil Steril.* 2024 Dec;122(6):993–1001.
44. Martel RA, Lee MB, Schadwell A, Siavoshi M, Kwan L, Miller J, Leonard C, Roman RA, Armstrong A, Kroener L. Aneuploidy rates and likelihood of obtaining a usable embryo for transfer among in vitro fertilization cycles using preimplantation genetic testing for monogenic disorders and aneuploidy compared with in vitro fertilization cycles using preimplantation genetic testing for aneuploidy alone. *Fertil Steril.* 2024 Dec;122(6):993–1001.
45. Rezazadeh Valojerdi M, Eftekhari-Yazdi P, Karimian L, Hassani F, Movaghar B. Vitrification versus slow freezing gives excellent survival, post warming embryo morphology and pregnancy outcomes for human cleaved embryos. *J Assist Reprod Genet.* 2009 Jun;26(6):347–54. doi: 10.1007/s10815-009-9318-6. Epub 2009 Jun 10. PMID: 19513822; PMCID: PMC2729856.
46. Devine K, Richter KS, Jahandideh S, Widra EA, McKeeby JL. Intramuscular progesterone optimizes live birth from programmed frozen embryo transfer: a randomized clinical trial. *Fertil Steril.* 2021 Sep;116(3):633–43.
47. Gaikwad S, Garrido N, Cobo A, Pellicer A, Remohi J. Bed rest after embryo transfer negatively affects in vitro fertilization: a randomized controlled clinical trial. *Fertil Steril.* 2013 Sep;100(3):729–35.
48. Friedler S, Glasser S, Azani L, Freedman LS, Raziel A, Strassburger D, Ron-El R, Lerner-Geva L. The effect of medical clowning on pregnancy rates after in vitro fertilization and embryo transfer. *Fertil Steril.* 2011 May;95(6):2127–30.
49. SART. All SART member clinics—2022 retrieval and transfer tables. https://www.sartcorsonline.com/EmbryoOutcome/PublicSARTOutcomeTables. Accessed November 30, 2024.
50. Pirtea P, De Ziegler D, Tao X, Sun L, Zhan Y, Ayoubi JM, Seli E, Franasiak JM, Scott RT Jr. Rate of true recurrent implantation failure is low: results of three successive frozen euploid single embryo transfers. *Fertil Steril.* 2021 Jan;115(1):45–53.
51. Gill P, Ata B, Arnanz A, Cimadomo D, Vaiarelli A, Fatemi HM, Ubaldi FM, Garcia-Velasco JA, Seli E. Does recurrent implantation failure exist? Prevalence and outcomes of five consecutive euploid blastocyst transfers in 123,987 patients. *Hum Reprod.* 2024 May 2;39(5):974–80.
52. Steiner N, Shrem G, Tannus S, Dahan SY, Balayla J, Volodarsky-Perel A, Tan SL, Dahan MH. Effect of GnRH agonist and letrozole treatment in women with recurrent implantation failure. *Fertil Steril.* 2019 Jul;112(1):98–104.
53. Lessey BA, Dong A, Deaton JL, Angress D, Savaris RF, Walker SJ. Inflammatory changes after medical suppression of suspected endometriosis for implantation failure: preliminary results. *Int J Mol Sci.* 2024 Jun 22;25(13):6852.
54. Ameho S, Klutstein M. The effect of chronic inflammation on female fertility. *Reproduction.* 2025 Mar 3;169(4):e240197.
55. Vexø LE, Stormlund S, Landersoe SK, Jørgensen HL, Humaidan P, Bergh C, Englund ALM, Klajnbard A, Bogstad JW, Freiesleben NC, Zedeler A, Prætorius L, Andersen AN, Løssl K, Pinborg A, Nielsen HS. Low-grade inflammation is negatively associated with live birth in women undergoing IVF. *Reprod Biomed Online.* 2023 Feb;46(2):302–11.
56. Ojo OA, Nwafor-Ezeh PI, Rotimi DE, Iyobhebhe M, Ogunlakin AD, Ojo AB. Apoptosis,

inflammation, and oxidative stress in infertility: A mini review. *Toxicol Rep.* 2023 Apr 13;10:448–62.
57. Li X, Luan T, Wei Y, Zhang J, Zhou L, Zhao C, Ling X. Association between the systemic immune-inflammation index and GnRH antagonist protocol IVF outcomes: a cohort study. *Reprod Biomed Online.* 2024 May;48(5):103776.
58. Albert AB, Corachán A, Juárez-Barber E, Cozzolino M, Pellicer A, Alecsandru D, Cervelló I, Ferrero H. Association of insulin resistance with in vitro fertilization outcomes in women without polycystic ovarian syndrome: potential improvement with metformin treatment. *Hum Reprod.* 2025 Aug 1;40(8):1562–69.
59. Vexø LE, Stormlund S, Landersoe SK, Jørgensen HL, Humaidan P, Bergh C, Englund ALM, Klajnbard A, Bogstad JW, Freiesleben NC, Zedeler A, Prætorius L, Andersen AN, Løssl K, Pinborg A, Nielsen HS. Low-grade inflammation is negatively associated with live birth in women undergoing IVF. *Reprod Biomed Online.* 2023 Feb;46(2):302–11.
60. Xie J, Yan L, Cheng Z, Qiang L, Yan J, Liu Y, Liang R, Zhang J, Li Z, Zhuang L, Hao C, Wang B, Lu Q. Potential effect of inflammation on the failure risk of in vitro fertilization and embryo transfer among infertile women. *Hum Fertil (Camb).* 2020 Sep;23(3):214–22.

## CHAPTER 8

1. Ameho S, Klutstein M. The effect of chronic inflammation on female fertility. *Reproduction.* 2025 Mar 3;169(4):e240197.
2. Rohleder N. Acute and chronic stress induced changes in sensitivity of peripheral inflammatory pathways to the signals of multiple stress systems—2011 Curt Richter Award Winner. *Psychoneuroendocrinology.* 2012 Mar;37(3):307–6.
3. Liu YZ, Wang YX, Jiang CL. Inflammation: the common pathway of stress-related diseases. *Front Hum Neurosci.* 2017 Jun 20;11:316.
4. Rizza RA, Mandarino LJ, Gerich JE. Cortisol-induced insulin resistance in man: Impaired suppression of glucose production and stimulation of glucose utilization due to a postreceptor defect of insulin action. *J. Clin. Endocrinol.* Metab. 1982;54:131–38.
5. Black PH. Stress and the inflammatory response: a review of neurogenic inflammation. *Brain Behav Immun.* 2002 Dec;16(6):622–53.
6. Schliep KC, Mumford SL, Silver RM, Wilcox B, Radin RG, Perkins NJ, Galai N, Park J, Kim K, Sjaarda LA, Plowden T, Schisterman EF. Preconception perceived stress is associated with reproductive hormone levels and longer time to pregnancy. *Epidemiology.* 2019 Nov;30 Suppl 2(Suppl 2):S76–S84.
7. Stephens MA, Mahon PB, McCaul ME, Wand GS. Hypothalamic-pituitary-adrenal axis response to acute psychosocial stress: effects of biological sex and circulating sex hormones. *Psychoneuroendocrinology.* 2016 Apr;66:47–55.
8. Zanettoullis AT, Mastorakos G, Vakas P, Vlahos N, Valsamakis G. Effect of stress on each of the stages of the IVF procedure: a systematic review. *Int J Mol Sci.* 2024 Jan 5;25(2):726.
9. Mínguez-Alarcón L, Williams PL, Souter I, Ford JB, Hauser R, Chavarro JE; Earth Study Team. Perceived stress and markers of ovarian reserve among subfertile women. *Reprod Biomed Online.* 2023 Jun;46(6):956–64.
10. Pal L, Bevilacqua K, Santoro NF. Chronic psychosocial stressors are detrimental to ovarian reserve: a study of infertile women. *J Psychosom Obstet Gynaecol.* 2010 Sep;31(3):130–39.
11. Crosswell AD, Lockwood KG. Best practices for stress measurement: How to measure psychological stress in health research. *Health Psychol Open.* 2020 Jul 8;7(2):2055102920933072.
12. Lynch CD, Sundaram R, Maisog JM, Sweeney AM, Buck Louis GM. Preconception stress increases the risk of infertility: results from a couple-based prospective cohort study—the LIFE study. *Hum Reprod.* 2014 May;29(5):1067–75.
13. Li J, Long L, Liu Y, He W, Li M. Effects of a mindfulness-based intervention on fertility quality of life and pregnancy rates among women subjected to first in vitro fertilization treatment. *Behav Res Ther.* 2016 Feb;77:96–104.
14. Pascoe MC, Thompson DR, Jenkins ZM, Ski CF. Mindfulness mediates the physiological markers of stress: Systematic review and meta-analysis. *J Psychiatr Res.* 2017 Dec;95:156–78.
15. Pascoe MC, Thompson DR, Ski CF. Yoga, mindfulness-based stress reduction and stress-related physiological measures: A meta-analysis. *Psychoneuroendocrinology.* 2017 Dec;86:152–68.

16. Yadav A, Tiwari P, Dada R. Yoga and lifestyle changes: a path to improved fertility—a narrative review. *Int J Yoga*. 2024 Jan–Apr;17(1):10–19.
17. Dumbala S, Bhargav H, Satyanarayana V, Arasappa R, Varambally S, Desai G, Bangalore GN. Effect of yoga on psychological distress among women receiving treatment for infertility. *Int J Yoga*. 2020 May–Aug;13(2):115–19.
18. Patel V, Menezes H, Menezes C, Bouwer S, Bostick-Smith CA, Speelman DL. Regular mindful yoga practice as a method to improve androgen levels in women with polycystic ovary syndrome: a randomized, controlled trial. *J Am Osteopath Assoc*. 2020 Apr 14.
19. Domar AD, Meshay I, Kelliher J, Alper M, Powers RD. The impact of acupuncture on in vitro fertilization outcome. *Fertil Steril*. 2009 Mar;91(3):723–26.
20. Zhong Y, Zeng F, Liu W, Ma J, Guan Y, Song Y. Acupuncture in improving endometrial receptivity: a systematic review and meta-analysis. *BMC Complement Altern Med*. 2019 Mar 13;19(1):61.
21. Kim J, Lee H, Choi TY, Kim JI, Kang BK, Lee MS, Joo JK, Lee KS, You S. Acupuncture for poor ovarian response: a randomized controlled trial. *J Clin Med*. 2021 May 18;10(10):2182.
22. Smith CA, de Lacey S, Chapman M, Ratcliffe J, Norman RJ, Johnson NP, Boothroyd C, Fahey P. Effect of acupuncture vs sham acupuncture on live births among women undergoing in vitro fertilization: a randomized clinical trial. *JAMA*. 2018 May 15;319(19):1990–98.
23. Martins MV, Peterson BD, Almeida VM, Costa ME. Direct and indirect effects of perceived social support on women's infertility-related stress. *Hum Reprod*. 2011 Aug;26(8):2113–21.
24. Lateef OM, Akintubosun MO. Sleep and reproductive health. *J Circadian Rhythms*. 2020 Mar 23;18:1.
25. Dzierzewski JM, Donovan EK, Kay DB, Sannes TS, Bradbrook KE. Sleep inconsistency and markers of inflammation. *Front Neurol*. 2020 Sep 16;11:1042.
26. Reutrakul S, Van Cauter E. Sleep influences on obesity, insulin resistance, and risk of type 2 diabetes. *Metabolism*. 2018 Jul;84:56–66.
27. Kloss JD, Perlis ML, Zamzow JA, Culnan EJ, Gracia CR. Sleep, sleep disturbance, and fertility in women. *Sleep Med Rev*. 2015 Aug;22:78–87.
28. Zhao J, Chen Q, Xue X. Relationship between sleep disorders and female infertility among US reproductive-aged women. *Sleep Breath*. 2023 Oct;27(5):1875–82.
29. Minguez-Alarcon L, Souter I, Williams PL, Ford JB, Hauser R, Chavarro JE, Gaskins AJ; Earth Study Team. Occupational factors and markers of ovarian reserve and response among women at a fertility centre. *Occup Environ Med*. 2017;74:426–31.
30. Reiter RJ, Mayo JC, Tan DX, Sainz RM, Alatorre-Jimenez M, Qin L. Melatonin as an antioxidant: under promises but over delivers. *J Pineal Res*. 2016 Oct;61(3):253–78.
31. Monteleone P, Fuschino A, Nolfe G, Maj M. Temporal relationship between melatonin and cortisol responses to nighttime physical stress in humans. *Psychoneuroendocrinology*. 1992;17(1):81–86.
32. Caetano G, Bozinovic I, Dupont C, Léger D, Lévy R, Sermondade N. Impact of sleep on female and male reproductive functions: a systematic review. *Fertil Steril*. 2021 Mar;115(3):715–31.
33. Eryilmaz OG, Devran A, Sarikaya E, Aksakal FN, Mollamahmutoğlu L, Cicek N. Melatonin improves the oocyte and the embryo in IVF patients with sleep disturbances, but does not improve the sleeping problems. *J Assist Reprod Genet*. 2011; 28(9): 815–20.
34. Mills J, Kuohung W. Impact of circadian rhythms on female reproduction and infertility treatment success. *Curr Opin Endocrinol Diabetes Obes*. 2019 Dec;26(6):317–21.
35. Zhao P, Jungheim ES, Bedrick BS, Wan L, Jimenez PT, McCarthy R, Chubiz J, Fay JC, Herzog ED, Sutcliffe S, England SK. Sleep variability and time to achieving pregnancy: findings from a pilot cohort study of women desiring pregnancy. *Fertil Steril*. 2025 Jul;124(1):113–20.
36. Cortés-Gallegos V, Castañeda G, Alonso R, Sojo I, Carranco A, Cervantes C, Parra A. Sleep deprivation reduces circulating androgens in healthy men. *Arch Androl*. 1983;10:33–37.
37. Zhong O, Liao B, Wang J, Liu K, Lei X, Hu L. Effects of sleep disorders and circadian rhythm changes on male reproductive health: a systematic review and meta-analysis. *Front physiol*. 2022;13:913369.
38. Wise LA, Rothman KJ, Wesselink AK, Mikkelsen EM, Sorensen HT, McKinnon CJ, Hatch EE. Male sleep duration and fecundability in a North American preconception cohort study. *Fertil Steril*. 2018;109:453–59.
39. Irwin MR. Sleep and inflammation: partners in sickness and in health. *Nat Rev Immunol*. 2019 Nov;19(11):702–15.

40. Stocker LJ, Macklon NS, Cheong YC, Bewley SJ. Influence of shift work on early reproductive outcomes: a systematic review and meta-analysis. *Obstet Gynecol.* 2014 Jul;124(1):99–110.
41. Stocker LJ, Macklon NS, Cheong YC, Bewley SJ. Influence of shift work on early reproductive outcomes: a systematic review and meta-analysis. *Obstet Gynecol.* 2014 Jul;124(1):99–110.
42. Minguez-Alarcon L, Souter I, Williams PL, Ford JB, Hauser R, Chavarro JE, Gaskins AJ; Earth Study Team. Occupational factors and markers of ovarian reserve and response among women at a fertility centre. *Occup Environ Med.* 2017;74:426–31.
43. Infante-Rivard C, David M, Gauthier R, Rivard GE. Pregnancy loss and work schedule during pregnancy. *Epidemiology.* 1993;4:73–75.
44. Liang Z, Liu J. Sleep behavior and self-reported infertility: a cross-sectional analysis among U.S. women. *Front Endocrinol (Lausanne).* 2022;13:818567–818567.
45. Borghouts LB, Keizer HA. Exercise and insulin sensitivity: a review. *Int J Sports Med.* 2000 Jan;21(1):1–12.
46. World Health Organization. *WHO Guidelines on Physical Activity and Sedentary Behaviour.* Geneva: World Health Organization; 2020.
47. Mussawar M, Balsom AA, Totosy de Zepetnek JO, Gordon JL. The effect of physical activity on fertility: a mini-review. *F S Rep.* 2023 Apr 14;4(2):150–58.
48. Paquin J, Lagacé JC, Brochu M, Dionne IJ. Exercising for insulin sensitivity—is there a mechanistic relationship with quantitative changes in skeletal muscle mass? *Front Physiol.* 2021 May 12;12:656909.
49. Richter EA, Derave W, Wojtaszewski JF. Glucose, exercise and insulin: emerging concepts. *J Physiol.* 2001 Sep 1;535(Pt 2):313–22.
50. Wise LA, Rothman KJ, Mikkelsen EM, Sørensen HT, Riis AH, Hatch EE. A prospective cohort study of physical activity and time to pregnancy. *Fertil Steril.* 2012;97:1136–42.e4.
51. De Souza MJ, Van Heest J, Demers LM, Lasley BL. Luteal phase deficiency in recreational runners: evidence for a hypometabolic state. *J Clin Endocrinol Metab.* 2003;88:337–46.
52. Williams NI, Leidy HJ, Hill BR, Lieberman JL, Legro RS, De Souza MJ. Magnitude of daily energy deficit predicts frequency but not severity of menstrual disturbances associated with exercise and caloric restriction. *Am J Physiol Endocrinol Metab.* 2015;308:E29–39.
53. Cerqueira É, Marinho DA, Neiva HP, Lourenço O. Inflammatory effects of high and moderate intensity exercise—a systematic review. *Front Physiol.* 2020 Jan 9;10:1550.
54. Patten RK, Boyle RA, Moholdt T, Kiel I, Hopkins WG, Harrison CL, et al. Exercise interventions in polycystic ovary syndrome: a systematic review and meta-analysis. *Front Physiol.* 2020;11:606.
55. Sõritsa D, Mäestu E, Nuut M, Mäestu J, Migueles JH, Läänelaid S, Ehrenberg A, Sekavin A, Sõritsa A, Salumets A, Ortega FB, Altmäe S. Maternal physical activity and sedentary behaviour before and during in vitro fertilization treatment: a longitudinal study exploring the associations with controlled ovarian stimulation and pregnancy outcomes. *J Assist Reprod Genet.* 2020 Aug;37(8):1869–81.
56. McNulty KL, Elliott-Sale KJ, Dolan E, Swinton PA, Ansdell P, Goodall S, Thomas K, Hicks KM. The effects of menstrual cycle phase on exercise performance in eumenorrheic women: a systematic review and meta-analysis. *Sports Med.* 2020 Oct;50(10):1813–27.
57. Oosthuyse T, Bosch AN. The effect of the menstrual cycle on exercise metabolism: implications for exercise performance in eumenorrhoeic women. *Sports Med.* (2010) 40(3): 207–27.
58. Romero-Moraleda B, Coso JD, Gutiérrez-Hellín J, Ruiz-Moreno C, Grgic J, Lara B. The influence of the menstrual cycle on muscle strength and power performance. *J Hum Kinet.* 2019 Aug 21;68:123–33.
59. Lebrun CM, McKenzie DC, Prior JC, Taunton JE. Effects of menstrual cycle phase on athletic performance. *Med Sci Sports Exerc.* 1995 Mar;27(3):437–44.
60. Jones BP, L'Heveder A, Bishop C, Kasaven L, Saso S, Davies S, Chakraverty R, Brown J, Pollock N. Menstrual cycles and the impact upon performance in elite British track and field athletes: a longitudinal study. *Front Sports Act Living.* 2024 Feb 20;6:1296189.
61. Boxem AJ, Blaauwendraad SM, Mulders AGMGJ, Bekkers EL, Kruithof CJ, Steegers EAP, Gaillard R, Jaddoe VWV. Preconception and early-pregnancy body mass index in women and men, time to pregnancy, and risk of miscarriage. *JAMA Netw Open.* 2024 Sep 3;7(9): e2436157.

## CHAPTER 9

1. Pitsavos C, Panagiotakos DB, Tzima N, Lentzas Y, Chrysohoou C, Das UN, Stefanadis C. Diet, exercise, and C-reactive protein levels in people with abdominal obesity: the ATTICA epidemiological study. *Angiology*. 2007 Apr–May;58(2):225–33.
2. Camilleri M. Leaky gut: mechanisms, measurement and clinical implications in humans. *Gut*. 2019 Aug;68(8):1516–26.
3. Leigh SJ, Uhlig F, Wilmes L, Sanchez-Diaz P, Gheorghe CE, Goodson MS, Kelley-Loughnane N, Hyland NP, Cryan JF, Clarke G. The impact of acute and chronic stress on gastrointestinal physiology and function: a microbiota-gut-brain axis perspective. *J Physiol*. 2023 Oct;601(20):4491–538.
4. Qi X, Yun C, Pang Y, Qiao J. The impact of the gut microbiota on the reproductive and metabolic endocrine system. *Gut Microbes*. 2021 Jan-Dec;13(1):1–21.
5. Cao W, Fu X, Zhou J, Qi Q, Ye F, Li L, Wang L. The effect of the female genital tract and gut microbiome on reproductive dysfunction. *Biosci Trends*. 2024 Jan 30;17(6):458–74.
6. Homma H, Hoy E, Xu DZ, Lu Q, Feinman R, Deitch EA. The female intestine is more resistant than the male intestine to gut injury and inflammation when subjected to conditions associated with shock states. *Am J Physiol Gastrointest Liver Physiol*. 2005;288:G4660150–G472.
7. O'Riordan KJ, Collins MK, Moloney GM, Knox EG, Aburto MR, Fülling C, Morley SJ, Clarke G, Schellekens H, Cryan JF. Short chain fatty acids: Microbial metabolites for gut-brain axis signalling. *Mol. Cell. Endocrinol*. 2022, 546, 111572.
8. Wang MY, Sang LX, Sun SY. Gut microbiota and female health. *World J Gastroenterol*. 2024 Mar 28;30(12):1655–62.
9. Garmendia JV, De Sanctis CV, Hajdúch M, De Sanctis JB. Microbiota and recurrent pregnancy loss (RPL); more than a simple connection. *Microorganisms*. 2024 Aug 10;12(8):1641.
10. Patel N, Patel N, Pal S, et al. Distinct gut and vaginal microbiota profile in women with recurrent implantation failure and unexplained infertility. *BMC Women's Health*. 2022;22:113.
11. Wen L, Duffy A. Factors influencing the gut microbiota, inflammation, and type 2 diabetes. *J Nutr*. 2017 Jul;147(7):1468S–1475S. doi: 10.3945/jn.116.240754. Epub 2017 Jun 14. PMID: 28615382; PMCID: PMC5483960.
12. Dinu M, Asensi MT, Pagliai G, Lotti S, Martini D, Colombini B, Sofi F. Consumption of ultra-processed foods is inversely associated with adherence to the Mediterranean diet: a cross-sectional study. *Nutrients*. 2022;14:2073.
13. Aleman RS, Moncada M, Aryana KJ. Leaky gut and the ingredients that help treat it: a review. *Molecules*. 2023 Jan 7;28(2):619.
14. Tristan Asensi M, Napoletano A, Sofi F, Dinu M. Low-grade inflammation and ultra-processed foods consumption: a review. *Nutrients*. 2023 Mar 22;15(6):1546.
15. Paray BA, Albeshr MF, Jan AT, Rather IA. Leaky gut and autoimmunity: an intricate balance in individuals health and the diseased state. *Int J Mol Sci*. 2020 Dec 21;21(24):9770.
16. Yang X, Liu W, Zhuo Y, Luo T, Wu D, Hua L. Intermittent fasting in female reproduction: A double-edged sword. *Nutr Rev*. 2025 Jun 30:nuaf107.
17. Velissariou M, Athanasiadou CR, Diamanti A, Lykeridou A, Sarantaki A. The impact of intermittent fasting on fertility: A focus on polycystic ovary syndrome and reproductive outcomes in Women-A systematic review. *Metabol Open*. 2025 Jan 6;25:100341.
18. Chawla S, Beretoulis S, Deere A, Radenkovic D. The window matters: A systematic review of time restricted eating strategies in relation to cortisol and melatonin secretion. *Nutrients*. 2021 Jul 23;13(8):2525.
19. Hosseini B, Berthon BS, Saedisomeolia A, Starkey MR, Collison A, Wark PAB, Wood LG. Effects of fruit and vegetable consumption on inflammatory biomarkers and immune cell populations: a systematic literature review and meta-analysis. *Am J Clin Nutr*. 2018 Jul 1;108(1).136–55.
20. Grieger JA, Grzeskowiak LE, Bianco-Miotto T, Jankovic-Karasoulos T, Moran LJ, Wilson RL, Leemaqz SY, Poston L, McCowan L, Kenny LC, Myers J, Walker JJ, Norman RJ, Dekker GA, Roberts CT. Pre-pregnancy fast food and fruit intake is associated with time to pregnancy. *Hum Reprod*. 2018 Jun 1;33(6):1063–70.
21. Willis SK, Wise LA, Wesselink AK, Rothman KJ, Mikkelsen EM, Tucker KL, et al. Glycemic load, dietary fiber, and added sugar and fecundability in 2 preconception cohorts. *Am J Clin Nutr*. 2020; 112:27–38.
22. U.S. Department of Agriculture and U.S. Department of Health and Human Services. Food

sources of dietary fiber. Dietary Guidelines for Americans, 2020–2025. 9th ed. 2020 Dec. dietaryguidelines.gov.
23. Chung Y, Melo P, Pickering O, Dhillon-Smith R, Coomarasamy A, Devall A. The association between dietary patterns and risk of miscarriage: a systematic review and meta-analysis. *Fertil Steril.* 2023 Aug;120(2):333–57.
24. Salas-Huetos A, Bulló M, Salas-Salvadó J. Dietary patterns, foods and nutrients in male fertility parameters and fecundability: a systematic review of observational studies. *Hum Reprod Update.* 2017 Jul 1;23(4):371–89.
25. Braga DP, Halpern G, Setti AS, Figueira RC, Iaconelli A Jr, Borges E Jr. The impact of food intake and social habits on embryo quality and the likelihood of blastocyst formation. *Reprod Biomed Online.* 2015 Jul;31(1):30–38.
26. Hoek J, Schoenmakers S, Baart EB, Koster MPH, Willemsen SP, van Marion ES, Steegers EAP, Laven JSE, Steegers-Theunissen RPM. Preconceptional maternal vegetable intake and paternal smoking are associated with pre-implantation embryo quality. *Reprod Sci.* 2020 Nov;27(11):2018–28.
27. Institute of Medicine. *Dietary Reference Intakes: The Essential Guide to Nutrient Requirements.* Washington, DC: National Academies Press; 2006.
28. Hruby A, Jacques PF. Dietary protein and changes in biomarkers of inflammation and oxidative stress in the Framingham Heart Study Offspring cohort. *Curr Dev Nutr.* 2019 Mar 28;3(5):nzz019.
29. Jinno M, Takeuchi M, Watanabe A, Teruya K, Hirohama J, Eguchi N, Miyazaki A. Advanced glycation end-products accumulation compromises embryonic development and achievement of pregnancy by assisted reproductive technology. *Hum Reprod.* 2011 Mar;26(3):604–10.
30. Lee DH, Tabung FK, Giovannucci EL. Association of animal and plant protein intakes with biomarkers of insulin and insulin-like growth factor axis. *Clin Nutr.* 2022 Jun;41(6):1272–80.
31. Chavarro JE, Rich-Edwards JW, Rosner BA, Willett WC. Protein intake and ovulatory infertility. *Am J Obstet Gynecol.* 2008 Feb;198(2):210.e1–7.
32. Bouvard V, et al. Carcinogenicity of consumption of red and processed meat. *Lancet Oncol.* 2015;16:1599–600.
33. Martín-Manchado L, Moya-Yeste AM, Sánchez-Sansegundo M, Hurtado-Sánchez JA, Gil-Miralles RA, Tuells J, Zaragoza-Martí A. Associations of nutritional status and dietary habits with the development of female infertility. A case-control study. *Front Nutr.* 2024 Oct 9;11:1476784.
34. Braga DP, Halpern G, Setti AS, Figueira RC, Iaconelli A Jr, Borges E Jr. The impact of food intake and social habits on embryo quality and the likelihood of blastocyst formation. *Reprod Biomed Online.* 2015 Jul;31(1):30–38.
35. Salas-Huetos A, Bulló M, Salas-Salvadó J. Dietary patterns, foods and nutrients in male fertility parameters and fecundability: a systematic review of observational studies. *Hum Reprod Update.* 2017 Jul 1;23(4):371–89.
36. Salas-Huetos A, Bulló M, Salas-Salvadó J. Dietary patterns, foods and nutrients in male fertility parameters and fecundability: a systematic review of observational studies. *Hum Reprod Update.* 2017 Jul 1;23(4):371–89.
37. Gaskins AJ, Nassan FL, Chiu YH, Arvizu M, Williams PL, Keller MG, Souter I, Hauser R, Chavarro JE; EARTH Study Team. Dietary patterns and outcomes of assisted reproduction. *Am J Obstet Gynecol.* 2019 Jun;220(6):567.e1–567.e18.
38. Sajadi Hezaveh Z, Sikaroudi MK, Vafa M, Clayton ZS, Soltani S. Effect of egg consumption on inflammatory markers: a systematic review and meta-analysis of randomized controlled clinical trials. *J Sci Food Agric.* 2019 Dec;99(15):6663–70.
39. Thomas MS, Huang L, Garcia C, Sakaki JR, Blesso CN, Chun OK, Fernandez ML. The effects of eggs in a plant-based diet on oxidative stress and inflammation in metabolic syndrome. *Nutrients.* 2022 Jun 19;14(12):2548.
40. Hruby A, Jacques PF. Dietary protein and changes in biomarkers of inflammation and oxidative stress in the Framingham Heart Study Offspring Cohort. *Curr Dev Nutr.* 2019 Mar 28;3(5):nzz019.
41. Chavarro JE, Rich-Edwards JW, Rosner BA, Willett WC. Protein intake and ovulatory infertility. *Am J Obstet Gynecol.* 2008 Feb;198(2):210.e1–7.
42. Gaskins AJ, Nassan FL, Chiu YH, Arvizu M, Williams PL, Keller MG, Souter I, Hauser R, Chavarro JE; EARTH Study Team. Dietary patterns and outcomes of assisted reproduction. *Am J Obstet Gynecol.* 2019 Jun;220(6):567.e1–567.e18.

43. Kim K, Yisahak SF, Nobles CJ, Andriessen VC, DeVilbiss EA, Sjaarda LA, Alohali A, Perkins NJ, Mumford SL. Low intake of vegetable protein is associated with altered ovulatory function among healthy women of reproductive age. *J Clin Endocrinol Metab.* 2021;106:e2600–e2612.
44. Haudum C, Lindheim L, Ascani A, Trummer C, Horvath A, Münzker J, Obermayer-Pietsch B. Impact of short-term isoflavone intervention in polycystic ovary syndrome (PCOS) patients on microbiota composition and metagenomics. *Nutrients.* 2020 Jun 1;12(6):1622.
45. Unfer V, Casini ML, Gerli S, Costabile L, Mignosa M, Di Renzo GC. Phytoestrogens may improve the pregnancy rate in in vitro fertilization-embryo transfer cycles: a prospective, controlled, randomized trial. *Fertil Steril.* 2004;82:1509–13.
46. Chavarro JE, Mínguez-Alarcón L, Chiu YH, Gaskins AJ, Souter I, Williams PL, Calafat AM, Hauser R; EARTH Study Team. Soy intake modifies the relation between urinary bisphenol A concentrations and pregnancy outcomes among women undergoing assisted reproduction. *J Clin Endocrinol Metab.* 2016 Mar;101(3):1082–90.
47. Beaton LK, McVeigh BL, Dillingham BL, Lampe JW, Duncan AM. Soy protein isolates of varying isoflavone content do not adversely affect semen quality in healthy young men. *Fertil Steril.* 2010 Oct;94(5):1717–22.
48. Reed KE, Camargo J, Hamilton-Reeves J, Kurzer M, Messina M. Neither soy nor isoflavone intake affects male reproductive hormones: an expanded and updated meta-analysis of clinical studies. *Reprod Toxicol.* 2021 Mar;100:60–67.
49. Oh DY, Talukdar S, Bae EJ, Imamura T, Morinaga H, Fan W, Li P, Lu WJ, Watkins SM, Olefsky JM. GPR120 is an omega-3 fatty acid receptor mediating potent anti-inflammatory and insulin-sensitizing effects. *Cell.* 2010;142:687–98.
50. Kim K, Browne RW, Nobles CJ, Radin RG, Holland TL, Omosigho UR, Connell MT, Plowden TC, Wilcox BD, Silver RM, Perkins NJ, Schisterman EF, Nichols CM, Kuhr DL, Sjaarda LA, Mumford SL. Associations between preconception plasma fatty acids and pregnancy outcomes. *Epidemiology.* 2019 Nov;30 Suppl 2(Suppl 2):S37–S46.
51. Mumford SL, Browne RW, Kim K, Nichols C, Wilcox B, Silver RM, Connell MT, Holland TL, Kuhr DL, Omosigho UR, Perkins NJ, Radin R, Sjaarda LA, Schisterman EF. Preconception plasma phospholipid fatty acids and fecundability. *J Clin Endocrinol Metab.* 2018 Dec 1;103(12):4501–10.
52. Mumford SL, Chavarro JE, Zhang C, Perkins NJ, Sjaarda LA, Pollack AZ, Schliep KC, Michels KA, Zarek SM, Plowden TC, Radin RG, Messer LC, Frankel RA, Wactawski-Wende J. Dietary fat intake and reproductive hormone concentrations and ovulation in regularly menstruating women. *Am J Clin Nutr.* 2016 Mar;103(3):868–77.
53. Nehra D, Le HD, Fallon EM, Carlson SJ, Woods D, White YA, Pan AH, Guo L, Rodig SJ, Tilly JL, Rueda BR, Puder M. Prolonging the female reproductive lifespan and improving egg quality with dietary omega-3 fatty acids. *Aging Cell.* 2012 Dec;11(6):1046–54.
54. Fritsche KL. The science of fatty acids and inflammation. *Adv Nutr.* 2015 May 15;6(3):293S–301S.
55. Gaskins AJ, Nassan FL, Chiu YH, Arvizu M, Williams PL, Keller MG, Souter I, Hauser R, Chavarro JE; EARTH Study Team. Dietary patterns and outcomes of assisted reproduction. *Am J Obstet Gynecol.* 2019 Jun;220(6):567.e1–567.e18.
56. Iwata NG, Pham M, Rizzo NO, Cheng AM, Maloney E, Kim F. Trans fatty acids induce vascular inflammation and reduce vascular nitric oxide production in endothelial cells. *PLoS One.* 2011;6(12):e29600.
57. Wise LA, Wesselink AK, Tucker KL, Saklani S, Mikkelsen EM, Cueto H, Riis AH, Trolle E, McKinnon CJ, Hahn KA, Rothman KJ, Sørensen HT, Hatch EE. Dietary fat intake and fecundability in 2 preconception cohort studies. *Am J Epidemiol.* 2018 Jan 1;187(1):60–74.
58. Willis SK, Wise LA, Wesselink AK, Rothman KJ, Mikkelsen EM, Tucker KL, Trolle E, Hatch EE. Glycemic load, dietary fiber, and added sugar and fecundability in 2 preconception cohorts. *Am J Clin Nutr.* 2020 Jul 1;112(1):27–38.
59. Aghaei B, Moradi F, Soleimani D, Moradinazar M, Khosravy T, Samadi M. Glycemic index, glycemic load, dietary inflammatory index, and risk of infertility in women. *Food Sci Nutr.* 2023 Aug 9;11(10):6413–24.
60. Chung Y, Melo P, Pickering O, Dhillon-Smith R, Coomarasamy A, Devall A. The association between dietary patterns and risk of miscarriage: a systematic review and meta-analysis. *Fertil Steril.* 2023 Aug;120(2):333–57.

61. Salvaleda-Mateu M, Rodríguez-Varela C, Labarta E. Do popular diets impact fertility? *Nutrients*. 2024 May 31;16(11):1726.
62. Lasa JS, Zubiaurre I, Soifer LO. Risk of infertility in patients with celiac disease: a meta-analysis of observational studies. *Arq Gastroenterol*. 2014 Apr–Jun;51(2):144–50.
63. Ulven SM, Holven KB, Gil A, Rangel-Huerta OD. Milk and dairy product consumption and inflammatory biomarkers: an updated systematic review of randomized clinical trials. *Adv Nutr*. 2019 May 1;10(suppl 2):S239–S250.
64. Qi X, Zhang W, Ge M, Sun Q, Peng L, Cheng W, Li X. Relationship between dairy products intake and risk of endometriosis: a systematic review and dose-response meta-analysis. *Front Nutr*. 2021 Jul 22;8:701860.
65. Kim K, Wactawski-Wende J, Michels KA, Plowden TC, Chaljub EN, Sjaarda LA, Mumford SL. Dairy food intake is associated with reproductive hormones and sporadic anovulation among healthy premenopausal women. *J Nutr*. 2017 Feb;147(2):218–26.
66. Hauser R, Chavarro JE; EARTH Study Team. The association of protein intake (amount and type) with ovarian antral follicle counts among infertile women: results from the EARTH prospective study cohort. *BJOG*. 2017 Sep;124(10):1547–55.
67. Nestel PJ, Mellett N, Pally S, Wong G, Barlow CK, Croft K, Mori TA, Meikle PJ. Effects of low-fat or full-fat fermented and non-fermented dairy foods on selected cardiovascular biomarkers in overweight adults. *Br J Nutr*. 2013 Dec;110(12):2242–49.
68. Afeiche M, Williams PL, Mendiola J, Gaskins AJ, Jørgensen N, Swan SH, Chavarro JE. Dairy food intake in relation to semen quality and reproductive hormone levels among physically active young men. *Hum Reprod*. 2013 Aug;28(8):2265–75.
69. Salas-Huetos A, Bulló M, Salas-Salvadó J. Dietary patterns, foods and nutrients in male fertility parameters and fecundability: a systematic review of observational studies. *Hum Reprod Update*. 2017 Jul 1;23(4):371–89.
70. Arnone D, Chabot C, Heba AC, Kökten T, Caron B, Hansmannel F, Dreumont N, Ananthakrishnan AN, Quilliot D, Peyrin-Biroulet L. Sugars and gastrointestinal health. *Clin Gastroenterol Hepatol*. 2022 Sep;20(9):1912–24.e7.
71. Hatch EE, Wesselink AK, Hahn KA, Michiel JJ, Mikkelsen EM, Sorensen HT, Rothman KJ, Wise LA. Intake of sugar-sweetened beverages and fecundability in a North American preconception cohort. *Epidemiology*. 2018 May;29(3):369–78.
72. Machtinger R, Gaskins AJ, Mansur A, Adir M, Racowsky C, Baccarelli AA, Hauser R, Chavarro JE. Association between preconception maternal beverage intake and in vitro fertilization outcomes. *Fertil Steril*. 2017 Dec;108(6):1026–33.
73. Efrat M, Stein A, Pinkas H, Unger R, Birk R. Sugar consumption is negatively associated with semen quality. *Reprod Sci*. 2022 Oct;29(10):3000–3006.
74. Kearns ML, Reynolds CM. The impact of non-nutritive sweeteners on fertility, maternal and child health outcomes: a review of human and animal studies. *Proceedings of the Nutrition Society*. 2024;83(4):1–13.
75. Cho NA, Klancic T, Nettleton JE, Paul HA, Reimer RA. Impact of food ingredients (aspartame, stevia, prebiotic oligofructose) on fertility and reproductive outcomes in obese rats. *Obesity (Silver Spring)*. 2018 Nov;26(11):1692–95.
76. Xu Y, Nisenblat V, Lu C, Li R, Qiao J, Zhen X, Wang S. Pretreatment with coenzyme Q10 improves ovarian response and embryo quality in low-prognosis young women with decreased ovarian reserve: a randomized controlled trial. *Reprod Biol Endocrinol*. 2018 Mar 27;16(1):29.
77. Nie X, Dong X, Hu Y, Xu F, Hu C, Shu C. Coenzyme Q10 stimulate reproductive vatality. *Drug Des Devel Ther*. 2023 Aug 30;17:2623–37.
78. Lafuente R, González-Comadrán M, Solà I, López G, Brassesco M, Carreras R, Checa MA. Coenzyme Q10 and male infertility: a meta-analysis. *J Assist Reprod Genet*. 2013 Sep;30(9):1147–56.
79. Meng X, Zhang J, Wan Q, Huang J, Han T, Qu T, Yu LL. Influence of vitamin D supplementation on reproductive outcomes of infertile patients: a systematic review and meta-analysis. *Reprod Biol Endocrinol*. 2023 Feb 3;21(1):17. doi: 10.1186/s12958-023-01068-8. PMID: 36737817.
80. Stanhiser J, Jukic AMZ, McConnaughey DR, Steiner AZ. Omega-3 fatty acid supplementation and fecundability. *Hum Reprod*. 2022 May 3;37(5):1037–46.
81. Zhang J, Jia H, Diao F, Ma X, Liu J, Cui Y. Efficacy of dehydroepiandrosterone priming in

women with poor ovarian response undergoing IVF/ICSI: a meta-analysis. *Front Endocrinol (Lausanne).* 2023 Jun 9;14:1156280.
82. Yong W, Ma H, Na M, Gao T, Zhang Y, Hao L, Yu H, Yang H, Deng X. Roles of melatonin in the field of reproductive medicine. *Biomed Pharmacother.* 2021 Dec;144:112001.
83. Lu X, Wu Z, Wang M, Cheng W. Effects of vitamin C on the outcome of in vitro fertilization–embryo transfer in endometriosis: a randomized controlled study. *J Int Med Res.* 2018 Nov;46(11):4624–33.
84. Ruder EH, Hartman TJ, Reindollar RH, Goldman MB. Female dietary antioxidant intake and time to pregnancy among couples treated for unexplained infertility. *Fertil Steril.* 2014 Mar;101(3):759–66.
85. Henmi H, Endo T, Kitajima Y, Manase K, Hata H, Kudo R. Effects of ascorbic acid supplementation on serum progesterone levels in patients with a luteal phase defect. *Fertil Steril.* 2003 Aug;80(2):459–61.
86. Zhou X, Shi H, Zhu S, Wang H, Sun S. Effects of vitamin E and vitamin C on male infertility: a meta-analysis. *Int Urol Nephrol.* 2022 Aug;54(8):1793–805.
87. Cicek N, Eryilmaz OG, Sarikaya E, Gulerman C, Genc Y. Vitamin E effect on controlled ovarian stimulation of unexplained infertile women. *J Assist Reprod Genet.* 2012;29:325–28.
88. Bahadori MH, Sharami SH, Fakor F, Milani F, Pourmarzi D, Dalil-Heirati SF. Level of vitamin E in follicular fluid and serum and oocyte morphology and embryo quality in patients undergoing IVF treatment. *J Fam Reprod Health.* 2017;11:74–81.
89. Kavtaradze N, Dominguez CE, Rock JA, Parthasarathy S, Murphy AA. Vitamin E and C supplementation reduces endometriosis related pelvic pain. *Fertil Steril.* 2003;80:221–22.
90. Zhou X, Shi H, Zhu S, Wang H, Sun S. Effects of vitamin E and vitamin C on male infertility: a meta-analysis. *Int Urol Nephrol.* 2022 Aug;54(8):1793–805.
91. Bennett M. Vitamin B12 deficiency, infertility and recurrent fetal loss. *J Reprod Med.* 2001 Mar;46(3):209–12. PMID: 11304860.
92. Rastegar Panah M, Jarvi K, Lo K, El-Sohemy A. Vitamin B12 is associated with higher serum testosterone concentrations and improved androgenic profiles among men with infertility. *J Nutr.* 2024 Sep;154(9):2680–87.
93. Merviel P, James P, Bouée S, Le Guillou M, Rince C, Nachtergaele C, Kerlan V. Impact of myo-inositol treatment in women with polycystic ovary syndrome in assisted reproductive technologies. *Reprod Health.* 2021 Jan 19;18(1):13.
94. Mohammadi S, Eini F, Bazarganipour F, Taghavi SA, Kutenaee MA. The effect of myo-inositol on fertility rates in poor ovarian responder in women undergoing assisted reproductive technique: a randomized clinical trial. *Reprod Biol Endocrinol.* 2021 Apr 23;19(1):61.
95. Azizi M, Cheraghi E, Soleimani Mehranjani M. Effect of myo-inositol on sperm quality and biochemical factors in cryopreserved semen of patients with asthenospermia. *Andrologia.* 2022 Nov;54(10):e14528.
96. Thakker D, Raval A, Patel I, Walia R. N-acetylcysteine for polycystic ovary syndrome: a systematic review and meta-analysis of randomized controlled clinical trials. *Obstet Gynecol Int.* 2015; 2015:817849. doi: 10.1155/2015/817849.
97. Amin AF, Shaaban OM, Bedlawy MA. N-acetyl cysteine for treatment of recurrent unexplained pregnancy loss. *Reprod Biomed Online.* 2008 Nov;17(5):722–26. doi: 10.1016/s1472-6483(10)60322-7. PMID: 18983759.
98. Li X, Wang Z, Wang H, Xu H, Sheng Y, Lian F. Role of N-acetylcysteine treatment in women with advanced age undergoing IVF/ICSI cycles: a prospective study. *Front Med (Lausanne).* 2022 Oct 4;9:917146.
99. Anastasi E, Scaramuzzino S, Viscardi MF, Viggiani V, Piccioni MG, Cacciamani L, Merlino L, Angeloni A, Muzii L, Porpora MG. Efficacy of N-acetylcysteine on endometriosis-related pain, size reduction of ovarian endometriomas, and fertility outcomes. *Int J Environ Res Public Health.* 2023 Mar 7;20(6):4686.
100. Zhou Z, Cui Y, Zhang X, Zhang Y. The role of N-acetyl-cysteine (NAC) orally daily on the sperm parameters and serum hormones in idiopathic infertile men: a systematic review and meta-analysis of randomised controlled trials. *Andrologia.* 2021 Mar;53(2):e13953.
101. Zarean E, Tarjan A. Effect of magnesium supplement on pregnancy outcomes: a randomized control trial. *Adv Biomed Res.* 2017;6:109.
102. Kapper C, Oppelt P, Ganhör C, Gyunesh AA, Arbeithuber B, Stelzl P, Rezk-Füreder M.

Minerals and the menstrual cycle: impacts on ovulation and endometrial health. *Nutrients.* 2024 Mar 29;16(7):1008.
103. Garner TB, Hester JM, Carothers A, Diaz FJ. Role of zinc in female reproduction. *Biol Reprod.* 2021;104:976–94.
104. Mier-Cabrera J, Aburto-Soto T, Burrola-Méndez S, Jiménez-Zamudio L, Tolentino MC, Casanueva E, Hernández-Guerrero C. Women with endometriosis improved their peripheral antioxidant markers after the application of a high antioxidant diet. *Reprod Biol Endocrinol.* 2009;7:54.
105. Pieczyńska J, Grajeta H. The role of selenium in human conception and pregnancy. *J Trace Elem Med Biol.* 2015;29:31–38.
106. Shukla S, Shrivastava D. Nutritional deficiencies and subfertility: a comprehensive review of current evidence. *Cureus.* 2024 Aug 8;16(8):e66477.
107. Lima LG, Santos AAMD, Gueiber TD, Gomes RZ, Martins CM, Chaikoski AC. Relation between selenium and female fertility: a systematic review. *Rev Bras Ginecol Obstet.* 2022 Jul;44(7):701–9.
108. Jasoni CL, Romanò N, Constantin S, Lee K, Herbison AE. Calcium dynamics in gonadotropin-releasing hormone neurons. *Front Neuroendocrinol.* 2010;31:259–69.
109. Chen X, Zhao H, Lv J, Dong Y, Zhao M, Sui X, Cui R, Liu B, Wu K. Calcium ionophore improves embryonic development and pregnancy outcomes in patients with previous developmental problems in ICSI cycles. *BMC Pregnancy Childbirth.* 2022;22:894.
110. Najib FS, Poordast T, Mahmudi MS, Shiravani Z, Namazi N, Omrani GR. Does vitex agnus-castus L. have deleterious effect on fertility and pregnancy outcome? An experimental study on rats for prediction of its safety. *J Pharmacopuncture.* 2022 Jun 30;25(2):106–13.

## CHAPTER 10

1. Hauptman M, Woolf AD. Childhood ingestions of environmental toxins: what are the risks? *Pediatr Ann.* 2017 Dec 1;46(12):e466–e471.
2. Allori M, Franzago M, Stuppia L, Garagna S, Ubaldi FM, Zuccotti M, Rienzi L. Endocrine-disrupting chemicals, gut microbiota, and human (in)fertility—it is time to consider the triad. *Cells.* 2022 Oct 22;11(21):3335.
3. Eepho OI, Bashir AAM, Oniyide AA, Aturamu A, Owolabi OV, Ajadi IO, Fafure AA, Ajadi MB, Areloegbe SE, Olaniyi KS. Modulation of GABA by sodium butyrate ameliorates hypothalamic inflammation in experimental model of PCOS. *BMC Neurosci.* 2023;24:62.
4. Stathori G, Hatziagapiou K, Mastorakos G, Vlahos NF, Charmandari E, Valsamakis G. Endocrine-disrupting chemicals, hypothalamic inflammation and reproductive outcomes: a review of the literature. *Int J Mol Sci.* 2024 Oct 22;25(21):11344.
5. Messerlian C, Williams PL, Ford JB, Chavarro JE, Mínguez-Alarcón L, Dadd R, Braun JM, Gaskins AJ, Meeker JD, James-Todd T, Chiu YH, Nassan FL, Souter I, Petrozza J, Keller M, Toth TL, Calafat AM, Hauser R; EARTH Study Team. The Environment and Reproductive Health (EARTH) study: a prospective preconception cohort. *Hum Reprod Open.* 2018 Feb;2018(2):hoy001.
6. Srnovršnik T, Virant-Klun I, Pinter B. Polycystic ovary syndrome and endocrine disruptors (bisphenols, parabens, and triclosan)—a systematic review. *Life (Basel).* 2023 Jan 4;13(1):138.
7. Buck Louis GM, Sundaram R, Sweeney AM, Schisterman EF, Maisog J, Kannan K. Urinary bisphenol A, phthalates, and couple fecundity: the Longitudinal Investigation of Fertility and the Environment (LIFE) study. *Fertil Steril.* 2014;101:1359–66.
8. Stathori G, Hatziagapiou K, Mastorakos G, Vlahos NF, Charmandari E, Valsamakis G. Endocrine-disrupting chemicals, hypothalamic inflammation and reproductive outcomes: a review of the literature. *Int J Mol Sci.* 2024 Oct 22;25(21):11344.
9. Whitworth KW, Haug LS, Baird DD, Becher G, Hoppin JA, Skjaerven R, Thomsen C, Eggesbo M, Travlos G, Wilson R, Longnecker MP. Perfluorinated compounds and subfecundity in pregnant women. *Epidemiology.* 2012 Mar;23(2):257–63.
10. Xu J, Wang Q, Jiao X, Kong P, Chen S, Yang W, Liu W, Li K, Teng X, Guo Y. Association between perfluorooctanoic acid-related poor embryo quality and metabolite alterations in human follicular fluid during IVF: a cohort study. *Environ Health Perspect.* 2025 Jun;133(6):67017.
11. Zhang Y, Mustieles V, Wang YX, Sun Y, Agudelo J, Bibi Z, Torres N, Oulhote Y, Slitt A, Messerlian C. Folate concentrations and serum perfluoroalkyl and polyfluoroalkyl substance

concentrations in adolescents and adults in the USA (National Health and Nutrition Examination Study 2003–16): an observational study. *Lancet Planet Health.* 2023 Jun;7(6):e449–e458.
12. Fenton SE, Ducatman A, Boobis A, DeWitt JC, Lau C, Ng C, Smith JS, Roberts SM. Per- and polyfluoroalkyl substance toxicity and human health review: current state of knowledge and strategies for informing future research. *Environ Toxicol Chem.* 2021 Mar;40(3):606–30.
13. Henley DV, Lipson N, Korach KS, Bloch CA. Prepubertal gynecomastia linked to lavender and tea tree oils. *N Engl J Med.* 2007 Feb 1;356(5):479–85.
14. Ramsey JT, Li Y, Arao Y, Naidu A, Coons LA, Diaz A, Korach KS. Lavender products associated with premature thelarche and prepubertal gynecomastia: case reports and endocrine-disrupting chemical activities. *J Clin Endocrinol Metab.* 2019 Nov 1;104(11):5393–405.
15. Henriques MC, Loureiro S, Fardilha M, Herdeiro MT. Exposure to mercury and human reproductive health: a systematic review. *Reprod Toxicol.* 2019 Apr;85:93–103.
16. Winder C. Lead, reproduction and development. *Neurotoxicology.* 1993;14:303–17.
17. Zhai Q, Narbad A, Chen W. Dietary strategies for the treatment of cadmium and lead toxicity. *Nutrients.* 2015 Jan 14;7(1):552–71.
18. Bloom MS, Fujimoto VY, Steuerwald AJ, Cheng G, Browne RW, Parsons PJ. Background exposure to toxic metals in women adversely influences pregnancy during in vitro fertilization (IVF). *Reprod Toxicol.* 2012;34:471–81.
19. Rafati Rahimzadeh M, Rafati Rahimzadeh M, Kazemi S, Moghadamnia AA. Cadmium toxicity and treatment: an update. *Caspian J Intern Med.* 2017 Summer;8(3):135–45.
20. Ha S, Sundaram R, Buck Louis GM, Nobles C, Seeni I, Sherman S, et al. Ambient air pollution and the risk of pregnancy loss: a prospective cohort study. *Fertil Steril.* 2018;109:148–53.
21. Zeng L, Zhou C, Xu W, Huang Y, Wang W, Ma Z, et al. The ovarian-related effects of polystyrene nanoplastics on human ovarian granulosa cells and female mice. *Ecotoxicol Environ Saf.* 2023;257:114941.
22. Wan S, Wang X, Chen W, Wang M, Zhao J, Xu Z, et al. Exposure to high dose of polystyrene nanoplastics causes trophoblast cell apoptosis and induces miscarriage. *Part Fibre Toxicol.* 2024;21(1):13.
23. Chiu YH, Williams PL, Mínguez-Alarcón L, Gillman M, Sun Q, Ospina M, Calafat AM, Hauser R, Chavarro JE. Comparison of questionnaire-based estimation of pesticide residue intake from fruits and vegetables with urinary concentrations of pesticide biomarkers. *J Expo Sci Environ Epidemiol.* 2018 Jan;28(1):31–39.
24. Albadrani MS, Aljassim MT, El-Tokhy AI. Pesticide exposure and spontaneous abortion risk: a comprehensive systematic review and meta-analysis. *Ecotoxicol Environ Saf.* 2024 Oct 1;284:117000.
25. Adena MA, Gallagher HG. Cigarette smoking and the age at menopause. *Ann Hum Biol.* 1982;9:121–30.
26. Practice Committee of the American Society for Reproductive Medicine. Smoking and infertility: a committee opinion. *Fertil Steril.* 2018 Sep;110(4):611–18.
27. Golding J, Gregory S, Northstone K, Pembrey M, Watkins S, Iles-Caven Y, Suderman M. Human transgenerational observations of regular smoking before puberty on fat mass in grandchildren and great-grandchildren. *Sci Rep.* 2022 Jan 21;12(1):1139.
28. Wetendorf M, Randall LT, Lemma MT, Hurr SH, Pawlak JB, Tarran R, Doerschuk CM, Caron KM. E-cigarette exposure delays implantation and causes reduced weight gain in female offspring exposed in utero. *J Endocr Soc.* 2019;3:1907–16.
29. Mumford SL, Flannagan KS, Radoc JG, et al. Cannabis use while trying to conceive: a prospective cohort study evaluating associations with fecundability, live birth and pregnancy loss. *Hum Reprod.* 2021;36:1405–15.
30. Klonoff-Cohen HS, Natarajan L, Chen RV. A prospective study of the effects of female and male marijuana use on in vitro fertilization (IVF) and gamete intrafallopian transfer (GIFT) outcomes. *Am J Obstet Gynecol.* 2006;194:369–76.
31. Nassan FL, Arvizu M, Minguez-Alarcon L, et al. Marijuana smoking and markers of testicular function among men from a fertility center. *Hum Reprod.* 2019; 34:715–23.
32. Ryan KS, Bash JC, Hanna CB, Hedges JC, Lo JO. Effects of marijuana on reproductive health: preconception and gestational effects. *Curr Opin Endocrinol Diabetes Obes.* 2021 Dec 1;28(6):558–65.
33. Tharmalingam J, Gangadaran P, Rajendran RL, Ahn BC. Impact of alcohol on inflammation,

immunity, infections, and extracellular vesicles in pathogenesis. *Cureus.* 2024 Mar 25;16(3):e56923.
34. Wang HJ, Zakhari S, Jung MK. Alcohol, inflammation, and gut-liver-brain interactions in tissue damage and disease development. *World J Gastroenterol.* 2010 Mar 21;16(11):1304–13.
35. Gill J. The effects of moderate alcohol consumption on female hormone levels and reproductive function. *Alcohol Alcohol.* 2000;35:417–23.
36. Anwar MY, Marcus M, Taylor KC. The association between alcohol intake and fecundability during menstrual cycle phases. *Hum Reprod.* 2021 Aug 18;36(9):2538–48.
37. Høyer S, Riis AH, Toft G, Wise LA, Hatch EE, Wesselink AK, Rothman KJ, Sørensen HT, Mikkelsen EM. Male alcohol consumption and fecundability. *Hum Reprod.* 2020 Apr 28;35(4):816–25.
38. Rossi BV, Berry KF, Hornstein MD, Cramer DW, Ehrlich S, Missmer SA. Effect of alcohol consumption on in vitro fertilization. *Obstet Gynecol.* 2011 Jan;117(1):136–42.
39. Gaskins AJ, Rich-Edwards JW, Williams PL, Toth TL, Missmer SA, Chavarro JE. Prepregnancy caffeine and caffeinated beverage intake and risk of spontaneous abortion. *Eur J Nutr.* 2018 Feb;57(1):107–17.
40. Lawson CC, LeMasters GK, Levin LS, Liu JH. Pregnancy hormone metabolite patterns, pregnancy symptoms, and coffee consumption. *Am J Epidemiol.* 2002;156(5):428–37.
41. American College of Obstetricians and Gynecologists. ACOG committee opinion no. 462: moderate caffeine consumption during pregnancy. *Obstet Gynecol.* 2010 Aug;116(2 Pt 1):467–68.
42. Rao M, Xia W, Yang J, Hu LX, Hu SF, Lei H, Wu YQ, Zhu CH. Transient scrotal hyperthermia affects human sperm DNA integrity, sperm apoptosis, and sperm protein expression. *Andrology.* 2016;4(6):1054–63.
43. McKinnon CJ, Joglekar DJ, Hatch EE, Rothman KJ, Wesselink AK, Willis MD, Wang TR, Mikkelsen EM, Eisenberg ML, Wise LA. Male personal heat exposures and fecundability: A preconception cohort study. *Andrology.* 2022 Nov;10(8):1511–21. doi: 10.1111/andr.13242. Epub 2022 Aug 11. PMID: 35924639; PMCID: PMC9588744.
44. Garolla A, Torino M, Sartini B, Cosci I, Patassini C, Carraro U, Foresta C. Seminal and molecular evidence that sauna exposure affects human spermatogenesis. *Hum Reprod.* 2013 Apr;28(4):877–85.
45. Wise LA, Cramer DW, Hornstein MD, Ashby RK, Missmer SA. Physical activity and semen quality among men attending an infertility clinic. *Fertil Steril.* 2011 Mar 1;95(3):1025–30.
46. Dore J-F, Chignol M-C. Laptop computers with Wi-Fi decrease human sperm motility and increase sperm DNA fragmentation. *Fertil Steril.* 2012;97(4):e12.
47. Wise LA, Cramer DW, Hornstein MD, Ashby RK, Missmer SA. Physical activity and semen quality among men attending an infertility clinic. *Fertil Steril.* 2011 Mar 1;95(3):1025–30.

# Index

1,4-dioxane, 297
17-OHP (17-hydroxyprogesterone), 86
2-butoxyethanol, 299
21-hydroxylase, 86

acne, 65, 85
ACTH (adrenocorticotropic hormone), 22, 30, 193
acupuncture, 199, 274
adenomyosis, 88, 96–97, 165, 173
ADH (antidiuretic hormone), 23
adhesions, 93, 100
adrenal fatigue, 86
adrenal glands, 21, 25, 29, 30, 68, 86–87
advice
  for adrenal supplements, 87
  for after conception, 146–49
  for checking cervical position, 115
  for cycle tracking, 311–15
  for doctor visits, 14–15, 350–53
  for embryo transfer, 179–80
  for exercise plan, 209–10, 277–79
  for food, 221, 228, 229–30, 231
  for healing gut, 240–44, 284–85
  for healthy habits, 309–10
  for intercourse, 142–46
  for irregular cycles, 67, 69
  for microplastics, 259
  for miscarriage, 130, 149
  for MRIs, 73
  for removing toxins in life, 264–69
  for rhythm method, 120
  for sleep, 203–4, 275–77
  for starting to get pregnant, 128–29, 133–38
  for stress reduction, 200, 274–75
  for supplements, 244
  for tracking basal body temperature (BBT), 111–12
  for using ovulation predictor kits (OPKs), 116
AFC (antral follicle count), 47–48, 155
age
  biological clock and, 41
  egg freezing and, 58, 59
  egg quality and, 52–54
  in embryo transfer success, 180, 181
  gut microbiome and, 218
  IVF and, 173, 176, 177, 178
  paternal, 160
  pregnancy wait time and, 129
  related infertility, 161
AGEs (advanced glycation end products), 222
air pollution, 258, 269, 291, 296, 302
alcohol, 26, 218, 240–41, 262–63, 269, 280, 291, 302
alpha-linolenic acid (ALA), 233
amenorrhea, 67, 68, 75
American College of Obstetricians and Gynecologists (ACOG), 46
AMH (anti-müllerian hormone), 46, 47, 49–51, 55, 155
ammonia, 299
anatomy
  of adenomyosis, 96
  of endometriosis, 100
  of fibroids, 95
  normal reproductive, 89, 139, 155–56
ancestry tests, 136
androgen resistance syndrome, 29
androgens, 81, 82, 85, 86
androstenedione, 82

aneuploidy, 176, 177
animal fat, 225
animal protein, 222, 241, 280, 281
anovulation, 67–87, 75–78, 88
antagonist protocol, 174, 181
anti-inflammatory medications, 11
anti-müllerian hormone (AMH). *See* AMH (anti-müllerian hormone)
antibiotics, 92
antioxidants, 57, 160, 220, 283, 293
antral follicle count (AFC). *See* AFC (antral follicle count)
APS (antiphospholipid syndrome), 164
artificial insemination. *See* IUI (intrauterine insemination)
artificial sweetener, 218, 231, 292
Asherman syndrome, 88, 92, 93–94
attrition, in IVF, 175–77
autoimmune disease
   celiac disease as, 17
   diminished ovarian reserve and, 45
   as extreme inflammation, 8, 13–15
   Graves' disease as, 77
   Hashimoto's disease as, 76
   hypothalamic anovulation and, 70
   premature ovarian insufficiency (POI) and, 79
   recurrent pregnancy loss and, 16, 162, 164–65
avocado oil
   choosing, 227
   in recipes, 320–22, 323–26, 329–32, 335–37, 339, 341

Baked Tofu recipe, 337–38
balanced translocation, 162
basal body temperature (BBT), 109–12, 121, 123, 311–12
BBQ Chickpeas recipe, 323–24
beans, 320–21, 331, 334–35, 336–37
beets, 284, 293
BHA (butylated hydroxyanisole), 297
Billings method, 122, 123
Billings, Evelyn, 122
Billings, John, 122
biochemical pregnancy, 149
biological clock, 41, 56–58
biotin supplements, 30–31
birth control pills
   effectiveness of, 124
   experiences with, 65–66
   light bleeding and, 92
   menstrual cycle on, 37
   vs natural family planning (NFP), 119
   ovarian reserve and, 51
   for PCOS, 84
   post–birth control pill syndrome, 65–66
   stopping, 130–32
birth defects, 134, 136, 149, 155–56, 161, 162, 163–64

bisphenol A (BPA). *See* BPA (bisphenol A)
Black Bean Taco Bowl recipe, 336–37
blastocysts, 175, 179
bleeding
   abnormal, 88–90, 94
   heavy, 88, 94–97
   light, 88, 92–94
blood sugar, 30, 227
body mass index (BMI), 209
bone density, 29
bottled water, 257
boundaries, 198
BPA (bisphenol A), 251
brain
   endocrine-disrupting chemicals (EDCs) impacts on, 249
   as hormone control center, 22, 24, 25
   mass as cause of abnormal prolactin, 73
   mass as cause of hypothalamic anovulation, 70, 72
breast growth, 29, 73, 74
breast sensitivity, 118
breastfeeding, 75
broccoli, 323–24, 329, 339
Broccoli and Peanut Tofu recipe, 329
bromelain enzyme, 221
butter, 226, 227, 229, 338, 340, 342
butternut squash, 325–26, 336–37
Butternut Squash Curry Soup recipe, 325–26

cadmium, 256–57
caffeine, 128, 204, 263, 275
calcium, 137, 239
calendar method, 108–9, 311
calorie restriction, 70, 72, 192
cancer, 16, 26, 84, 88, 97
candles, 288, 296, 297
cannabis, 180, 248, 262, 269, 291, 302, 310
canned food, 251
carbohydrates, 227–29, 243, 281
Carrot and Lentil Gnocchi recipe, 328
carrots, 328, 331, 340
cauliflower, 320–21, 331, 336–37, 339
celiac disease, 17, 165, 229
cellular damage, 41, 52
cervical mucus
   monitoring of (CCM), 112–14, 123, 141, 143, 312–13
   at ovulation, 34, 36
   progesterone's impact on, 26
   in two-day method, 121–22
cervical position, 115, 313
cervical stenosis, 88
chickpeas, 322–24, 326–27
childhood factors, 218
chlorine bleach, 299
cholesterol, 225
choline, 137, 222
chromosomes, 52, 53, 162, 176

# INDEX

circadian rhythm, 201, 219
cleaning products, 270, 288, 297, 300–301
Clomid (clomiphene citrate), 169, 170, 174
clothing, 297
clotting disorders, 164
coenzyme Q10 (CoQ10). *See* CoQ10 (coenzyme Q10)
coffee, 252, 266, 269, 290, 291, 294, 302, 310
complex carbohydrates, 227, 280
conception, 143–49
condoms, 119
congenital adrenal hyperplasia (CAH), 68, 86–87
contraception
  effectiveness chart for, 123–24
  hormonal, 51, 92
  intercourse and FAM in, 141
  options, 119
  stopping, 130–33
conventional fertilization, 175
copper IUDs, 51, 124, 133
CoQ10 (coenzyme Q10), 232, 304, 305, 306, 307, 308
Cornbread-and-Herb Stuffing recipe, 343–44
corpus luteum, 34, 108
cortisol, 30, 86, 193–95, 201, 206
coverline in cycle tracking, 111, 112
cranberries, 344
cycle syncing, 314–15
cycle tracking
  after birth control pill use, 132
  apps, 106
  basal body temperature (BBT), 109–12
  basics of, 106–7
  calendar method, 108–9
  cervical mucus monitoring (CCM), 112–14
  cervical position, 115
  to detect issues, 71, 79
  as a fertility awareness method, 58, 105
  guide for, 311–15
  mid-luteal progesterone levels in, 117–18
  natural family planning (NFP) and, 119–23
  ovulation predictor kit (OPK), 115–17
  symptothermal method using, 123

dairy, 229–30, 241, 243, 280, 281, 285
dehydroepiandrosterone (DHEA). *See* DHEA (dehydroepiandrosterone)
dementia, 79
Depo-Provera, 124, 132
depression, 85
DHEA (dehydroepiandrosterone), 29–30, 234, 306
DHEAS (dehydroepiandrosterone sulfate), 29–30, 82
diabetes, 16, 162, 228
diethanolamine (DEA), 298
diminished ovarian reserve (DOR), 44–45, 54–55, 79, 88, 100, 102, 117

docosahexaenoic acid (DHA), 233
doctors
  on cycle tracking, 105
  dismissive experiences with, 127
  experiences with, 151–52
  preconception visits, 133–34
  preparing to visit, 352–53
  responding to inflammation symptoms, 14–15
  what to expect at fertility appointment, 349–52
donor eggs, 80, 183
donor embryos, 183
donor sperm, 172, 173, 183
dopamine, 204–5
dryer sheets, 288, 296
due dates, 147–48
dysmenorrhea, 98–102

E1 (estrone). *See* estrone (E1)
E2 (estradiol). *See* estradiol (E2)
E3 (estriol). *See* estriol (E3)
Early Day Rules, 122
eating disorders, 70
eggs
  diminished ovarian reserve, 44–45
  donor, 80, 173, 183
  fertilization of, 138–39
  fertilization window of, 107
  in follicular phase, 33
  freezing, 43, 57–60
  implantation, 146
  main discussion, 42–43
  maturing in cycle, 25
  ovarian reserve testing, 154–55
  during ovulation, 33–34
  in PCOS, 81
  quality of, 51–54
  quality vs quantity, 41, 54–55
  retrieval, 58–59, 174–75
  running out of, 39–40
  supplements for poor quality, 307–8
  testing for number of, 45–51
eggs, chicken, 222, 281
eicosapentaenoic acid (EPA), 233
elimination phase, 240–42
embryo transfer, 178–80, 181, 182, 355–56, 358–59
endocrine disease, 162–63
endocrine disrupters, 248–53, 256
endocrine-disrupting chemicals (EDCs), 248–53
endometrial lining, 84, 92–94
endometrial protection, 84, 85
endometriomas, 102
endometriosis
  as an inflammatory disease, 161, 165
  as cause of painful periods, 98, 99–102
  dairy and, 229

# INDEX

endometriosis (*cont.*)
  endocrine-disrupting chemicals
    impact on, 250
  IVF and, 173
  supplements for, 305
endometritis, 88, 91–92
endometrium, 32–33
endorphins, 23
Environmental Working Group, 267, 297, 300
essential fatty acids, 225
essential oils, 254
estimated gestational age (EGA), 148
estradiol (E2)
  in birth control pills, 37
  low in hyperprolactinemia, 74
  low in hypothalamic dysfunction, 72
  in menstrual cycle, 32
  in ovarian failure, 80
  in ovarian reserve testing, 47, 48–49, 155
  overview, 25
  in ovulation evaluation, 154
  in predicting ovulation, 116
  *See also* estrogen
estriol (E3), 25
  *See also* estrogen
estrobolome, 216
estrogen
  cardiovascular function and, 208
  cervical mucus and, 112
  cervical position and, 115
  clearing of, 249
  dominance, 28
  in frozen embryo transfer, 179
  introduction to, 24
  low, and hypothalamic amenorrhea, 70
  main discussion, 25
  metabolism in gut, 216
  from ovaries, 78
  at ovulation, 33–34
  in PCOS, 81
  production of, 22
  replacement of, 79–80
  soy and, 224
estrone (E1), 25, 84
  *See also* estrogen
ethinyl estradiol, 37, 131
euploidy, 176, 181
exercise
  excess, 70, 192, 206
  menstrual cycle and, 314, 315
  plan for, 277–79
  for reducing inflammation, 204–10

fallopian tubes, 138–39, 140, 158, 173
FAM (fertility awareness methods)
  basal body temperature (BBT), 109–12
  benefits of, 105
  calendar method, 108–9
  cervical mucus monitoring (CCM), 112–14
  cervical position, 115
  intercourse and, 141
  mid-luteal progesterone levels in, 117–18
  natural family planning based on, 119–23
  overview of tracking, 106–7
  ovulation predictor kit (OPK), 115–17
family history of disease, 135
family planning, 55, 119–25
fasting, 219
fatigue, 6, 9–10, 25, 80, 159, 213, 215, 216, 314
fats, dietary, 225–27, 243, 281, 283
fecundability, 53–54
fermented foods, 284
fertility
  age and, 41, 51–54
  awareness methods (FAM), 105, 141
  clinics, 152
  impact of endocrine-disrupting chemicals on, 250
  information for planning, 46–47
  signs of, 118
  testing and evaluation, 153–157
  window, 106, 110, 122, 140, 141
fertility doctors, 16, 17, 19, 37–38
fertility treatments, 19, 37–38, 43, 167–86
fertilization, 138–39
FHA (functional hypothalamic amenorrhea), 70
fiber, 217–18, 220–21, 227, 253, 281, 282, 283–84, 293
fibroids, 88, 94–95, 250
fight-or-flight response, 30, 193
fish, 222, 254–55, 259, 281, 289, 292, 293
flea treatments, 260, 267, 290, 296
folate, 136, 138, 253
folic acid, 136, 137, 138, 231–32, 244, 304
follicular phase
  body temperature in, 110
  exercise in, 207, 208, 315
  long, 68, 71, 72
  in menstrual cycle, 31
  normal, 106–7
  overview, 33
food choices
  anti-inflammatory diet, 280–86
  fighting inflammation with, 218–31
  for healing your gut, 240–44
  meal ideas overview, 319–20
  menstrual cycle and, 314, 315
  overview of, 214, 218–19
  recipes, 320–44
  for reducing toxins, 265–66, 291–93
  reducing toxins from, 289, 300
formaldehyde, 297, 298, 299
FORT-T (Forty and Over Treatment Trial), 171
fragrances, 252, 268, 290, 296, 298, 299
frozen embryo transfers (FETs), 179, 181, 182

# INDEX

fructose, 220
fruits and vegetables, 220–21, 243, 260, 261, 280, 281, 282–83, 292–93
FSH (follicle-stimulating hormone)
    in birth control pill function, 131
    in egg freezing, 58
    estrogen and, 25, 37
    in hypothalamic amenorrhea, 70
    in hypothalamic dysfunction, 71
    impaired by hyperprolactinemia, 73, 74
    in IVF, 174
    in men, 159
    in menstrual cycle, 32, 33, 69
    in ovarian failure, 79
    in ovarian reserve testing, 47, 48, 154–55
    overview, 22
    in ovulation, 42, 45
    for ovulation induction, 169
    in PCOS, 81
    prolactin and, 29
FSH/LH, 169, 170, 174
functional hypothalamic amenorrhea (FHA). *See* FHA (functional hypothalamic amenorrhea)

galactorrhea, 73, 74
genetics
    disease and IVF, 173
    egg quality and, 52, 53
    gut microbiome and, 218
    in recurrent pregnancy loss, 162
    screening, 134–36, 186
    sperm quality and, 159
gestational carriers, 173, 183
GH (growth hormone), 22
ginger, 284
glucose, 81, 83, 206, 208
gluten, 229, 241, 280, 285
glycemic index (GI), 227, 228
GnRH (gonadotropin-releasing hormone), 31–32, 69, 70, 71, 159, 174, 181, 249
gonadotropins, 170–71, 202, 211
    *See also* FSH (follicle-stimulating hormone); LH (luteinizing hormone)
Graves' disease, 77
Green Bean Casserole recipe, 341–42
green beans, 338, 341–42
green tea, 284, 293, 310
GUS (β- glucuronidase), 216, 249
gut health, 214–16
gut microbiome, 12, 215, 216–18, 224

habit tracker, 309–10
hair growth, 85, 87
hair loss, 10, 77, 78, 85
Hashimoto's disease, 76
hCG (human chorionic gonadotropin), 27, 34–35, 130, 146–47, 166, 174
headaches, 10, 74, 80, 216

health risks, 15–16
heart disease, 16, 79
heat, 264, 269
heavy metals, 254–57
HEPA filters, 258, 267, 290, 296
high blood pressure, 16
high-intensity interval training (HIIT), 206, 208
    *See also* exercise
Homemade Cranberry Sauce recipe, 344
hormonal contraception, 51, 92, 119, 311
    *See also* birth control pills
hormone dysfunction
    as cause of irregular cycles, 68–69
    chronic inflammation and, 12, 23
    endocrine disease and, 162–63
    from endocrine-disrupting chemicals (EDCs), 252–53
    from essential oils, 254
    leaky gut and, 215
hormone replacement, 74, 76, 77, 78, 79–80
hormones
    balancing, 24
    biotin affecting, 30–31
    birth control and, 37
    as communication system, 20–21
    other important, 28–30
    production and function of, 21–23
    reproductive, 24–28
    suppression of, 88, 96
    *See also* specific hormones
HPO axis, 21, 25, 38, 202, 262
HSG (hysterosalpingogram), 90, 94, 155
hyperprolactinemia, 68, 73–74
hyperthyroidism, 68, 77–78
hypothalamic amenorrhea (HA), 68, 70–71, 169, 170, 173, 192
hypothalamic anovulation, 69–70
hypothalamic dysfunction, 68
hypothalamic-pituitary-adrenal (HPA) axis, 193
Hypothalamic-Pituitary-Ovarian (HPO) axis. *See* HPO axis
hypothalamus, 21, 22, 23, 30, 31, 68, 69–70, 201, 249
hypothyroidism, 68, 76–77
hysterosalpingogram (HSG). *See* HSG (hysterosalpingogram)
hysteroscopy, 91, 94, 156, 184

imaging, diagnostic, 69, 90–91, 93, 94, 95, 96, 99, 155–56, 174–75, 178–79
immune system, 23, 27, 216–17
immunizations, 134
implantation window, 26, 28, 106, 139, 146–47, 221
in vitro fertilization (IVF). *See* IVF (in vitro fertilization)
infections, 88, 93, 218

infertility
  affecting the couple, 349
  birth control and, 133
  as a disease and health marker, 14–16
  gut microbiome and, 217
  main causes of, 157–61
  ovulation induction medication for, 170–71
  polyps and, 90–91
  rising rates of, 6–8
  sleep impact on, 200–202
  stress and, 195
  supplements for unexplained, 307
  as symptom of hyperprolactinemia, 74
  treatment embryo transfer, 178–82
  treatment in vitro fertilization, 173–78
  treatment intrauterine insemination, 171–73
  treatment lifestyle changes, 185–86
  treatment ovulation induction, 168–71
  treatment surgery, 184–85
  treatment third-party reproduction, 182–84
  unexplained, 4, 166–67
inflammation
  in adenomyosis, 96
  autoimmune disease as, 13–15
  autoimmune thyroid diseases and, 77
  chronic, 9–12, 15–16, 23, 30, 38, 44, 191, 213, 215–16
  contributors to, 66
  egg quality and, 52, 56
  estrogen as anti-inflammatory, 25
  from high insulin levels, 81, 83
  hypothalamic function and, 70
  impact on hormones, 69
  infertility and, 7–8
  introduction to, 5–6
  IVF and, 185
  menstrual cycle and, 35
  in ovulation and implantation, 27
  POI and, 79
  in recurrent pregnancy loss, 162
  reducing before pregnancy, 128–29
  reducing with exercise, 204–10
  sleep and, 200–202
  uterine, 91–92
inositol, 305
insomnia, 77, 78
insulin, 30, 194
insulin resistance
  fasting and, 219
  from high glycemic index foods, 227
  inflammation and, 12
  leaky gut and, 215
  low carbohydrate diets and, 228
  metformin improving, 171
  in PCOS, 81, 83, 84, 85
  pregnancy loss and, 13
  sleep deprivation and, 201
  strength training and, 206

intercourse
  advice for, 142–46
  in infertility definition, 6
  pain with, 10, 99
  prolactin and, 73
  timing of, 109, 114, 116, 120, 121, 122, 123, 140
interpregnancy interval, 129–30
intestines, 215
intracytoplasmic injection (ICSI), 159, 175
iodine, 137
iron, 137
isobutane, 298
isoflavones, 224
IUDs (intrauterine devices), 39, 51, 93, 124, 132–33
IUI (intrauterine insemination), 38, 159, 169, 171–73, 354
IVF (in vitro fertilization)
  biological goal of, 43
  egg freezing and, 59
  embryo transfer, 178–80
  exercise during, 206–7
  fallopian tubes and, 158
  overview, 173–75
  polyps and, 90
  pregnancy attempt timing and, 55
  questions to ask after failed cycle, 357–58
  questions to ask before, 354–55
  reciprocal, 173, 183
  success rates, 181
  timing of, 129
  as treatment option, 85, 168, 170, 171, 173–84

journaling, 198, 274, 275

kale, 322–23, 325–26
key facts, 18, 38, 61, 103, 125, 150, 187, 211–12, 245, 270
kitchens, 266, 290, 291–92, 293–95

L-arginine, 309
L-carnitine, 309
lactational amenorrhea, 75
laparoscopy, 156, 184–85
last menstrual period (LMP), 148
laundry balls, 259, 267, 290, 296
lead, 255–56, 257, 267, 290
leaky gut, 215–16
legumes, 227, 320–21, 328, 331, 334–35, 336–37
lemon, 284, 300
letrozole (Femara), 169, 170, 174, 181
LH (luteinizing hormone)
  basal body temperature (BBT) and, 110
  in birth control pill function, 131
  in hypothalamic dysfunction, 71
  in men, 159

in menstrual cycle, 32, 34
overview, 22, 69
in ovulation evaluation, 154
in ovulation predictor kit (OPK), 116, 117
in PCOS, 81
progesterone and, 26, 27
prolactin and, 29
libido, 29, 34, 74, 80, 118
lifestyle interventions
for adenomyosis, 96–97
for endometriosis, 100
for hypothalamic amenorrhea (HA), 70–71
for hypothalamic dysfunction, 72
impact on egg quality, 57
impact on inflammation, 17–18
impact on sperm quality, 160
improving sleep, 200–204
in IVF, 185
as overlooked, 16
for PCOS, 85, 102, 170
for removing toxins, 264–69
for starting to get pregnant, 128–29
for stress, 191–93
liver disease, 16, 26
lubrication, 144–45
Lupron protocol, 174, 179, 181
lupus, 165
luteal phase
defect (LPD), 68, 88, 162–63, 170, 206
exercise in, 207, 208, 315
normal, 107, 108
overview, 31, 32, 34–35
progesterone in, 117–18
short, 71, 72, 169
supplements for short, 306
lymph nodes, 118

magnesium, 237–38, 244, 304
malabsorption, 70
marijuana. *See* cannabis
medications
antibiotics, 92
for endometriosis, 100
fertility, 117
gut microbiome and, 218
hyperprolactinemia and, 73, 74
in IVF, 173–74
Mucinex, 114
for ovulation induction, 168–71, 179
for PCOS, 83
meditation, 197, 204, 274, 275, 276, 277
meiosis, 52
melatonin, 201, 204, 234, 276, 304, 305, 306, 307, 308
menopause, 26, 29, 44, 45, 78–80, 250
*See also* ovarian failure
menses phase, 31, 32–33, 36, 122, 207, 208, 314
menstrual cycle
assessing normality of, 35–37, 106–7, 108

causes of irregular, 67–87
cramping and pain in, 36–37
DHEAS in, 30
EDCs impact on, 249
hormonal control of, 24–26
length, 45
overview of, 31–35
overview of irregular, 65–67
syncing exercise to, 207–209
testosterone in, 29
tips and sheet for tracking, 311–15
mercury, 254–55, 289, 292, 293
metabolic by-products, 52–53
metabolism, 29, 75, 76, 77, 83, 204
metformin, 83, 171
methylated folate, 138
microplastics, 258–59, 267, 298
milk production, 74
*See also* prolactin (PRL)
mindfulness, 196–97, 274
*See also* meditation
Minestrone Soup recipe, 334–35
miscarriage
experiences of, 3–4, 127
how to know if, 149
insulin resistance and, 13
progesterone and, 28
rate of, 53
recurrent, 161–66
trying again after, 130
mitochondria, 52, 56
mittelschmerz, 34, 118
MRIs, 69, 73, 74, 96, 156
MSH (melanocyte-stimulating hormone), 23
Mucinex, 114
MUFAs (monounsaturated fatty acids), 225, 226
Müllerian anomalies, 163–64
muscle mass, 29, 83, 277
myo-inositol (MI), 83, 84, 236–37
myocardial infarction, 16
myometrium, 96

NAC (N-acetylcysteine), 237, 305, 306, 307, 308
Natalie's Christmas Spaghetti recipe, 324–25
natural cleaning products, 300–301
natural family planning (NFP), 119–24
nature time, 274, 275
NSAIDs (nonsteroidal anti-inflammatory drugs), 11
nutrition phase, 242–43

obesity, 26, 84, 250
OHSS (ovarian hyperstimulation syndrome), 174, 182
omega-3 fatty acids, 137, 222, 225, 227, 233, 244, 280, 304, 306
omega-6 fatty acids, 225, 227

# INDEX

omega-9 fatty acids, 225
OPK (ovulation predictor kit), 115–17, 141
organ meat, 257, 292
organic produce, 221, 243, 257, 260, 265, 281, 289, 292
orgasm, female, 144
Orilissa, 181, 359
osteoporosis, 79
ovarian failure, 26, 39–40, 68, 69, 78–80
ovarian hyperstimulation syndrome (OHSS). *See* OHSS (ovarian hyperstimulation syndrome)
ovarian reserve
    diminished ovarian reserve (DOR), 44–45
    egg quality and, 54–55
    in IVF, 173
    overview, 42–43
    stress and, 194
    supplements for low, 306
    testing, 45–51, 154–155
ovarian vault analogy, 42–43
ovaries
    in HPO axis, 21
    ovarian torsion, 207
    polycystic, 82, 85
    production of hormones from, 25, 78
    progesterone from, 28
    responding to LH, 27
    testosterone from, 29
    tumors, 26, 29
ovulation
    basal body temperature (BBT) signs of, 110
    causes of irregular cycles of, 67–87
    cervical position in, 115
    egg reserve and, 42–43
    estrogen and, 25, 26
    evaluation of, 154
    follicular phase preparing for, 33
    induction, 71, 72, 74, 83, 85, 168–71, 179, 354
    intercourse timing and, 140
    within menstrual cycle, 33–34
    other signs, 118
    ovulatory dysfunction, 68, 158
    as part of menstrual cycle, 22, 31
    predicted by cervical mucus, 112–14
    predictor kit (OPK), 115–17, 141, 142, 314
    progesterone and, 26–28, 117–18
    questions to ask before induction, 354
    suppression of, 101
    tracking, 106–7, 108
oxytocin, 23

pain during menstruation, 36–37, 94, 98–102
pancreas, 30
parabens, 297, 299
pasta, 324–25, 332, 333, 334–35
Pasta and Courgette Tofu Marinara recipe, 332
Pasta Salad recipe, 333

PCOS (polycystic ovary syndrome)
    as cause of irregular cycle, 66, 68, 81–85
    EDC impact on, 250
    estrogen in, 26
    insulin resistance and, 12, 30
    IVF and, 173
    ovulation and, 28
    ovulation induction medication for, 169, 170, 171
    supplements for, 305
    testosterone in, 29
    time-restricted eating and, 219
PdG (pregnanediol 3-glucuronide), 117–18
perfluorinated compounds (PFCs). *See* PFCs (perfluorinated compounds)
perimenopause, 26, 79
personal time, 196
pesticides, 259–60
PFCs (perfluorinated compounds), 252–53
PGT (preimplantation genetic testing), 134–35, 176, 177, 179
phthalates, 252, 268, 298, 299
phytoestrogens, 224
pineapple, 221
pituitary gland
    in anovulation, 68, 70, 72–75
    function of, 21, 22, 23
    gonadotropins released by, 32, 33
    thyroid hormones and, 29
placenta, 25, 27–28
plant protein, 222–24, 280, 281
plastics, 251, 252, 258–59, 266, 267, 290, 291, 294
PMS (premenstrual syndrome), 34, 308
POI (premature ovarian insufficiency), 46, 79
polycystic ovary syndrome (PCOS). *See* PCOS (polycystic ovary syndrome)
polypectomy, 91
pregnancy
    after ovulation, 34–35
    as cause of hyperprolactinemia, 73
    confirming with tests, 146–47
    determining due date, 147–48
    with endometriosis, 161
    fertility awareness methods (FAM) supporting, 105
    immune system during, 27
    length of, 147–48
    loss, 3–4, 13, 14
    odds with POI, 80
    preconception doctor visits, 133–34
    progesterone and, 26
    recurrent loss of, 161–66
    retained tissue from, 88
    before starting to try, 128–29
    timing of, 41, 55, 129–30
    while breastfeeding, 75
pregnanediol 3-glucuronide (PdG). *See* PdG (pregnanediol 3-glucuronide)

preimplantation genetic testing (PGT). *See* PGT (preimplantation genetic testing)
premature ovarian insufficiency (POI). *See* POI (premature ovarian insufficiency)
premenstrual syndrome (PMS), 34, 308
PRL (prolactin). *See* prolaction (PRL)
processed foods, 218, 280
products, personal, 267–68, 291, 295, 296, 297–99
progesterone
  in birth control pill use, 131
  contraception, 124
  glucose and, 208
  impact on endometrial lining, 92
  implantation window controlled by, 139
  IUDs, 132–33
  levels at ovulation, 110
  in luteal phase, 34, 117–18
  in menstrual cycle, 24, 26–28, 32, 33
  miscarriage and, 166
  in ovulation evaluation, 154
  in PCOS, 82
  production of, 22
  taken with estrogen, 80
  vaginal, 179
progestins, 131
prolactin (PRL), 22, 29, 72–74, 75, 154, 162
proteins, 221–24, 243
psoriasis, 165
puberty, 249
PUFAs (polyunsaturated fatty acids), 225

questions for doctors, 353–56

receipts, 251, 269, 291, 302
recipes, 320–44
reciprocal IVF, 173, 183
  *See also* IVF (in vitro fertilization)
recurrent implantation failure (RIF), 217
recurrent pregnancy loss (RPL), 161–66, 173
refined carbohydrates, 227–28, 280
rheumatoid arthritis, 165
rhythm method, 120, 123
Roasted Broccoli recipe, 339
Roasted Carrots recipe, 340
Roasted Cauliflower recipe, 339
Roasted Cauliflower Tacos recipe, 320–21
Roasted Okra recipe, 341
rubella (MMR) vaccine, 134

saline infusion sonogram (SIS), 90, 94, 155
same-sex couples, 183
saturated fats, 225, 226
scar tissue, 93
SCH (subchorionic hematoma), 149
scrotum, 264, 269, 291, 302
seaweed, 284
second opinions, 353–56
seed oils, 227

selenium, 238–39, 308
self-advocacy, 46–47, 349–59
semen analysis, 156–57, 172
septum, uterine, 149
serotonin, 204–5
sex hormone binding globulin (SHBG), 84
sex of child, 143
sex positions, 143–44
sex selection, 173
SHBG (sex hormone binding globulin). *See* sex hormone binding globulin (SHBG)
Sheehan syndrome, 68, 74
Shettles method, 143
shift work, 202
SIS (saline infusion sonogram). *See* saline infusion sonogram (SIS)
Sjögren's syndrome, 165
sleep, 73, 200–202, 218, 275–77
smoking, 261, 269, 291, 302
*So Now What?* (Manikowski), 186
social time, 199–200, 275
sodium laureth sulfate (SLES), 298, 299
sodium lauryl sulfate (SLS), 298, 299
sono-HSG (sono-hysterosalpingography), 155
soy, 224
  *See also* tofu
sperm, 142, 152, 158–60, 171–72, 202, 224, 229, 248, 264, 308–9
spotting, 88, 90–92, 118
  *See also* bleeding
stain protectors, 253, 267, 270, 290, 296
standard days method, 120–21, 123
strength training, 205–6, 208, 277–79
stress
  cortisol, 30
  estrogen and, 26
  exercise and, 204–5
  gut microbiome and, 218
  hypothalamic anovulation and, 70
  insulin resistance and, 83
  journaling for managing, 198
  management of, 193–200
  plan for reducing, 274–75
stretching, 275
stroke, 16
subchorionic hematoma (SCH). *See* SCH (subchorionic hematomoa)
sugar, 218, 220, 230–31, 243, 280, 281, 292
sunscreen, 299
supplementation phase, 244
supplements, 26, 30–31, 87, 231–39, 304–9
surgery, 93, 95, 97, 99, 100–101, 163, 184–85
Sweet Potato Bowl with Cashew Curry Sauce recipe, 335–36
Sweet Potato Chickpea Curry recipe, 326–27
sweet potatoes, 323–24, 326–27, 335–36
symptoms
  of abnormal estrogen, 26
  of adenomyosis, 97

symptoms (cont.)
  of congenital adrenal hyperplasia (CAH), 87
  of endometriosis, 99, 101
  of endometritis, 92
  of high progesterone, 27
  of hyperprolactinemia, 74
  of hyperthyroidism, 77, 78
  of hypothalamic amenorrhea (HA), 71
  of hypothalamic dysfunction, 72
  of hypothyroidism, 76, 77
  of inflammation, 9–11
  of luteal phase, 34
  menstrual, 24–25
  of ovarian failure, 80
  of PCOS, 81, 85
  of Sheehan syndrome, 74
  of uterine fibroids, 95
  of uterine polyps, 91
symptothermal method, 123
systemic sclerosis, 165

T3 (triiodothyronine), 29, 75
T4 (thyroxine), 29, 75
tacos, 320–21
Tahini Kale Salad recipe, 322–23
Teflon, 253, 266, 290
testes, 21, 157, 158, 264
testosterone, 29, 81, 82, 84, 154, 159, 202, 224
THC (delta-9-tetrahydrocannabinol), 262
  *See also* cannabis
therapy, 274
third-party reproduction, 182–84
Three-Bean Chili recipe, 331
thyroid disease, 162, 165
thyroid gland, 21, 29, 68, 75–78, 249
thyroid hormones, 29
time-restricted eating, 219
tofu, 325–26, 329, 332, 335–36, 337–38
toluene, 298
total motile sperm (TMS), 157, 172
toxins
  from behaviors, 261–63, 302
  checklist for, 303
  eliminating exposure to, 128, 264–69, 270, 289–300
  environmental contaminants, 258–60
  estrogen and, 26
  exposure self-assessment, 286–89
  gut microbiome and, 218
  heavy metals, 254–57
  overview, 165, 247–48
TPO (thyroid peroxidase), 76
tracking apps, 106, 108–9
trans fats, 225–26
translocation, balanced, 162
transvaginal ultrasound (TVUS), 95, 155
triclosan, 298, 299
trigger shots, 147

TSH (thyroid-stimulating hormone), 22, 29, 75–78, 154
Tunnel Pasta recipe, 330
turmeric, 284, 293
two-day method, 121–22, 123

ubiquinol, 232
ultrasound, 90, 148, 149, 154, 174–75, 178–79
unsaturated fats, 225, 226
urine, 116
uterus
  uterine birth defects, 163–64
  uterine cycle, 32
  uterine fibroids, 94–95, 250
  uterine health, 161
  uterine lining, 32–33, 34, 37, 307
  uterine polyps, 88, 90–91
  uterine septum, 149, 163

vaccines, 134
vaginal atrophy, 88
vaping, 261–62, 269, 291, 302
varicella (chickenpox) vaccine, 134
vas deferens, 152
vasectomy, 152
vegetables. *See* fruits and vegetables
Veggie Stir-Fry recipe, 321–22
vigorous exercise, 205, 206
  *See also* exercise; inflammation
vinegar, 300–301
vitamin A, 137, 222
vitamin B12, 137, 222, 236, 280
vitamin B7 (biotin), 30–31
vitamin B9, 136, 137, 231–32
vitamin B9 (folic acid), 136, 137
vitamin C, 137, 235, 305, 306, 307, 308, 309
vitamin D, 137, 222, 232–33, 244, 280, 304
vitamin E, 222, 235–36, 305, 306, 307, 308, 309
vitamins, general, 129, 136–38
  *See also* supplements
vitex, 239–40

walking, 275
  *See also* exercise
water, 257, 259, 289, 295
weight
  gain, 77, 80, 85, 208–9
  loss, 70, 77, 78, 80
whole foods, 220–21
whole grains, 227

X-ray dye test, 155

yoga, 198–99, 274, 276
  *See also* exercise; stress

zinc, 238, 304, 305, 306, 308